Contents

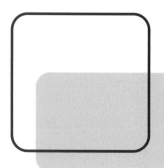

Acknowledgements

The authors would like to thank our husbands Scott and Simon, and our children Sophie, William and Tom for their support and encouragement throughout the writing process. Thanks also to Rick Jackman, Sue Stuart, Claire Davies, Janet Dodson, Megan Reilly and Barbara DiNicoli for their continued professional advice.

Every effort has been made to trace the copyright holders of quoted material. The authors and publishers would like to thank the following for kind permission to reproduce illustrations:

Fig 9.13, © a4stockphotos/Fotolia.com; Fig 8.12, © Adrienne Hart-Davis/Science Photo Library; Fig 3.13, © Alison Bowden/Fotolia.com; Fig 3.23, © Ashley Cooper/Alamy; Fig 8.4, the Assured Food Standards Agency; Fig 11.6, © bens-world.org/Fotolia.com; Fig 5.1, © Bill Brandt/Getty Images; Fig 10.4, BSI Product Services; Fig 11.20, © BSIP/Science Photo Library; Fig 11.19, © CDC/Science Photo Library; Fig 9.6, the Citizens Advice Bureau; Fig 6.14, © CORBIS; Fig 6.19, Crown copyright; Fig 9.22, © D. Ducouret/Fotolia.com; Fig 4.8, © Danny Hooks/ Fotolia.com; Fig 10.2, © David J. Green/Alamy; Fig 6.20, the Department of Health; Fig 8.6, © Dima/Fotolia.com; Figs 6.18 and 11.10, © Dino O./ Fotolia.com; Fig 11.7, © Dr Kari Lounatmaa/Science Photo Library; Fig 9.5, the Home Builders Federation Ltd; Fig 9.16, © Ewa Walicka/Fotolia.com; Fig 4.5a, © Fairtrade Foundation; Fig 9.14, © foodfolio/ Alamy; Fig 11.24, the Food Standards Agency; Fig 8.3, Freedom Food; Fig 10.11, © Gérard Delattre/ Fotolia.com; Fig 3.15, © govicinity/ Fotolia.com; Fig 4.6, © Grégory Delattre/Fotolia.com; Fig 9.5, the Home Builders Federation Ltd; Figs 8.1, 9.11 and 11.2, Ingram Publishing; Fig 10.3, Intertek; Fig 10.10, © JackF/ Fotolia.com; Fig 3.16, © Janine Wiedel Photolibrary/Alamy; Fig 11.17, © Jean-Claude Drillon/Fotolia.com; Fig 3.20, © Jean-François DESSUP/ Fotolia.com; Fig 3.24, © Joe Gough/Fotolia.com; Fig 3.22, © Keith Nolan/Fotolia.com; Fig 4.3, © Kerioak/ Fotolia.com; Fig 10.8, © Kirsty Pargeter/Fotolia.com; Fig 3.6, © L. R. Scott/Fotolia.com; Fig 11.14, © L Shat/ Fotolia.com; Fig 9.8, © Lansera/ Fotolia.com; Fig 11.1, © Lucky Dragon/Fotolia.com; Fig 9.25, © mediablitzimages (uk) Limited/Alamy; Fig 11.5, © Medical-on-Line/Alamy; Fig 3.21, © moira lovell/Alamy; Fig 8.8, © Monika Korzeniec/Fotolia.com; Fig 10.12, © Natalia Bratslavsky/Fotolia.com; Fig 11.4, © Oleg Kozlov/Fotolia.com; Fig 3.19, © Paul Glendell/Alamy; Fig 9.2, © Peter Girling/Fotolia.com; Figs 2.1, 3.3, 6.10, 6.11, 7.1 and 8.5, Photodisc; Fig 6.12, © PHOTOTAKE Inc./Alamy; Fig 10.6, © Realimage/Alamy; Figs 10.7 and 10.9, © rgbdigital.co.uk/ Fotolia.com; Fig 11.15, Sam Bailey/Hodder Education; Fig 4.5b, © Soil Association (2004); Fig 4.2, © Stockbyte/ Photolibrary.com; Fig 6.15, © Terence Mendoza/Fotolia.com; Fig 8.7, © Vangelis Thomaidis/Fotolia.com; Fig 6.4, © vario images GmbH & Co.KG/Alamy; Fig 8.2, the Vegetarian Society; Fig 9.24, © Xavier HORVILLE/ Fotolia.com; Fig 10.1, © Yanik Chauvin/Fotolia.com; Fig 11.9, © Yuriy Rozanov/Fotolia.com

Crown copyright material is reproduced with the permission of the Controller of HMSO and the Queen's Printer for Scotland.

Figure 6.3 is taken from the Health Survey for England. Copyright © 2008. Re-used with permission of The Information Centre. All rights reserved.

The organisation that puts information at the heart of decision making in health and social care

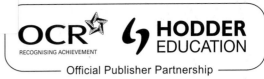

Official Publisher Partnership

OCR
Home Economics for AS

Food, nutrition and health today

Alexis Rickus
Bev Saunder

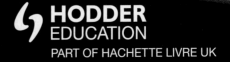

HODDER
EDUCATION
PART OF HACHETTE LIVRE UK

Orders: please contact Bookpoint Ltd, 130 Milton Park, Abingdon, Oxon OX14 4SB. Telephone: (44) 01235 827720. Fax: (44) 01235 400454. Lines are open from 9.00–5.00, Monday to Saturday, with a 24-hour message answering service. You can also order through our website www.hoddereducation.co.uk.

British Library Cataloguing in Publication Data
A catalogue record for this title is available from the British Library

ISBN: 978 0340 968031

First Published 2008
Impression number   10 9 8 7 6 5 4 3 2 1
Year   2014 2013 2012 2011 2010 2009 2008

Cover photo © Dmitri Vervitsiotis.
Typeset by Dorchester Typesetting Group Ltd
Illustrations by Oxford Designers and Illustrators
Printed in Great Britain for Hodder Education, part of Hachette Livre UK, 338 Euston Road, London NW1 3BH by Martins the Printers, Berwick upon Tweed.

Society and Health

This unit matches AS Unit: Society and Health (G001) from your course.

DEMOGRAPHY

Learning objectives

By the end of this chapter you will be able to:

- explain the factors that influence the population patterns and trends in the UK
- identify how these patterns and trends will impact the structure of our society in the future.

Introduction

Population is defined as the number of people inhabiting a specified area or space, as measured by some kind of **census**.

Demography is the study of the characteristics of human populations, such as its size, growth and vital statistics. In this chapter you will study the factors that influence the population patterns and trends in the UK, and consider the implications of these patterns and trends for the structure of society in the future.

It is **estimated** that by 2040 one in four people will be a pensioner. By that time just half the population will be under 45 years old. Official population **projections** for the UK suggest that the population will reach 63.6 million people. By that time there will be 12.2 million pensioners.

Population patterns

The graph below shows the number of people living in the UK under the age of 16 and over the age of 65 between 1971 and 2003. It also shows the projected number of people likely to be living in the UK under the age of 16 and 65 and over between 2003 and 2021 (Source: Social Trends).

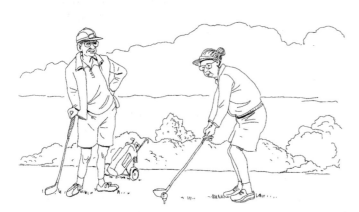

Figure 1.1 *These people are over 65*

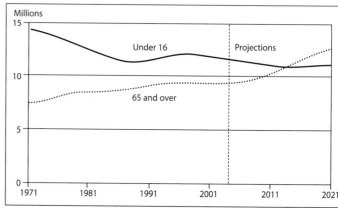

Figure 1.2 *People in the UK under the age of 16 and over the age of 65*

What does the graph above tell us about changing population patterns in the UK?

Describe what the graph suggests will happen to our population pattern over the next ten years.

Population patterns and trends

There are several important factors that influence population patterns and trends. Here are the key ones:

Declining fertility rates

Fertility rate means the ratio of live births and is expressed per 1000 population per year. There has been a decline in fertility rates in recent years with fewer babies being born. In the UK in the 1950s women had an average of 2.5 children, while the rate is now 1.7, and some forecasts suggest it may continue to fall.

The table below shows the national averages for ten European countries.

Ireland:	1.99
France:	1.90
Norway:	1.81
Sweden	1.75
UK:	1.74
Netherlands:	1.73
Germany:	1.37
Italy:	1.33
Spain:	1.32
Greece:	1.29
Source: Eurostat	

Children born per woman in 2004

Declining mortality rates

Mortality rate is the ratio of deaths and is expressed per 1000 population per year. There has been a decline in mortality rates as people are living longer. The increasing population has largely been the result of increased life expectancy.

Although mortality rates in Britain have fallen over time, the UK still has the highest child death rate among the 24 richest countries in the world.

Research mortality rates in other countries round the world and discuss what you find out.

ASSESSMENT HINT!

Discuss means to review the facts and figures that you discover and then to make your own commentary on what you have found.

Migration into the UK

Immigration is the migration into a place or a country of which you are not a native in order to settle there. More people than ever before are migrating into the UK. Some immigrants come to Britain seeking asylum to escape from repressive regimes in their own countries, while some come to achieve a better life for themselves and their family.

The working-age population

The UK's working-age population is falling in size. The proportion of the population aged 65 and over will increase as the large numbers of people born after the Second World War and during the 1960s baby boom become older. The working-age population will fall in size as the baby boomers move into retirement and are replaced by the relatively smaller generations of people who have been born since the mid-1970s.

The role of women in society

More women are choosing to have children later in life and are therefore having fewer children. Many women are choosing to remain childless. One quarter of women in the UK are opting to have no children at all. Effective contraception methods that are widely and easily available make considered choice possible for all women.

The desire for material possessions has meant that some people are delaying having children until they have accumulated a number of possessions, such as a car or a house, or have fulfilled ambitions to travel.

Advances in hygiene and medicine

Advances in hygiene and medicine over the last two hundred years have reduced the mortality rate, particularly the infant mortality rate. This is the death rate during the first year of life. In addition, people are living longer. Drug treatments have been developed for previously fatal conditions and preventative medicine involving immunisation programmes has reduced the incidence of life-threatening conditions. Improved diagnostic equipment can enable doctors to detect conditions more quickly and accurately which makes treatment likely to be more effective. New surgical procedures can now extend life where it would previously have been impossible. Improved diet and a greater understanding of the health risks involved in smoking and lack of exercise have improved life expectancy for many people.

Religious beliefs

Religious beliefs which previously may have had an influence on birth rates do not have such a strong influence today. For instance, some Catholic women use contraception and have abortions despite the Catholic Church advising against both of these.

Cultural expectations

Birth rate is the ratio of total live births expressed as the number of live births per 1000 of the population per year. It is now considered acceptable to have a small family – one or two children – and very large families are considered unusual. Limited family size is usually more economically viable. More women are choosing to have children later in life and are therefore having fewer children and many women are choosing to remain childless. Women in the UK are generally better educated than in the past when it was accepted that when they married their role was to be primarily a wife and mother. When women invest time and effort in their education and career they may choose not to have children.

Activity 3

Review

1. Create a table with social, economic and health as column headings.
2. Place each of the factors influencing population patterns into the most appropriate category.
3. Choose the two most important factors affecting population trends in the UK.
4. Explain how these two factors have influenced trends.

Implications for society

The possible implications of the changing population can be divided into three areas.

Implications for individuals

Increased life expectancy

Life expectancy continues to increase in the UK. Retirement is a time to look forward to as the individual can enjoy more years of active retirement. The enduring stereotype of the frail elderly person is completely outdated. There are many more leisure activities to pursue and opportunities to travel for the retired. The retired population makes a significant contribution to society by completing voluntary work – working in hospitals, as school governors and unpaid carers. However, for some people increased life expectancy and dwindling financial resources restrict opportunity.

Greater need for health care

Inevitably, increasing age will result in the need for greater health care and it may result in longer waiting lists for hospital treatment. There are more very old people who are dependent on others. Advances in health care do not bring resistance to neurological diseases such as Alzheimer's disease. The rising cost of medical treatments and the growing number of people that will require care creates a **burden of dependency** on the working population. The burden of dependency means that the working population will have to pay more tax and National Insurance to support those unable to work and provide the services they need.

More people living alone

The way in which we live our lives is also changing. More people are living alone for longer periods during their lives. This is due to both choice and circumstances, but as age increases the elderly may need care from outside the family. In 2005 a total of 7 million people lived alone compared to 3 million in 1971 (Source: Social Trends 37). Those living alone may need social care. Studies suggest that elderly people can suffer abuse or neglect from their carers when living alone.

Increased retirement age

The retirement age has been raised to ensure people make more contributions through earnings to a pension. During our working lives we will be expected to make more savings to schemes that will supplement our income on retirement. Taxation may be increased to fund the need for more state pensions. The type of jobs individuals do may change with increasing age as more people may choose part-time work or flexible working patterns in later years.

Increased ownership of goods and demand for services

The ownership of goods and demand for services is continuing to rise. Expenditure on leisure services is increasing. The elderly are wealthier than previous generations and have higher expectations as they grew up during the post-war period of growing affluence.

Implications for the family

Smaller families

The falling birth rate has contributed to smaller families. The average family size in the UK is expected to continue declining. Smaller families have contributed to a rise in the standard of living for many; with fewer mouths to feed there is more money to spend on luxury items.

Fewer primary schools

Demand for schools in some areas is threatened by the falling birth rate. Many primary schools in rural areas are under threat of closure as falling rolls reduces their viability. This will mean greater travelling distances to school for some children and closure of the village school in some rural communities.

Changes to caring roles

Caring roles in the family are changing. Both male and female family members may have to care for elderly relatives at some point. Grandparents have a more active role in childcare and caring for other elderly relatives. The contribution the elderly make to the economy as unpaid carers is worth £10 billion per year (Source: Carers UK 2004). Families are increasingly mobile and move home for better employment opportunities. This can create problems for elderly relatives who live alone without family support nearby.

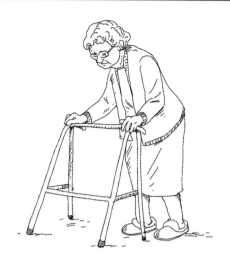

Figure 1.3 *This person may need care and support*

Implications for society

The government uses a census every ten years to gather information on the population to help with social planning.

Increased demand and cost for social and health care

An ageing population may increase demand for places in care homes and put more pressure on voluntary services, such as meals on wheels and home helps.

The government must also consider that an increasing number of older people want to stay at home but require some social and health care. In some communities there could be a shortage of carers. The cost of care in the community must be met. At present the government makes a significant contribution to the long-term personal care of the elderly, but this cost will increase. In addition, the number of people claiming welfare benefits may rise which will increase the tax burden for the working population.

More dependency on the working population

The **dependency ratio** is increasing. The dependency ratio tells us how many young people (under 16) and older people (over 64) depend on those people who are of working age (16 to 64). A high dependency ratio is not good news. In the future it may become harder to maintain the current standard of living for the dependent population because the workforce is shrinking.

Increased need for housing

More specialist accommodation will be required – retirement flats, bungalows, residential and sheltered accommodation. Much of the existing housing stock is not adequate. In 2004, 21% of housing stock failed to give adequate thermal comfort in England. Households with the lowest income are more likely to live in poor quality accommodation (Source: Social Trends 37).

Influence on culture

Poverty still exists in the UK, but most elderly people are wealthier, healthier and better educated than previous generations. There are more old people than young, and our media, culture and values will be influenced by this change. There is a growing need for social activities and leisure pursuits that engage the elderly in every community.

A shortage of young people

There will be a shortage of young people as the fertility rate is declining and the required **replacement level** is not being met. The replacement level is the number of births per woman required to replace the existing population. This is estimated to be 2.1 children per woman; in 2005 the replacement level in England was 1.8 children per woman (Source: Social Trends 37). Immigration is the possible solution to this problem. More labour is required for essential services including nurses, plumbers, fruit pickers and catering staff. There needs to be a considered public debate about immigration.

Greater mobility

People are moving. Some parts of the UK have higher concentrations of older people and this can affect local services. In coastal areas of the UK there are disproportionately high numbers of elderly people. Many people now choose to retire overseas and Mediterranean destinations are popular with many affluent Europeans. This movement puts more pressure on health services and housing needs in those areas.

Age of the workforce

The average age of the British workforce is rising and fewer young people are entering the labour market.

Many people are choosing not to retire, making the average age of the workforce older. There is increasing evidence of discrimination and **ageism** in the workplace. Ageism is stereotyping against individuals because of their age. October 2006 regulations made it illegal to discriminate against someone in employment or training on the grounds of age.

Increased poverty

The gap between the wealthy and poor remains immense. There are a significant number of elderly people who are living in poverty, and it is estimated that 20% of pensioners in the UK live in poverty. This is due to the state pension being inadequate, means testing complex and many old people living in housing which is too expensive to maintain (Source: BBC Action Network, 28 April 2006).

Activity 4

Check your understanding

1. Check your understanding of the meaning of the following key terms:

demography	fertility rate	mortality rate
birth rate	infant mortality	population
migration	rate	census
burden of	replacement level	
dependency	dependency ratio	ageism

Activity 5

Review

1. The future structure of society: individuals. Identify two key terms and search out newspaper articles which discuss the issues.
2. The future structure of society: family. Again, identify two key terms and search out newspaper articles which discuss the issues.
3. Are there differing views on these issues or do all experts agree on the implications for changes in population structure?

Exam-style questions

The graph below shows life expectancy in years at retirement in the UK since 1981.

It shows the number of additional years both men and women can expect to live after retiring at 65 years.

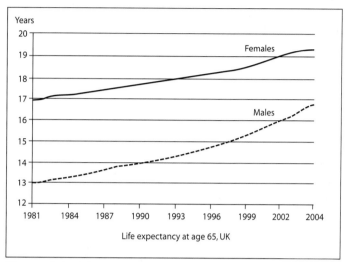

Figure 1.4 *Life expectancy at age 65, UK*

Source: Office for National Statistics and Government Actuary's Department, 2006

1 With reference to the graph above, what does the trend in this graph suggest for the life expectancy at retirement for men and women?   (1 mark)

2 State how many years after retirement men and women can expect to live.   (2 marks)

3 Give two reasons why people live longer nowadays.   (2 marks)

4 Describe the possible effects of an increasing number of elderly people on society.   (10 marks)

(Total of 15 marks)

Family and society

Learning objectives

By the end of this chapter you will be able to:

- give the definition of a household and family
- understand the functions of the family
- identify the different types of families and household groups and the possible implications of change
- understand statistical data related to household and family structures
- identify basic human needs and the needs of individuals, households and families
- explain the factors which affect our standard of living.

Introduction

This chapter begins with two very important definitions of the family and a household. It is important to distinguish between a family and a household because the government provides statistical information based upon these two terms. Therefore an understanding of these terms will help you interpret data from government sources.

You will then explore how the function of the family is changing and how the diversity of family and household groups is expanding. The possible impact of change will be investigated. A major upheaval in attitudes towards the social acceptability of different family or household groups is occurring. To help develop your understanding of the issues you will examine statistical data on households and families.

In the final section you will investigate basic human needs and the factors that may affect the standard of living for households and families.

What is a family?

In the UK a wide variety of social arrangements exist. Defining a family is difficult as there are many exceptions to virtually every definition.

A **family** can be defined as a social unit connected by blood, marriage or adoption.

The family is a vital social unit in almost every society. Many people spend their lives within a family and place a high value on it. There are many different types of family in the UK. They are essential in terms of economic organisation, the socialisation of children and cultural identity.

What is a household?

A **household** can be defined as one person living alone or a group of people who share the same address and living arrangements.

Virtually all families live in a household but *not* all households are families. A single elderly person living alone is classed as a household. A married couple without children can also be classified as a household.

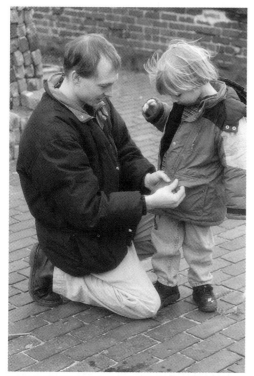

Figure 2.1 *A one-parent family with a male parent*

types identified are one-person and one-family households. Family households are divided into those with dependent children (under the age of 18 in full-time education), those with non-dependent children, couples with no children and lone parents.

Great Britain	Percentages				
	1971	1981	1991	2001	2006
One person	6	8	11	12	12
One-family household					
Couple with no children	19	20	25	25	25
Dependent children	52	47	53	39	37
Non-dependent children only	10	10	12	9	8
Lone parent with dependent and non-dependent children	4	6	9	12	12
All people in private households (millions)	53.4	53.9	54.1	56.4	57.1

Source: Census, Labour Force Survey, Office for National Statistics, 2006

Activity 2

Review

1. With reference to the table above, how many people lived in private households in 2006?
2. What has happened to the percentage of one-family households with dependent children since 1991?
3. What has happened to the percentage of couples with no children since 1971?
4. How does this data support the claim that most households still contain children?

Activity 1

Group discussion

Read the following description which shows how one person has lived in several different types of household.

As a child Tom lived with both his parents. When he was five his parents divorced and he lived with his mother. A few years later his mother remarried and Tom lived with his mother and stepfather.

Tom did well at school and decided to study at university away from home, where he shared a house with some friends.

After finishing his studies, Tom lived with his girlfriend for three years and they had a baby. Last year they split up and Tom decided to move back home to his mother and stepfather. While living at home he was able to save enough money to buy a flat and he moved in last week.

How many different household types can you identify?

Tom lived in a family household three times. Can you identify them?

The table below shows the different types of household in Great Britain since 1971 as percentages. The two

Functions of the family

The family unit has many very important functions. It provides a place where strong relationships are formed. These relationships satisfy our emotional needs for love and security. The family stabilises sexual and reproductive functions. It provides a secure, safe place for children to be raised. The socialisation of children starts within the family. **Socialisation** is the process in which a child learns to fit into their social environment. This process can take many years but starts at home with parents.

The family provides its members with a cultural identity, a position in society and a set of values and beliefs. A cultural identity gives an individual a feeling of belonging to a social group with the same attitudes, behaviour and values. This is important to communities with a strong sense of cultural or religious identity.

The family home provides shelter and protection. The actual address provides a base to access health, education and welfare services, such as registration for a school place, GP surgery and Department for Work and Pensions (DWP) benefits. Family members provide care and support for each other.

The family provides financial resources for its members, particularly when they are young. The basic needs for food and clothing are met due to the provision of financial resources.

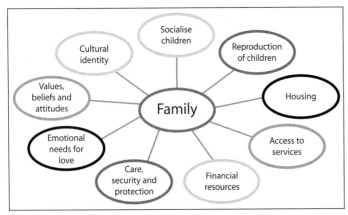

Figure 2.2 *Summary of the key functions of the family*

Activity 3

Review and group discussion

Write a sentence to explain how the family fulfils each function shown in Figure 2.2.

Discuss what circumstances may exist where a family is unable to fulfil its functions.

Discuss which of these functions may be completed by the state.

Structures of families and households

There are many different types of family and household. The structure of families and households are changing. For example, the number of single-person households is increasing. Many single women with increased earning power are choosing to live alone. You will now look at the different types of household and family group.

Nuclear family

The nuclear family usually consists of two generations living together – parents and children. They do not have daily contact with other family members, such as grandparents; contact becomes a matter of choice.

Extended family

The extended family usually consists of three generations living together in the same household or living very close to other family members. They have daily contact with other family members and support each other.

Reconstituted (step) family

The reconstituted family consists of a family unit in which one or both parents have been previously married and have children from that relationship. There will be a step parent for each child.

Lone parent family

The lone parent family is formed from a single male or female parent and dependent children living together. The most common reason for a lone parent family is divorce, separation or one partner's unwillingness to marry or cohabit.

Gay and lesbian family

A same-sex couple living together as a family with children.

Single person household

A person living on their own. A significant number of these households are female.

Multiperson household

A group of people living together in one household.

Changes in household and family group composition

There have been many changes in society which have affected the family and household structure. The significance of some of these changes has been exaggerated by the media, in particular the number of teenage pregnancies and lone parents. It is important to consider the fact that couples living with children (dependent and non-dependent) still made up the largest family type in the UK in 2006. The key changes and their possible impact will now be explored.

Changing nature of the extended family

The traditional extended family is declining. Greater mobility, higher standards of living and the emergence of the welfare state have contributed to the decline of the extended family. Many families are becoming self-contained and self-reliant units. Today most families with dependent children live in nuclear families, and due to developments in technology, links between family members are maintained. However, with the rising cost of residential care, inadequacy of some pension provision and childcare costs, it has been suggested that there will be a return to several generations living together under one roof. Grandparents may become live-in childminders if both parents work.

Changing roles within the family

The roles within the family are changing. Traditionally, the male role was to provide for the family and the female was to care for the family. Women are now much more likely to be working, making a significant contribution to the family income. Some men have taken over the traditional female domestic role and are 'househusbands'. There is evidence to suggest that there is some division of household tasks between men and women. Yet, the main responsibility for childcare and housework is more likely to be taken by women.

Changes in legislation have aimed to provide greater equality between the employment rights of men and women. However women earn on average much less than men. Women are more likely to be employed in caring, clerical or service industries which are often less well paid.

The table below is from the UK 2005 Time Use survey. It shows the time spent on activities by both males and females each day. The figures are based on averages calculated over seven days.

	Hours and minutes per day	
	Males	Females
Sleep	8.04	8.18
Resting	0.43	0.48
Personal care	0.40	0.48
Eating and drinking	1.25	1.19
Leisure		
Watching TV/DVD and listen to radio/music	2.50	2.25
Social life and entertainment/culture	1.22	1.32
Hobbies and games	0.37	0.23
Sport	0.13	0.07
Reading	0.23	0.26
All leisure	5.25	4.53
Employment and study	3.45	2.26
Housework	1.41	3.00
Childcare	0.15	0.32
Voluntary work and meetings	0.15	0.20
Travel	1.32	1.22
Other	0.13	0.15

Notes: People aged 16 and over
Source: Office for National Statistics, 2006

Activity 4

Group discussion
With reference to the table above, what are the three main activities carried out by people?
How much time is spent on housework each day?
Who spends the most time on housework?
Make a list of ten household tasks. In pairs discuss if they should be completed by females, males or shared.

Smaller family size

The number of births has declined since 1901. However, there were sharp increases in births after the First and Second World Wars. These peaks are sometimes referred to as **baby booms**. During the 1960s there was a further peak. The 1960s were a time of high living standards for many, so the birth rate increased. When the large number of girls born in the 1960s reached childbearing age, a further peak occurred in the 1980s. The projections suggest that the number of births will remain stable.

The graph below shows the number of live births (babies showing signs of life at birth) in millions each year since 1901. It shows the significant peaks.

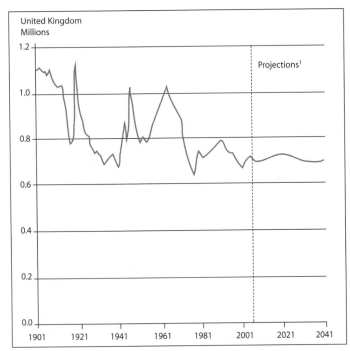

Figure 2.3 *Number of live births each year*

Data for 1901 to 1921 exclude Ireland, which was constitutionally a part of the UK during this period. Data from 1981 exclude the non-residents of Northern Ireland.

1 2004-based projections for 2006 to 2041.

Source: Office for National Statistics, 2006, Government Actuary's Department, General Register Office for Scotland and Northern Ireland Statistics and Research Agency

Activity 5

Group discussion

With reference to the graph above, what does the overall trend suggest about live births?

Approximately how many births were expected in 2006?

Explain the three key peaks in 1920, 1947 and 1964.

The reasons for the decline in births and the subsequent effect on family size are varied. The changing role of women in society and increased mobility of the population have undoubtedly contributed.

Developments in health care have reduced infant mortality so parents do not need to create large families to ensure that some children survive to adulthood. The widespread availability of contraception and accessibility of abortion has been significant in reducing family size. Some commentators suggest that society is more children-centred and more money and time are devoted to the upkeep and needs of the child. As a result, there are many smaller families with a higher standard of living.

Increase in childless women

The trend towards childlessness is expected to continue as more women make significant contributions to the labour market. The proportion of women who remain childless is rising steadily. Data from the Office for National Statistics in 2006 suggests that nearly one in five women, born in the mid-1960s and now in their forties, is childless. This compares to one in ten women born in the mid-1940s who were childless at the same age. These women will not have children who can care for them in later years and may have to rely upon the state for assistance.

Increase in older mothers

The average age for a first child was 27.3 years in 2005, which was three years older than in 1971 (Social Trends 37). The growth in the number of women continuing their education beyond 18 years has contributed to the rise in later marriage and child bearing. Research suggests that age-related fertility problems have increased as some women leave pregnancy until their mid-thirties. According to the Office for National Statistics, the over 35s now have the fastest growing birth rates. The number of women having babies in their 40s has nearly doubled in ten years.

The changing divorce rate

The increase in divorce is possibly the most significant factor to affect the family in the UK today. The Divorce Reform Act 1969 became effective in 1971 and led initially to a notable increase in the number of divorces. However, since 1993 the figures have remained relatively constant. Nearly half of all new marriages end in divorce and this may affect a significant number of children. Research has suggested that the effect of divorce on young children can cause emotional and behavioural problems. Children can blame themselves for the divorce and they may become withdrawn and feel insecure. Divorce can also lead to stress and depression in adults too. It can cause financial hardship and lead to extra demand for housing.

Marriages and divorces

The graph below shows the number of divorces, marriages and remarriages since 1950 in the UK. There is a sharp increase in divorces and remarriages in the early 1970s. The number of marriages has fallen steadily since this period.

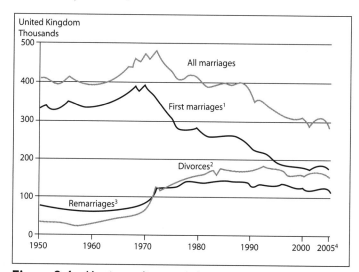

Figure 2.4 *Marriages, divorces and remarriages*

1 For both partners.

2 Includes annulments. Data for 1950 to 1970 for Great Britain only. Divorce was permitted in Northern Ireland from 1969.

3 For one or both partners.

4 Data for 2005 are provisional. Final figures are likely to be higher.

Source: Office for National Statistics, General Register Office for Scotland and Northern Ireland Statistics and Research Agency

Activity 6

Group discussion

Is a decline in the number of marriages important?

More step families

The number of remarriages for one or both partners has increased since the introduction of divorce legislation. Surveys suggest that two fifths of all marriages were remarriages in 2005. As children tend to stay with their mother when a relationship ends, they will form a new family on remarriage. Additionally, the data suggests more than 10 per cent of all families with dependent children were step families. Step families can offer greater stability and financial resources for individuals and households. However, in some cases step families can encounter problems. There could be tension and resentment of the new step parent or step brothers and sisters.

More cohabitation

Marriage remains the most common partnership in the UK, but as we have seen the number of marriages is in decline. **Cohabitation** is when a couple share an intimate relationship living together without being married. This is increasing. In 2005 24 per cent of non-married people under the age of 60 years were cohabiting which is almost twice as many as in 1986. There is some evidence to suggest that cohabiting arrangements are more likely to break down than marriages. If they do the consequences can be difficult to resolve. At present there is no straightforward legal answer to the division of assets and property. The significant increase in cohabiting arrangements has led the government to consider a review of the situation.

Increased births outside marriage

There has been a considerable rise in the number of children born outside marriage. In 2005 43 per cent of births occurred outside marriage (Social Trends 37). In different parts of the UK the number of births outside marriage varies. For example, in the North East of England 55 per cent of births happen outside marriage. Most births outside marriage are registered jointly, suggesting that the parents live together at the time of the birth of the child.

Increase in lone parent families

Lone parent families are formed due to divorce, separation, widowhood or births to single women outside marriage. The number of lone parents has increased. The number with dependent children has more than doubled from 3 per cent of households in 1971 to 7 per cent in 2006 (Social Trends 37). The causes of this increase may be attributed to many factors including the changes to divorce legislation and social acceptability of lone parent families. Families are constantly changing and lone parenthood for the majority is not a permanent state. The majority of these families are headed by women and can be disadvantaged by being more vulnerable to poverty. Lone parent families need affordable housing and in many cases childcare so the parent can work.

More non-dependent children living with parents

The number of adults living with their parents has increased. This may be due to the costs of higher education and the shortage of affordable housing. This creates a longer period of dependency on parents. Young men are more likely to live with their parents than young women. This change may bring a higher standard of living to these households.

Civil partnerships

A **civil partnership** is a legal relationship, which can be registered by two people of the same sex. It gives same-sex couples the ability to obtain legal recognition for their relationship. Couples in these relationships have the same tax, inheritance and pension rights as a civil marriage. The Adoption and Children Act 2002 modernised the adoption procedures and allowed single people and same-sex couples to adopt children. The impact of this change means that this type of family unit will become part of the diverse nature of UK families.

More one-person households

There are more one-person households. A significant number of pensioners live alone and these are usually females. Females tend to live longer and are more likely to live alone. Increased life expectancy has played a part in the rise in one-person households.

The rise in divorce and separation has also contributed to those at a younger age living alone. The age group 25 to 44 years has seen a significant increase in individuals living alone in recent years. The impact of this change means that there is a housing shortage for single people.

The table below shows the size of different households in Great Britain since 1971. It also shows the percentages number of each type of household.

Great Britain	Percentages				
	1971	1981	1991	2001[1]	2006[1]
One person	18	22	27	29	29
Two people	32	32	34	35	36
Three people	19	17	16	16	16
Four people	17	18	16	14	13
Five people	8	7	5	5	4
Six or more people	6	4	2	2	2
All households (=100%) (millions)	18.6	20.2	22.4	23.8	24.2
Average household size (number of people)	2.9	2.7	2.5	2.4	2.4

1 Data are at spring for 2001 and Q2 for 2006.

Source: Census, Labour Force Survey, Office for National Statistics, 2006

Activity 7

Group discussion

With reference to the table above, what does this data suggest about the trend in one-person households and four- and five-person households?

How many households (millions) were there in 2006?

What was the average household size in 2006?

Why are households becoming smaller?

Basic human needs

All human beings are born with needs that must be fulfilled. The root of all human motivation is to satisfy our needs. The need for food, warmth and shelter are essential for life and must be satisfied first. But we have other needs, the need to feel safe, be successful and be satisfied with life – and these must also be addressed.

Maslow's hierarchy of needs

The psychologist Abraham Maslow studied human behaviour and motivation. Maslow alleged that unsatisfied needs motivate people. He devised the structure of needs into a pyramid, which is called Maslow's hierarchy of needs.

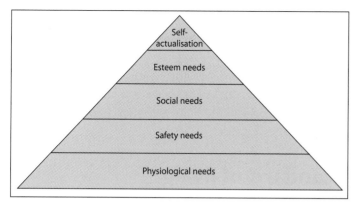

Figure 2.5 *Maslow's hierarchy of needs*

company	rules at school
food	friends
laugh at self	a home
shun social pressures	success at school
warm clothes in winter	laws in society
love from family	routines
good reputation at work	fashionable clothes
accepting of others	responsibility at work
mobile phones	club membership
comfortable with self	sleep

The physiological needs are situated at the base of the pyramid. These include food, warmth, sleep, shelter and sex. These needs are the most important. We must satisfy these needs before progressing to the next set of needs.

Safety needs include the need to feel safe and protected. They consist of the need for security and stability. This can be achieved by living in a society with a clearly defined set of values and laws. On top of this individuals can take measures to ensure they feel secure, such as fitting a burglar alarm.

Social needs consist of the need for love and a sense of belonging. This could be through social relationships in the family, with friends or at work.

The final two sets of needs are the high order needs. The esteem needs are the desire to achieve, acquire status and independence. They can be met through achievement at school and work.

The highest need, self-actualisation, is potentially the most difficult to achieve, and only a small proportion of the population achieve this need. To fulfil this need an individual must realise their potential and feel a sense of satisfaction and accomplishment in their achievement. They are accepting of others and content with themselves.

Activity 8

Review

Draw your own pyramid with plenty of space on each level.

Then look at the twenty terms below which could help to satisfy different needs.

Insert the terms into a position on your pyramid to show which set of needs you think they satisfy.

The needs of household and family groups

You have looked at individual needs and now you will examine the needs of households and families. Every family or household is different and will have slightly different needs.

You have seen that there are more single person households, more parents working and a greater number of older people in the community. But each community is different and it should meet a diversity of needs. It is the intention of the government to provide communities which will meet all our present and future needs.

> 'People are very clear about what they want from their communities – places that are safe, clean, friendly and prosperous, with good amenities such as education, health services, shopping and green spaces.'
>
> *The Egan Review: Skills for Sustainable Communities, April 2004*

The term 'sustainable communities' is used to describe a place where needs are met and opportunities provided. In these communities there will be a sense of belonging, trust and inclusion.

The needs of the households and family groups in the community are as follows:

- **Identity and inclusivity:** The UK is a multicultural society and communities consist of many different cultural groups, backgrounds and beliefs. There should be opportunities for everyone to engage in community activities and to feel a valued part of the community. A friendlier and more inclusive community may have lower levels of crime so it will feel a safer place for the residents.

- **Structure and organisation:** There needs to be an accepted set of values and beliefs within each community. This will give security, responsibility and confidence to family and household groups. Legislation to support and protect against antisocial behaviour, domestic violence, discrimination at work and maternity and paternity rights meet these needs. Local government provides many services including social housing, refuse collection, street lighting and cleaning, libraries, consumer protection and the care and support of children and vulnerable adults.

- **Safe, affordable places to live:** A range of affordable housing must be available to meet the needs of household and family groups. This creates a sense of place and people can feel they belong in the community. High quality and well designed housing that meets the needs of families and individuals is required. The housing should be an appropriate size, layout and design. The environment should have a balance between green public space and secure private space.

- **Employment opportunities:** The community must offer opportunities for people to work. The financial needs of families and households can be met by employment. Employment may also provide a sense of achievement and enjoyment. In addition, the community should provide training opportunities to families or households, as the skills people require may change over time.

- **Access to services:** Households and family groups require health care services, schools and social services. These services need to be high quality and accessible to all. Family and household groups may need voluntary and private organisations for advice, support and guidance. The community is a place for business and retail services. Family and household groups need to shop for food and clothes, and to buy services to maintain their home. The community should provide these services.

- **Transport systems:** Being able to travel and reach work, school, shops, relatives, friends and leisure facilities is very important for families and households. There must be a public transport structure as not everyone has their own transport. The opportunity for those wishing to walk or cycle safely should be available.

Activity 9

Review

Produce a written report describing your community. Consider the six key needs above and identify the strengths of your community and areas needing development.

Standard of living

A family or household's standard of living is determined by the financial resources that are left over after its basic needs are met. The remaining funds, if significant, allow households or families to enjoy a higher standard of living.

The standard of living in the UK has risen for the majority of people. It can be measured against income or against the quality of goods and services bought. Standard of living can also refer to the quality of life experienced by individuals. This is more subjective and relies upon personal judgement so it is difficult to measure. For the purpose of this discussion, we will use a materialistic definition.

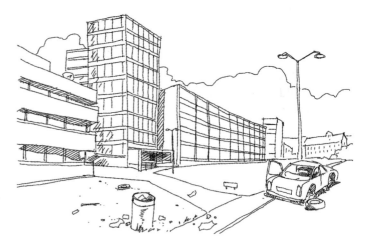

Figure 2.6 *A deprived community*

Standard of living is defined as a measure of the goods, services and luxuries available to an individual or household once the basic necessities are met.

Factors affecting standard of living

Financial resources available

Financial resources could include income from employment, welfare benefits and investments. Household and family groups with access to considerable financial resources are likely to have a higher standard of living. Alternatively, those with limited financial resources may have a lower standard of living.

The cost of running a home means that many households and family groups require more than one wage to maintain an acceptable standard of living. The reliance on two wages to buy and maintain a home means many households are increasing the risk of financial hardship should one of the wage earners become unable to work.

The number of people

The number of people in a household or family group can influence the standard of living. Large households need large incomes to maintain a high standard of living. The collective income of a large number of people living together could allow for a higher standard of living.

The number of dependents

The dependent members in a household or family group could include children, the elderly, the unemployed or the disabled. These individuals may only make a limited financial contribution but require a greater proportion of the resources. A household with many dependent members can have a lower standard of living if the financial resources do not meet their needs.

The profession or occupation of individuals

A household or family group with one or more high earning members may have a relatively high standard of living. Certain professions or occupations command greater salaries than others. A household or family group which depends upon its income from unskilled manual work or part-time work may not have a high standard of living, particularly if there are dependents in the group. The level of education may contribute towards the standard of living. Graduates can earn considerably more than non-graduates although this can be moderated by the repayment of student loans.

The health of individuals

Illness and disability can affect the earning potential of household and family members and subsequently the standard of living. The loss of earnings and the cost of illness can be a burden (prescription charges, special diets, heating the home all day and transport costs to hospital). A member of the household or family group may have to give up work to care for an ill child or relative, therefore reducing income further.

The geographical location

In some areas of the UK there are fewer employment opportunities so if unemployment is high the standard of living is likely to be affected. Living in a rural location can increase transport costs. Although the traditional north–south divide is slowly disappearing as many companies are deciding to relocate to cities outside the south east, there are certain parts of the UK where it is more expensive to buy property and basic necessities.

The amount of debt

According to recent research, the average family now spends more of its household income on repaying debts than at any time over the past ten years. Consumer borrowing using credit cards, motor and retail finance deals, overdrafts and unsecured personal loans has risen. A household or family group with substantial debt may have a lower standard of living as it will have less disposable income available than a debt-free household or family group.

The cost of housing

Meeting the cost of purchasing or renting a house can make a significant impact on the standard of living. House prices have increased considerably and mortgage repayments can be burdensome. If borrowing is linked to variable interest rates, then increases in interest rates can reduce the amount of money available to purchase other items and lower the standard of living.

The cost of maintaining a home can be expensive. Many people live in property that was constructed in the period after the Second World. Data from research suggests that 19 per cent of housing stock is even older and was constructed before 1919 (Social Trends 2006). This type of property is more likely to need repairs, be poorly insulated and be more expensive to heat in winter. This cost could burden a household or family group.

CHECK YOUR UNDERSTANDING

1 Check your understanding of the meaning of the following key terms:

socialisation	civil partnership	step family
households	baby boom	nuclear family
extended family	lone parent family	househusband
standard of living	family	cohabitation
sustainable communities	hierarchy of needs	human needs

2 Complete the following exercise using some of the key words and phrases above.

There are many different types of family in the UK. The _____ family is when three generations live together. It is an important _____ structure because it can provide a secure environment for the _____ of children. Due to greater mobility and different employment opportunities, the _____ is increasingly common.

Divorce has contributed to the rise in the number of _____ families and _____ families. The number of single person _____ has also increased. When a couple live together but are not married it is known as_____.

All behaviour is motivated by _____. Maslow devised a _____. The government believes the needs of households and families may be achieved by living in _____. The income of a household and the health of its members are just two factors that can affect the _____.

Exam-style questions

The table below shows the main types of household in Great Britain. The types are one-person households, one-family households, lone parent and unrelated adults living together. The percentages of each type of household are shown since 1971. The data also shows the percentages for the number of dependent and non-dependent children in family and lone parent households.

Great Britain	Percentages				
	1971	1981	1991	2001	2006
One person					
Under pensionable age	6	8	11	14	14
Over pensionable age	12	14	16	15	14
One-family households					
Couple with no children	27	26	28	29	28
1–2 dependent children	26	25	20	19	18
3+ dependent children	9	6	5	4	4
Non-dependent children only	8	8	8	6	7
Lone parent with					
Dependent children	3	5	6	7	7
Non-dependent children	4	4	4	3	3
2+ unrelated adults	4	5	3	3	3
All households 100% (millions)	18.6	20.2	22.4	23.8	24.2

Source: Adapted from Social Trends 37

1 With reference to the table above, how many households were there in Great Britain in 2006? (1 mark)

2 What does the trend suggest about one-person households? (1 mark)

3 What does the trend suggest about one-family households with dependent children? (1 mark)

4 Explain two reasons why non-dependent children may continue to live in a family household. (4 marks)

5 Describe what has happened to the number of lone parent households with dependent children since 1971. (2 marks)

6 Give three reasons for the trend in lone parent households. (3 marks)

7 Discuss the factors which can affect the standard of living of households and family groups. (8 marks)

(Total of 20 marks)

Key issues for society

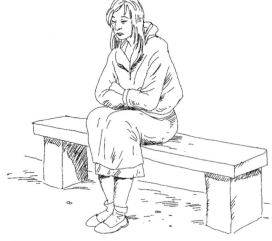

Figure 3.1 *The impact of poverty on the individual*

Introduction

In this chapter four key issues are explored:

- poverty
- employment and unemployment
- leisure
- housing and homelessness.

Each issue will be explained and, where relevant, the impact on individuals, households and society are described. Changing patterns of leisure and developments in housing design to meet changing needs are be investigated.

Poverty

The UK could be considered a wealthy country where many people enjoy a high standard of living. Yet for some this is simply not the case. Poverty really impacts upon their daily lives.

There are many definitions of poverty:

- **Poverty** is the state of being poor and lacking the means to provide material needs or comforts. It is a situation where resources are insufficient to meet individual needs.

- **Absolute poverty** is a state below which it is not possible to live a healthy life, being unable to afford sufficient food, clothing, warmth and shelter.
- **Relative poverty** is having resources below the average individual or family so that they are in effect excluded from what we would consider ordinary living patterns and activities.
- **The poverty trap** is the idea that once in poverty a person is often trapped in it. Being in poverty and being unable to escape from it is called the poverty trap.

Activity 1

Group discussion
What do you consider to be the most appropriate definition of poverty and why?

Causes of poverty

There are many causes of poverty. Here are the most common ones.

The cycle of deprivation

The cycle of deprivation causes poverty. This is where children who are born into poor families with backgrounds of social problems then go on to cohabit or marry one another, have children and the cycle begins again. People who are said to be in the cycle of deprivation may sometimes bring up their children in an inadequate manner, failing to give them the opportunities most children have. Often these people are unable or unwilling to find work and therefore have a low income.

The cycle of deprivation frequently occurs when at least three of the following are present: poor intellect, family instability, poorly educated children, poorly kept home and a large family.

Being dependent upon the state

People can become poor because they become dependent on the state for their income. They either cannot or will not work and find it very difficult to budget. This position may be due to the fault of the individual or it may be how a person has been brought up.

Lack of employment

Not being able to find work, particularly for prolonged periods of time, can result in poverty. Even paid employment does not necessarily lift people out of poverty if the work is short term or very low paid.

Lack of education

Factors such as lack of education or not having the required skills can defeat people who want to work. Access to better paid jobs requiring specialist skills or knowledge may be limited.

Caring for others

Some single parents are unable to work because there is no affordable childcare. This means that the money coming in to the family can be significantly reduced because of the cost of childcare. In addition, some people are unable to work because of family responsibilities such as caring for the disabled or elderly.

Being homeless

A homeless person may be unable to get work because they do not have a permanent address. This causes problems in obtaining benefits and opening a bank account.

Being elderly, sick or disabled

The elderly may no longer be fit to work and may be totally dependent on the state pension, which is a fixed amount. If they have no other income and no savings, they may well be living in poverty. The long-term sick or disabled may not be able to work because of their condition or they may only be able to access very low paid work. The standard of living of this group may well be very low as a result of their costs of living. For example, their heating bills may be higher than normal.

The poverty trap

Some people are born into deprivation and poverty and may never be able to escape because the area in which they live offers them limited opportunities and they may not have the financial capability to escape. People can be trapped in poverty, finding it difficult to get out.

The effects of poverty

Poverty can affect individuals, families and society. The effects of poverty can be as follows.

Deprivation

This means going without basics and necessities such as adequate heating, nourishing food and an effective means of transport. Individuals suffering poverty may not be adequately fed or clothed and may not be able to keep warm. Some may not even be properly housed.

Lack of leisure pursuits and activities

This can be particularly difficult for children who may not be able to participate in trips and activities at school. It may be difficult for them to join clubs which cost money, such as dancing, football or music lessons, or where a uniform is required like karate or guides. Children experiencing poverty are also less likely to go out, go on holiday and have 'treats' such as a trip to the cinema.

Stigma and lack of status

This can be particularly difficult for children who may not have the newest designer accessories such as mobile phones, handbags and trainers. They may be socially excluded if they cannot participate in a discussion about latest trends or the latest computer game. Children born into poverty may not excel at school and are more likely to truant. Those who suffer poverty are **marginalised** if they do not have access to basic equipment which most of society take for granted. An example of this would be a computer.

Inadequate housing conditions

People living in poverty may have to live in squalid conditions such as living in a damp house. There may be overcrowding if there are not enough bedrooms. Bathrooms may need to be shared with other families so the conditions may be unsanitary. In extreme cases they may become homeless.

Ill health

Lack of sufficient money may mean people living in poverty are unable to feed the family adequately. This can lead to poor health as can housing not being warm enough or being damp.

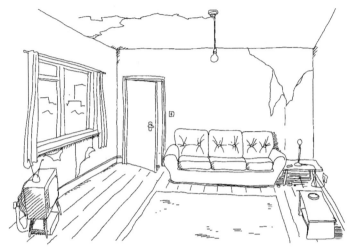

Figure 3.2 *Squalid housing conditions*

Locality

People living in poverty may be housed in deprived neighbourhoods. These deprived areas may have higher crime rates, poor performing schools and even fewer doctors. Some people in these areas could turn to crime and vandalism as they feel it is unfair that they are unable to have some of the material things that others have. Local authorities sometimes house 'problem families' in these areas who may then be ostracised by the local community because of antisocial behaviour. Areas where there is real poverty could easily become rundown. Businesses and shops may end up closing down due to a lack of custom.

Strain on individuals and relationships

Due to the difficult circumstances poorer people find themselves in there can often be arguments, frequently over money and budgeting. The result of deprivation can lead to mental and physical health problems. Self-esteem can become very low and individuals may suffer depression which can in turn cause behavioural problems and create the inability to socialise and communicate effectively with others. Some individuals can become withdrawn while others become aggressive. Relationships with other family members may also suffer.

Finances

People living in poverty will have limited money available to them. They may not be able to afford any luxuries and some may not even have sufficient funds for necessities. They may be tempted to take out loans with disreputable companies at high interest rates, which can often make the financial situation worse. Failure to pay service bills such as telephone, electricity and gas may mean they are disconnected. General living costs are often higher because of limited funds. This may mean that they are not able to take advantage of offers and bulk buying.

Social exclusion

Social exclusion is a situation where individuals, due to a lack of resources, are excluded from participating in aspects of society that the majority of us take for granted. Poverty can cause social exclusion because the very poor do not have the material wealth to participate in normal society. They may not have access to facilities for maintaining personal hygiene. They may not have acceptable clothing in which to present themselves.

Activity 2

Review
Summarise in a bulleted list the causes of poverty and the effects of poverty.

Activity 3

Research opportunity and group discussion
Go on to the website of a supermarket chain.
Imagine you only have £50 in your budget to spend on food this week for a family of four. How far can you make your £50 go? Decide what should go in your shopping basket.
Print off your food items and the cost.
Compare and discuss your findings.

Groups most at risk of poverty

Certain members of society are more at risk of poverty than others.

The unemployed

Advances in technology, increasing automation in industry and foreign competition have led over the years to a higher level of unemployment. The least skilled are more likely to be made unemployed. Being unemployed puts you at risk of poverty because the family may have to cope with a significantly reduced income.

The low paid

Low paid workers are often caught in the poverty trap. A low income may mean they find it difficult to budget, and in some cases they would actually earn more if they did not work and claimed benefits.

Single parent families

Over recent years there has been a growth in the divorce rate and an increase in single parenthood. Frequently the single parent is the mother and the extra cost of looking after children and the limited earning opportunities can push them into poverty.

The sick and disabled

Many sick and disabled people are unable to work. If this is the case, they may have to depend upon state benefits. This gives them a limited income to live on and may push them into poverty.

The elderly

Some elderly people, particularly those who may be reliant on the basic state pension, may be at risk from poverty. Poverty in old age is not something that happens to all pensioners. Those who are poor in old age are most likely to be the ones who earned least in their lifetimes. Therefore, the groups in poverty mentioned above – the low paid, single parent families, the disabled and the unemployed – are all likely to be poor in their old age.

Young teenagers

Teenagers, who have left home or have been required to leave home because of marital break-up or family tensions, may find they cannot afford to find a suitable place to live or have enough money to look after themselves adequately.

Ethnic minorities and refugees

This group of people may find themselves in this country with no money or possessions. It can take some time for them to settle and be eligible for any state benefits.

The illiterate and poorly educated

These are the groups of people who are least likely to get a well paid job, and therefore often have to accept low paid or unskilled work.

Activity 4

Practical opportunity

Read these extracts from *Nutrition and Diet in Lone Parent Families* by Elizabeth Dowler and Claire Calvert. They are statements from lone parents claiming income support.

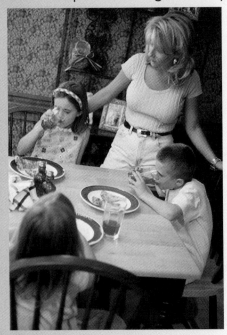

Figure 3.3   *A lone parent*

'I buy apples and bananas every fortnight. It's horrible when she has a banana and then says can I have an apple. And you've got to stop her because it's got to last.'
Lone mother, mid-20s, claiming income support with one young daughter

'He gets hot nourishing food inside him – he gets meat and veg I can't afford to buy, he gets a pudding. If I did a sandwich it would be jam. School holidays are a nightmare trying to give him that extra meal a day is impossible.
Lone mother, early 40s, claiming income support referring to son having free school meals

'The kids can't come and help themselves to food. They don't have access to milk just to drink. Milk goes on their cereal, their hot chocolate at night is mostly water.
Lone mother, mid-30s, claiming income support with two teenagers

Find out how much the basic income support for lone parents with dependent children is.

Plan an economical nutritious main course dish suitable for a lone parent and three dependent young children aged three, seven and nine. Itemise the cost of each ingredient. Then cost out the whole dish and work out the cost per portion.

Activity 5

Group discussion

This is a list of necessities taken from a survey devised to obtain information about poverty (J. Mack and S. Lansley, *Poor Britain*, 1985).

- new not second-hand clothes
- heating to warm areas of the house [even] if it is not cold
- enough bedrooms for every child over ten
- leisure equipment for children
- carpets in living rooms and bedrooms
- presents for friends and family once a year
- three meals a day for children
- toys for children
- refrigerator
- car
- a holiday away from home at least once a year for a week
- a television
- a garden
- a night out once a fortnight (adults)
- a warm waterproof coat
- a telephone
- a washing machine
- a packet of cigarettes every other day
- two pairs of all-weather shoes
- a best outfit for special occasions
- friends and family round for a meal once a month
- beds for everyone in the household
- a dressing gown
- celebrations on special occasions such as Christmas.

Place them in what you think should be the correct order of priority.

Discuss your findings.

Activity 6

Check your understanding

Check your understanding of the meaning of the following key terms:

poverty   **relative poverty**   **absolute poverty**
poverty trap   **cycle of deprivation**

Employment and unemployment

Employment is a person's regular trade or profession – in other words the job that they do.

Unemployment is the lack of employment or the inability to find work.

You are going to explore the changes within the employment market. Economic, demographic, social and technological developments have all contributed to the changing patterns of employment.

Yet for those who cannot find employment, the consequences can be challenging. The number of children living in workless households in the UK is the highest in Europe (Joseph Rowntree Foundation 2005). **Workless households** contain at least one person of working age but no one in employment. The effects of unemployment on households, families and society can be considerable and will be examined in detail later. First, you will consider the importance of employment.

The importance of employment

In the UK today over 30 million people are economically active (Social Trends 37). The **economically active** are people aged 16 years or over who are either employed or are unemployed but want to work. The **economically inactive** are those aged 16 years or over who are out of work, and are either not seeking work or unavailable to start work. They could be caring for relatives, unable to work due to long-term illness, early retirees or students.

In the UK there were more than 10 million working households in 2006 (Social Trends 37). The number of working households has increased since 1992. To fully understand the changes in employment patterns and impact of unemployment you need to explore the benefits of employment or work. Figure 3.4 shows the main benefits of employment.

Patterns of employment and unemployment

A brief historical perspective

The 1990s saw new technology replacing manpower. This in turn meant a loss of employment to those people employed in such industries. Examples of this are automated telephone systems to replace a person

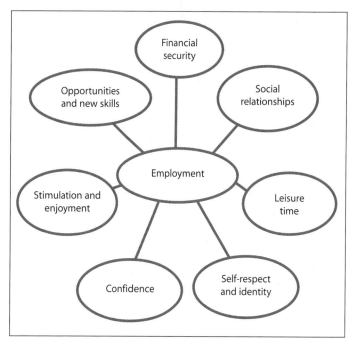

Figure 3.4 *The benefits of employment*

on the end of a phone. Banking was developed so that it could be done easily over the phone or the internet which meant fewer people in banks discussing banking issues face to face.

New technology has also brought about the growth of communication. For instance, the use of the internet has grown as people use it to book holidays, cutting out the middle man, the travel agents. Shopping online is also commonly used.

Service industries, such as hotels, catering and beauty therapy, have expanded resulting in an increase in employment in these areas.

Generally, there has been an increase in short-term contracts and short-term casual labour which has led to insecure employment.

Current facts and figures

According to the 'In work better off' paper published by the government in 2007, there are currently 2.6 million more people in jobs and more women, lone parents and disabled people working than ever before.

A number of factors have contributed to the highest employment in the UK's history:

- economic stability
- labour market flexibility
- employee rights
- active welfare to work programmes.

But there are still three million people of working age who have been on benefits for over a year. There are concentrations of worklessness in our cities, often close to thriving labour markets. There are nearly three million households in which no one is working; 1.7 million children are growing up in such families.

In July 2007, according to a press release from the government, the following patterns were recorded:

- There was a rise in employment to its highest ever level at 29.08 million.
- There has been a fall in unemployment and a further fall in the number of people on Jobseeker's Allowance.
- Vacancies remain very high. More than 10,000 new vacancies are placed at Jobcentres every working day and at least as many again come up through other recruitment channels.
- Redundancies are at a record low.
- The numbers on the main out-of-work benefits have fallen by 981,900 between May 1997 and November 2006.

According to research, the patterns of employment and unemployment in the UK today are dependent upon the following factors:

- **Education:** Young people are being encouraged to remain longer in education.
- **Age:** Older people are spending more years in retirement, a contributory factor to this being the increase in life expectancy. The work force is also older.
- **Gender:** More women than ever before are in paid employment. Male employees are most likely to be employed as managers or senior officials while female employees are more likely to be employed in administrative and secretarial work. Only the professional occupations, such as nurses, financial advisers and IT technicians, and occupations such as catering assistants, bar and supermarket staff are likely to be taken by both male and female employees.
- **Technology:** Employment in service industries continues to increase while employment in manufacturing continues to fall. There has been a continued shift in the UK from manufacturing to service-providing industries.
- **Contracts:** There has been a growth of part-time and temporary employment. Flexible working practices are a further development. Job sharing is very popular, particularly with women with dependent children.

- **Immigrants:** Many people seek employment opportunities in the UK from other parts of Europe. This is seen in rural areas where workers arrive for specific and often seasonal tasks such as fruit picking.
- **Job type:** The largest increase in employee jobs has been in the banking, finance and insurance industry, where the number of jobs doubled between June 1981 and June 2006 from 2.7 million to 5.4 million. There were also large increases in employee jobs in public administration, education and health (up by 40 per cent) and in the distribution, hotel and restaurant industries (up by 34 per cent). The extraction and production industries, made up of agriculture and fishing, energy and water, manufacturing and construction, showed a combined fall of 43 per cent from 8.2 million jobs in 1981 to 4.7 million jobs in 2006.
- **Self-employed:** There are 3.7 million self-employed people in the UK, accounting for 13 per cent of all those in employment. Men are more likely than women to be self-employed at 73 per cent of the total.

Figure 3.5 shows unemployment by gender in the UK from 1971 to 2006.

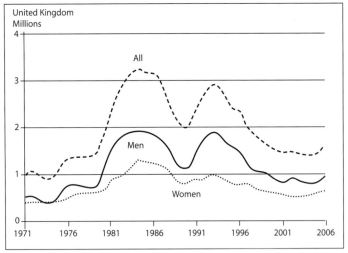

Figure 3.5 *Unemployment in the UK by gender, 1971–2006*

Activity 7

Review

Using the data in the graph above describe the trends of unemployment between 1990 and 2006.

Give reasons for these trends.

Groups vulnerable to unemployment

There are some groups in society which can encounter difficulties finding work. Sometimes it is factors beyond their immediate control that determine their chances of employment.

Young people

There are still a significant number of young people who are not economically active. The government started the New Deal schemes for different groups of people including young people who are unemployed and claiming benefit. New Deal schemes give help to the unemployed to find work, provide subsided employment opportunities and specialist training.

Although the New Deal for Young People for 18 to 24 year olds has helped to reduce the numbers, the problem of long-term unemployment among young people remains. Low achievers in school who enter the labour market with few skills or qualifications face an almost impossible task to find a sustainable job.

Ethnic minorities

Some ethnic groups can be more susceptible to unemployment. Research has found that young Caribbean men are more than twice as likely to be unemployed as young white men. In addition, Pakistani and Bangladeshi men are more likely to be unemployed than Caribbeans. Some ethnic groups may suffer discrimination.

Discrimination is the unfair treatment of a person or group on the basis of prejudice. Higher unemployment can be attributed to discrimination, underachievement at school or living in areas with fewer opportunities for work.

Disabled

Research suggests that the disabled who are economically active are twice as likely to be unemployed as non-disabled people. According to the Joseph Rowntree Foundation, for any level of qualification, disabled people are much more likely to be unemployed. The disabled are more likely to suffer discrimination when seeking employment from employers. This is despite the **Disability Discrimination Act 1995** which makes it unlawful to discriminate against disabled people in connection with employment.

Lone parents

There are many barriers which can prevent lone parents from working. The cost of childcare and loss of benefits may contribute to unemployment. The government has introduced 'in work' benefits and tax credits to make work more attractive to lone parents. Research suggests that these strategies are reducing the number of lone parents in poverty and claiming benefits. According to a Labour Force Survey in 2007, 60 per cent of lone parents aged 25 and over are working, up from 50 per cent a decade ago. In addition, a further 20 per cent are not working but would like to work.

Individuals over 50 years

Due to age discrimination, the opportunities can be limited for those over 50 if they become unemployed. Women in their fifties are much more likely to lack educational qualifications than men: 25 per cent lack qualifications compared to 18 per cent of men (Labour Force Survey, 2007). Older people are more likely to claim incapacity benefit. In February 2005 about 1.2 million incapacity benefit claimants in the UK, almost half the total, were aged between 50 and retirement age. Many older workers find it difficult to adjust and retrain for new employment opportunities.

The effects of unemployment

The effects of unemployment on individuals, households, families and society have been well researched. You will now examine the long-term effects of removing employment from individuals, households families and society.

Self-respect and identity

Employment gives us a sense of social identity. This is important to self-esteem and self-respect. Without employment an individual is more likely to feel worthless and have low self-esteem. Self-respect can also be lost by becoming dependent on state welfare benefits. Some individuals and families may feel embarrassed by this dependency. In some communities a stigma is attached to failure to work or a reliance on welfare benefits. **Social stigma** is severe social disapproval of personal characteristics or beliefs that go against cultural norms.

An unemployed individual may stay at home for longer periods of time. Changes in the roles within the family unit could cause conflict or stress. The unemployed individual may also be unwilling to take on a greater share of domestic chores to fill their available time. On the other hand, it may be possible to arrange role reversal where the unemployed member takes on more domestic responsibilities.

Confidence

Employment can give self-confidence while unemployment can remove confidence, possibly causing depression. A lack of self-confidence can reduce attempts to find employment. The unemployed person may blame others or feel guilty because of the inability to find work. From a feeling of inadequacy they might increase or take up smoking or drink large quantities of alcohol to escape the reality of the situation. Ultimately, in extreme cases they may become suicidal.

It is possible that children living in an environment where confidence is low will be affected. Their aspirations could be lowered and they may underachieve at school. Inevitably, this disheartening situation could affect their employment prospects.

Financial security

Financial security provides choices, opportunities and freedom. Unemployed individuals may worry about debt and the responsibility of feeding and clothing the family. Meeting the cost of paying the rent or the mortgage to maintain a roof over their head could be a further burden. Families and households might have to give up hobbies and leisure pursuits. A low income can contribute towards a poor diet, affecting health. Some people resort to gambling to seek a solution to financial problems.

When young people are unemployed they are more likely to remain dependent on their parents and continue living at home. This increases the risk of poverty for the family or household.

Stimulation and enjoyment

Many individuals who work have their time structured for them. The working day can be highly structured with a set start time, break times, lunchtimes and finish time. The unemployed can find it difficult to occupy themselves. The structuring of time is a psychological need, and evidence suggests that the unemployed have more disturbed sleep and anxiety than the employed. Work provides a sense of purpose, while being at home for long periods can cause boredom, especially if

coupled with a lack of financial resources to engage in activities and hobbies.

Opportunities and new skills

Employment provides the opportunity to learn and develop new skills. Many employers encourage their staff to take opportunities for skill development and training. In many employment sectors this is essential, such as communication technology and medical services. If employment is removed the individual could quickly feel out of touch with the skills needed in the workplace.

However, being unemployed can provide more opportunities. Many people choose to retrain, become self-employed or develop new skills by enrolling for further learning at college. They may even relocate to a different area where opportunities for employment are better.

Leisure time

Due to a lack of financial resources, the children of unemployed parents may not have the opportunity to use a computer at home or go on school trips. Families and households may have to manage without holidays, car ownership, consumer goods and leisure services. Research suggests that the unemployed watch more television and are less socially active outside the home. Their leisure activities tend to become more solitary.

Social relationships

Work provides friendships and supports existing relationships within the family. The removal of work can mean the loss of social contacts with friends and puts a strain on family relationships in times of difficulty. Tension in the home can cause mood swings and friction which can lead to arguments and, in extreme cases, violence and marital breakdown. An unemployed individual may not be willing to share their worries or concerns with their family who may be unaware of their state of mind.

Effects of unemployment on society

More social problems

Social problems include homelessness, poverty, increased crime, drug and alcohol abuse. Evidence suggests that in areas of high unemployment these problems increase. Young unemployed people with time on their hands and nothing to do may spend more time

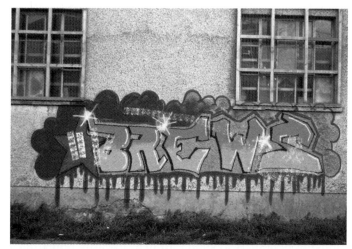

Figure 3.6 *Vandalism in a community with high unemployment*

in town centres or parks. There may be an increase in the incidence of petty crime and begging. Other more vulnerable members of the community may feel intimidated by the presence of large groups of young people.

If an individual loses their job, the likelihood of rent or mortgage arrears increases as does the risk of homelessness. The availability of affordable housing may be restricted in some communities. Housing and businesses may become neglected and rundown in appearance because of the lack of money to maintain and refurbish them.

Decline in the local economy

If unemployment is widespread, the economy of the whole community suffers as the unemployed have less money to spend. Access to basic services could be restricted and fewer food shops in the community could produce a 'food desert'. A **food desert** is a poor urban area where residents cannot afford to buy or have a limited choice of healthy food. Local businesses and services may suffer and close down due to reduced custom, increasing the problems for the unemployed in the area. Businesses that offer less essential services, such as restaurants, may disappear from an area completely. These businesses may be replaced in the high street by charity shops, betting shops and discount alcohol retailers.

More social exclusion and conflict in society

When the gap between the standard of living of the employed and unemployed becomes too wide, discontent can increase. This can cause social unrest and violence. It has been suggested that the inner city riots of the early 1980s were caused by a growing feeling of inequality between communities. In areas of high unemployment, divisions in communities increase and the prospect of equality disappears. Inequality is linked to social exclusion. Not having a job is considered to be one of the most profound forms of social exclusion. Employment provides financial resources to access many aspects of society.

Demand on health and voluntary services

The harmful effects of unemployment on mental and physical health are well documented. They include depression, self-harming behaviour, feelings of apathy, isolation and hopelessness. The health service needs to be equipped to deal with these issues in areas of high unemployment. There are higher mortality rates among the unemployed than the employed. Research suggests that the unemployed have significantly higher rates of GP consultations than those who are employed. Older workers are more vulnerable to stress from unemployment than younger workers.

Voluntary organisations which support the family are under more pressure in areas of high unemployment. Organisations which support and counsel the family or individuals are also in greater demand.

Demand for welfare benefits

Unemployment is a burden for the taxpayer. There is a loss of tax revenue, since people who are out of work do not pay taxes and those in work support the benefits system by paying taxes. Jobseeker's allowance, housing benefit and council tax benefit are most likely to be received by a person claiming assistance on the grounds of unemployment. If unemployed people are also ill the cost can escalate further.

Insecurity for those in work

When there is high unemployment in the community, the employed feel less secure. Workers are less willing to leave unsatisfactory jobs. Employers can take advantage of this situation. Employers may refuse pay rises, bring in unpopular changes to working practices or make less effort to retain workers. Both the employer and employee know there are plenty of potential employees who will accept the situation.

More scapegoating

The unemployed often need someone to blame for their predicament. A **scapegoat** is a person or group of people who are blamed for something that is not their fault. The most vulnerable groups in society are usually targeted, often immigrant workers or ethnic minorities.

Lower aspirations and opportunities

Children in areas of high unemployment may have less motivation to work hard at school. They may feel there is no prospect of achieving a job. Schools in areas of high unemployment may find it difficult to recruit staff and schools in areas of deprivation face challenging social issues which can affect the academic performance of children.

However, areas of high unemployment can have more opportunities for training and developing new skills. These opportunities may be offered in local colleges, job centres or increasingly with employers. Yet, access to training services and further employment opportunities can be harder for those who are out of work than for those who are in work.

Activity 8

Review

1. Describe how being unemployed could affect the following people:
   - a young school leaver
   - a middle-aged man who has worked in the same manufacturing industry for twenty years
   - a lone mother with two children.
2. List the main benefits of work.
3. Why can unemployment cause conflict in the household and society?

Support services available to the unemployed

The Department for Work and Pensions provides benefits for those seeking work. There are four main benefits:

● Jobseeker's allowance
Jobseeker's allowance (JSA) is available for those under retirement age who are out of work or working less than 16 hours a week on average. To qualify, claimants must be available for work, able to work and be actively seeking work. There are two different types of JSA: one is contribution based and the other is income

based. The contribution-based JSA is the higher of the two. National insurance contributions are required to qualify for JSA.

● Income support
Income support is available to people aged 16 to 59 years, who cannot work and do not have enough money to maintain a reasonable standard of living. Income support claimants may include lone parents, registered sick or disabled or carers for someone who is sick or elderly. The amount of savings is also taken into consideration.

● Housing benefit
Housing benefit is available to help towards rent from a private landlord or a housing association. **Council tax benefit** is help towards paying council tax.

● Job grants
Job grants are designed to help with the costs of moving from unemployment into work. The grant is a one-off payment which is free of tax and available to claimants of JSA and income support.

Government employment schemes

Local jobcentres provide government employment schemes. They employ employment service advisers. Some employment schemes are compulsory for people claiming jobseeker's allowance while others are voluntary.

Compulsory schemes
Jobseeker's allowance claimants must take part in certain schemes. Benefits may be stopped if an individual refuses to complete a scheme or training course. An employment service adviser (ESA) will organise a series of compulsory interviews and produce a jobseeker's agreement. This will provide a plan on how to find employment and will be reviewed with the ESA. The ESA will continue to support unemployed individuals until they find work.

Voluntary schemes
Some government schemes are voluntary but unemployed individuals are encouraged to join.

- **Work-based learning for adults:** This is for people aged 25 years and over who are unemployed for long periods. It offers focused training and help with developing the basic skills required for the labour market.

- **Programme centres or job clubs:** These centres offer training on the completion of CVs and preparation for interviews. They have facilities to help find employment, such as telephones, internet access, word processors, newspapers, stationery and photocopying facilities. They provide help and support to the long-term unemployed.

- **Work trials:** These schemes enable employers to try out unemployed people in a particular job for up to 15 working days while the person remains entitled to benefits. The aim is to encourage employers to consider employing the individual permanently when an appropriate vacancy arises.

- **Training schemes:** Training schemes for young people are government funded and provide work-based training. Most young people are not entitled to jobseeker's allowance or income support. These schemes may be their only source of income for the young unemployed as they will be paid a training allowance or a wage.

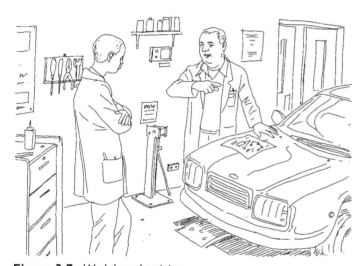

Figure 3.7 *Work-based training*

- **Apprenticeship programmes:** Apprenticeship programmes help young people leaving school or college to achieve vocational qualifications and skills. Subsequently, many apprentices are employed by their training organisation in engineering, construction, manufacturing, information technology, hospitality, care and financial services.

- **New Deal:** New Deals are a wide number of schemes for different groups of people who are unemployed and claiming benefit. They offer intensive support to find work, give subsidised employment opportunities and specialist training.

Activity 9

Check your understanding

Check your understanding of the meaning of the following key terms:

employment	**unemployment**
economically active	**scapegoat**
economically inactive	**New Deal**
social stigma	**social exclusion**
food desert	**jobseeker's**
employment service adviser	**allowance**
Disability Discrimination	**workless households**
Act 1995	**discrimination**

Leisure

Leisure interests and patterns are affected by many factors including age, class, gender, marital status, education, income, work and family commitments.

Leisure does not depend upon work but it is influenced by it. The higher the income the more spending power a person has on all things including leisure. Some leisure activities are more expensive than others while some are available at no cost at all.

Leisure time is important for people who work because it allows them the opportunity for recreation, rest and recuperation to restore energy levels. It can relieve stress and improve mental health and general well-being.

Definition of leisure

Leisure is the time used at a person's own discretion in a variety of ways once they have completed various duties such as study, domestic chores and work – it is the time left over. Most people find leisure enjoyable as they have freedom of choice in what to do. There are three main constraints to leisure choices:

- facilities in the area
- time
- available income to spend.

The changing patterns of leisure

There has been a marked change in the pattern of leisure over the last 20 years with a movement from spectator sports outside the home to domestic entertainments (TV, radio and video) and a steady increase in participant sport.

With working hours falling and work itself becoming less physically demanding, due to technology and automation, the need for leisure is becoming more urgent. Leisure can be used to develop skills and creativity and provide a sense of purpose.

The changing patterns of leisure in the UK today are dependent upon the following factors.

Employment

Research suggests that unemployed people generally spend more time watching television, reading and doing hobbies. No change was found in the amount of time spent in creative activities, playing games or in outdoor activities. Social life and going out decreased, as did participation in sport.

In all groups of people television viewing is the most popular leisure activity. Single people under the age of 30 spend less time watching television and more time socialising than older and married people.

Age

Age affects leisure activities because younger people tend to be more physically strong and active. Participation in sport is more usual in young people, and as age increases individuals are more likely to retain their interest in sport but more as a spectator.

Gender

Generally women have less leisure time than men because of their additional household responsibilities, particularly married women who are working with dependent children. Research tells us that 38 per cent of women and 54 per cent of men participate in physical activities.

Marriage or cohabitation

Married couples, or couples living together, are more likely to organise their leisure activities around their home.

Dependent children

The ages of children within a family may affect leisure activities. Many parents with young children spend less time socialising by themselves and more time socialising with their children. As the children get older this gives parents more opportunities to socialise by themselves or with other adults.

Education

The more educated usually watch less television and spend more time outside the home. They also tend to go the theatre and concerts more.

Income

The amount of money available in a household influences spending power and the amount of money available for leisure. Some leisure activities are more expensive than others. The cost of some leisure activities can limit participation, such as hang gliding, flying and skiing.

Time available

If an individual becomes unemployed they can become time rich but money poor. This can have an influence on which leisure activities they can continue to participate in. Many people work away from home during the week and come home for weekends, while others can spend a great deal of time commuting. This has an impact on what leisure activities they can participate in due to lack of time. In addition, they would need to allow time for rest and relaxation, as well as time to socialise and enjoy time with family and friends.

Location

Where an individual lives can also affect their leisure choices. Those in large population centres may have access to a much wider range of leisure facilities and opportunities than those living in rural populations. In a large city like Birmingham there are many theatres, museums, arenas, leisure centres, parks, restaurants and bars. Smaller towns and villages inevitably have more limited facilities and choices.

Holidays

Holidays are a popular leisure activity. The number of holiday trips taken abroad in 2005 has increased by 65 per cent since 1996. Spain has been the UK's favourite holiday destination since 1994, France being the second most popular. The UK has almost 6,500 visitor attractions, including country parks and farms, historic properties, theme parks, zoos, gardens, museums and galleries, and places of worship. These are very popular leisure pursuits. The most visited region in Britain by UK residents taking a holiday was the South West.

Activity 10

Research opportunity

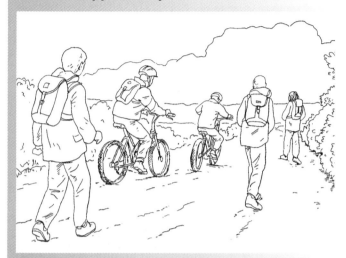

Figure 3.8 *Low-cost leisure activities*

Within your local area investigate what leisure activities there are that are either free or are available at a low cost.

Write up your findings.

Activity 11

Practical opportunity

Plan a range of low-cost food and drink which could be **made** for a picnic for a family consisting of two adults and two children, aged eight and ten. Do not spend more than £5 on ingredients for the whole picnic.

Cook one or two of the dishes in your next practical session.

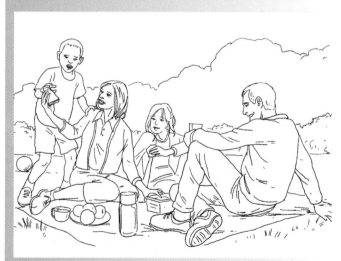

Figure 3.9 *The picnic*

Housing and homelessness

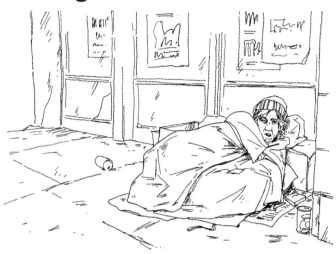

Figure 3.10 *Homelessness*

According to the charity Shelter more than one million children in Britain live in bad housing – enough to fill the cities of Edinburgh, Bath and Manchester – and more than one million homes in Britain are unfit for human habitation, and yet more than 90 per cent of these are occupied.

What is homelessness?

Homeless literally means having no home or haven, and **the Homeless** are described as people without a home. According to the Housing Act 1996 in England and Wales a homeless person is defined as:

'One who does not have accommodation available for his occupation in the UK or elsewhere which is not a moveable structure, or has accommodation which he cannot continue to occupy.'

Local authorities have an obligation to find accommodation for certain types of homeless people:

- pregnant women
- people with dependent children
- those who are vulnerable because of old age, mental illness or physical disability
- those who have vulnerable people in their household
- those who have lost their home as a result of an emergency.

OCR Home Economics

Activity 12

Group discussion

Read these four scenarios and discuss whether the local authority would house them under the Housing Act.

1. **Under 18 and being thrown out.** Jade is 17, lives with her mum, dad and two sisters. She is having loads of arguments with her mum who has said she has had enough of her and she is going to throw her out next week. Jade applies to the council as homeless.

2. **Pregnant and homeless.** Susan got divorced from her abusive husband and moved in with some friends. She discovered she was pregnant and as a consequence could not stay long with her friends as they told her she would have to leave. Susan applies to the council as homeless.

3. **Family evicted for non-payment of rent.** Derek and Dawn live in a rented flat. They took out a loan and went on holiday to Spain. Derek was unemployed and used his housing benefit to pay off the holiday loan instead of paying the rent. His landlord took him to court because he owed three months' rent. The court evicted them, so they applied to the council as homeless.

4. **Married with nowhere to live.** Sunitta and Harry got married last year and have been living with Sunitta's parents. They are both earning but cannot afford the rents in flats where they live and do not earn enough for a mortgage. They want somewhere of their own to live so apply to the council as homeless.

ASSESSMENT HINT!

Discuss means to investigate or examine by argument from more than one viewpoint, setting out factors to support, and not to support. It is not always necessary to come to a conclusion.

Our suggestions are at the back of the book.

Causes of homelessness

There are many and varied causes of homelessness. Here are the most common ones.

Eviction

Being evicted by the landlord would result in the loss of the home. This may be for a number of reasons such as rent arrears or the property being sold.

Loss of employment

Losing your job or being made redundant may mean that you lose your home. It could come with the job or it may be that you cannot afford to live there with the reduction in finances that losing a job may incur.

Health problems

Deteriorating mental or physical health may mean not being able to remain in your home. Some of these people may find themselves sleeping rough or in hostels.

Unable to be accommodated by parents, relatives or friends

For a variety of reasons people may be unable to be housed by family or friends. This could be due to lack of space or tensions between family members that make it difficult to live together happily.

Breakdown of relationship

Divorce or separation may result in one partner being unable to live in the home. There may be a variety of reasons for the break-up. The relationship may have been abusive which results in the partner – usually the woman – having to leave the home.

Mortgage or rent arrears

Being unable to pay the rent or mortgage may result in the home being repossessed. Repossession is to reclaim possession of something – in this case the house for failure to pay the instalments due.

Moving out of a home

There are many reasons why an individual may leave their home – coming out of an institution such as hospital, prison or residential home or returning from abroad. It may then be difficult to re-enter the housing market due to finances or personal circumstances.

Emergency such as fire or flooding

In July 2007 many areas of Britain, such as Tewkesbury in Gloucestershire, were badly affected by flooding. Many people were made homeless and faced a long period of time where they could not return and live safely in their home due to flood damage. This is an emergency situation where they were made homeless.

34

Limited housing supplies

Homelessness can be caused by a national shortage of adequate and suitable housing in the right places and available at the right price. Relationship breakdown, where one of the household leaves to set up another home, and single person households have also increased demands for available and suitable accommodation.

Activity 13

The use of data

Using the data in the figure below, name four causes of homelessness that may be included under 'Other reasons'.

ASSESSMENT HINT!

Review the data carefully. The first question on each of the examination papers is usually data which sets the context for some of the questions in section A.

Our suggestions are at the back of the book.

Activity 14

Practical opportunity

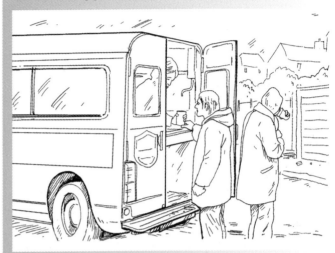

Figure 3.12 *A soup kitchen*

Devise your own recipe for a 'chunky' soup which could be served as a main meal in a soup kitchen for the homeless.
Calculate the cost of the soup and the cost per portion.
A suggestion for a soup is at the back of the book.

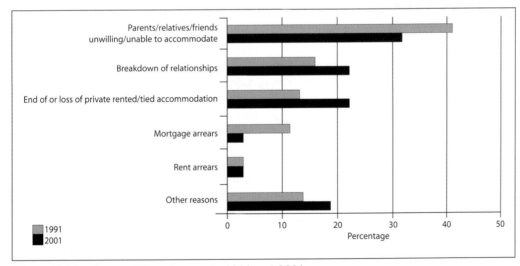

Figure 3.11 *Causes of homelessness in 1991 and 2001*

The effects of homelessness

According to the charity Shelter:
- One in 12 children in Britain is more likely to develop diseases such as bronchitis, tuberculosis (TB) or asthma because of bad housing.

- Homeless children living in bed and breakfast accommodation are twice as likely to be admitted to accident and emergency with burns and scalding.
- On average, homeless children miss out on a quarter of their schooling.

Another effect of homelessness on both individuals and families is that it is difficult to obtain mainstream services. If you do not have an address it is more difficult to obtain a job, open a bank account or claim benefits. There may also be difficulties in accessing social housing or private rented housing. Although people sleeping on the streets have a right to register with a doctor, it can be difficult to get medical treatment.

Here are some of the other common effects of homelessness.

Low self-esteem

Being without a home could in extreme cases result in the deterioration of mental and physical health which could lead to the loss of the ability to care for oneself adequately. It may also become apparent in children who could develop behavioural problems.

Limited access to health and hygiene

If people are living rough on the streets or in inadequate or crowded conditions, hygiene may be more difficult to maintain – access to toilets and hot running water. Their diet may be inappropriate because there may be limited facilities to prepare nutritious food.

Boredom

Individuals can suffer from boredom due to lack of facilities available, which can have an effect particularly on teenagers or young children. It may increase their chances of entering the criminal justice system, and it may also increase their chances of substance abuse.

Difficulties with relationships

The stress of being homeless can put a strain on relationships resulting in relationship disputes. The end-result could be that the relationship breaks down.

Increased dangers

Sleeping in a visible place can put you at risk from the general public. Women especially may be more at risk if they are in an area where there are people they don't know.

Lack of privacy

Children do not have their own space or area to do their homework. The high stress of living in one room can also increase the chances of non-accidental injury.

Activity 15

Review
Summarise in two bulleted lists the causes and effects of homelessness.

Activity 16

Research opportunity
Carry out some research on the internet to find out what support is available to homeless people. Here are some useful websites to start you off:
- www.shelter.org.uk
- www.bigissue.com
- www.centrepoint.org.uk
- www.crisis.org.uk
- www.housemate.org.uk

Produce an information sheet outlining what support is available.

Activity 17

Check your understanding
Check your understanding of the meaning of the following key terms:
repossession   the homeless   homeless

Housing

Shelter is a basic human need. Our home should provide adequate protection from the environment. It should also fulfil the needs for security, a place for relaxation and a sense of belonging to a community. It contributes to the quality of life experienced by individuals and families. The link between poor housing and ill health, underachievement at school and access to employment has been researched. Housing can provide opportunities and poor housing can remove them.

It is essential that housing is well designed and maintained. A high number of rundown and empty homes contributes to social problems in the community. These homes attract vandals, drug-users and burglars, they become overgrown and filled with rubbish. They are an eyesore, reducing the value of surrounding properties and removing any pride individuals have in their community.

It is important that the issues of design and maintenance are considered when constructing new homes. The design, layout and location of housing should meet the needs of individuals and families. Homes should be able to cope with changing needs and circumstances and not fall into disrepair when no longer fit for purpose.

The materials which houses are made of and the management of the resources in the home have major environmental implications. This issue is increasingly significant as we become more conscious of our 'environmental footprint'.

Types of housing

There are two main types of housing available in the UK:

- house or bungalow – these can be detached, semi-detached or terraced
- flat or maisonette – these can be purpose-built or exist as part of a property. A **flat** is a room or set of rooms located in a larger building. A **maisonette** is an apartment or flat on two levels with internal stairs, or which has its own entrance at street level.

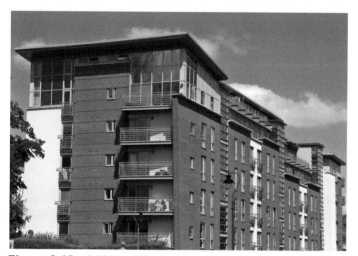

Figure 3.13 *A block of flats in Nottingham*

The type of home that people live in is usually reflected by the size and type of household and financial resources available. Overall 80 per cent of households in Great Britain live in a house or a bungalow (Social Trends, 2005). Families with dependent children are the largest group living in houses or bungalows. Lone parents and single person households are more likely to live in flats or maisonettes.

Activity 18

Research opportunity

Investigate the types of housing in your community. Produce a guide to the different properties and prices using information from estate agents, the local press or the internet.

There are two main housing options available:

- buying a home
- renting a home.

A home which is owned or being bought is referred to as owner-occupied. The owner is called the **owner occupier**. The number of owner-occupied homes reached 18.4 million in 2005, representing nearly three-quarters of all dwellings (Social Trends 37). A home can be rented from a registered social landlord (RSL), a local authority or a private landlord.

Renting from a registered social landlord

Registered social landlords (RSLs) are independent and non-profit-making. They are sometimes called housing associations and are important providers of social housing. **Social housing** is the term used to describe affordable homes provided by councils and RSLs. They receive some government funding to build homes and provide specialist housing for vulnerable groups. However, most of their income comes from rent. RSLs offer rented homes at affordable rates but some are sold through low-cost home ownership schemes.

Most RSLs are housing associations, but there are some trusts, co-operatives and companies. They vary in size – some are small and offer just a few homes while others offer thousands of homes. In 2005 2.2 million homes were rented from RSLs (Social Trends 37). They provide affordable homes for people with a housing need.

Rents are fixed by the government. RSLs work with local authorities to meet local housing needs. Most local authorities operate a waiting list for all council and RSL properties. Some RSLs can support individuals with specific needs. These groups include the elderly, young people, the disabled, people with learning difficulties, people rehabilitating from drug and alcohol problems and the homeless. Many RSLs are also involved in community initiatives to encourage employment, training and the regeneration of communities. They refurbish and improve old council house stock with the aim of reducing social exclusion in communities. They may offer community-based services including employment training, childcare facilities, credit unions, food co-operatives and community centres.

Individual and families have to apply to rent a property from a council or RSL. Applications are assessed and prioritised. 'Reasonable preference' is given to families who are homeless, living in very poor quality or overcrowded housing or have special welfare considerations, such as a disability. Other issues including medical needs, leaving prison, domestic abuse may be taken into consideration.

Homes can be allocated using the traditional point-based system. Applications are awarded points depending upon their circumstances. The number of points is used to judge the priority and a place on the housing waiting list. This system aims to ensure that housing is allocated to those in greatest need.

Activity 19

Research opportunity
Using the internet, investigate the points system for social housing offered by your local council.

Choice-based lettings may also be used to allocate housing. Once the local authority has received an application, families or individuals can bid for properties from a list advertised in the local press or on the council website. The property is allocated to the bidder with the highest priority and longest time on the waiting list.

Housing may be provided due to a referral. Some statutory and voluntary organisations including probation and social services may have arrangements with local authorities and request housing. The individuals and families in these situations could require urgent housing.

Renting from a private landlord

Most people rent from a private landlord at some time during their life. A private landlord is a person or company that owns property which is rented out to make a profit.

Private rented housing is a growing part of the housing market with almost 2.5 million homes in England rented from private landlords. Investing money in property has become more profitable and house prices have increased significantly in recent years. The increase in 'buy to let' investments has improved the quality of private rented housing and encouraged many smaller investors into the housing market.

Private renting has many advantages over owner-occupied housing. It is usually easy to access, as the process of buying a home can take months. There is a

good choice of private rented housing in some parts of the UK and landlords respond to change quickly. For example, there is more student accommodation in an area with a large university. Private rented housing is a particularly important resource for younger households who do not want the commitment of a mortgage. It supports the labour market as it allows easier mobility for employment.

Private rented housing can vary greatly in quality, size, price and services. The government improved the standard of private rented housing in the Housing Act 2004. It stipulates the health and safety standard of the property and the management standards through licensing.

A person renting a property is called a **tenant** and they have a tenancy agreement when renting a property. Private landlords usually let their property on an **assured short-hold tenancy**. These tenancies give the legal rights to the tenant to live in the accommodation for a period of time, usually for at least six months. Registered social landlords provide assured short-hold tenancies if the tenancy is temporary.

Housing tenure

The term **tenure** is used to describe the type of property held or lived in. This could be owner-occupied or rented.

The graph below shows trends in the different types of housing tenure since 1981.

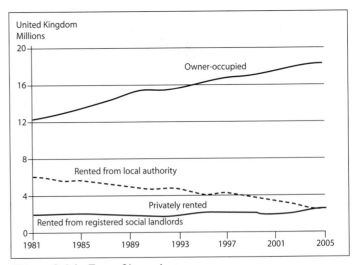

Figure 3.14 *Type of home by tenure*

Activity 20

Review

Using the data in the graph above, describe the housing trend since the early 1980s in the following:
- owner-occupied
- rented from local authorities
- rented from RSLs.

What are RSLs?

Buying a home

Buying a home is very expensive, but there are schemes available to help individuals and families buy a home.

Conventional home purchase

Buying a home is a major financial commitment which will involve many costs. These include a deposit, legal fees, stamp duty, land tax and searches. Even with secure employment it can be a financial challenge to meet these costs. Some people are able to purchase their home outright using savings, investments or an inheritance. However, the majority of individuals and families require a mortgage to buy a property.

A **mortgage** is a loan from a bank, building society or finance company used to buy a home. The mortgage term can vary, but it is usually 25 years. There are two main types of mortgage: a repayment mortgage and an interest-only mortgage. With a repayment mortgage, each month some of the capital and interest on the amount still outstanding is paid. During the first years payments are made up of more interest than capital. With an interest-only mortgage, you only pay interest to the lender and do not repay any of the capital until the end of the term. Instead payments are invested into a long-term savings plan which should clear the mortgage debt when it matures.

Failing to make regular mortgage repayments can result in repossession of the property by the bank or building society. **Repossession** is when the lender reclaims the property due to failure by the borrower to pay mortgage instalments.

For first-time buyers most lenders insist on a deposit of five or ten per cent of the purchase price. Some will lend 100 per cent of the price and will charge a higher interest rate or 'higher lending charge'.

Low-cost home ownership

To help individuals and families purchase a home, the government funds HomeBuy schemes. These are sometimes called shared ownership or shared equity schemes. A registered social landlord may also offer affordable home ownership options. Families and individuals can part-rent and part-buy a home. The schemes give those eligible the opportunity to purchase part of their home and begin building their own equity. These schemes are increasingly significant as the cost of purchasing a home in certain areas of the UK is beyond the reach of many families and individuals.

There are several factors that can influence whether the scheme is used to purchase a property. These factors include personal circumstances, where the individual lives and their employment status.

These are the main schemes:
- *New Build HomeBuy scheme*
  This is a government-funded shared ownership scheme. It allows families or individuals to buy a share of a property from a housing association, typically 50 per cent, and pay rent on the rest. A further share of the property can be purchased when it can be afforded. It is designed to help key workers and those first-time buyers considered to be in housing need to buy a home.

A **key worker** is someone who works in the public sector in an area where there is a high demand for housing.

Activity 21

Research opportunity

Using the internet or newspaper articles find out:
- who key workers are
- where they live
- why they are important.

- *Social HomeBuy scheme*
  Since the early 1980s, tenants of local councils with secure tenancies of at least two years' standing have been entitled to buy their home. The scheme, known as 'Right to Buy' was particularly popular during the 1980s when the housing market was stable and legislation encouraged tenants to purchase the home they lived in. It allows social housing tenants to buy a share in their current home at a considerable discount or to buy outright. In addition, the 'Right to Acquire' scheme is offered to some housing association tenants to buy their rented home at a discount.

● *Open Market HomeBuy*
   This is a government-supported scheme. It aims to help certain groups of people who cannot afford to buy a home on the open market to purchase a home. It provides access to additional money called an equity loan, which runs alongside a conventional mortgage.

Families or individuals initially buy 75 per cent of a property using a conventional mortgage. The remaining 25 per cent is met by an equity loan. The equity loan is split equally between the government and the mortgage lender. They will share in any rise or fall in the value of the property over the course of the loan. Interest rates on equity loans are low. When the last mortgage repayment is made, the lender's equity loan must be repaid.

Sheltered accommodation

With increasing age, the ability to live independently can become a challenge for some elderly people. There are several options available to those who feel unable to live completely independently, the most popular being sheltered accommodation.

The key characteristics of sheltered accommodation:
● A warden lives in the accommodation or nearby.
● Residents have an alarm system to contact the warden.
● Accommodation can be purchased or rented.

● 'Very sheltered housing' is for people with disabilities or the very frail. More personal care, specialised facilities and trained staff are available.
● Local authorities supply some accommodation but places are limited. Private companies and trusts are important providers.

Below is an advertisement for sheltered accommodation managed and owned by a private company, with the support of local social services.

Activity 22

Review

Discuss why Twilight Housing may appeal to an elderly person.

List the ways in which it aims to meet the physical, social and health needs of the elderly.

Identify the disadvantages of this particular accommodation.

Design of housing

The design of a house is important during different stages of the lifecycle of both individuals and household groups. It has been recognised for a long time that housing design should meet the needs the individuals and families.

Twilight Housing is situated three miles outside the town centre. The area is rural and there are some farm properties nearby. There is a regular bus service into the local town. The town provides a good selection of shops, weekly markets, transport, libraries, restaurants, a post office, doctors, churches and one supermarket.

Twilight Housing is mixed tenure. It is open to the fit and frail. Our aim is to provide a balance in the age and abilities among the residents. Some residents may require minimal care services whilst others may require a high level of personal care and support. Twilight Housing caters for all needs.

Twilight Housing consists of 30 high quality apartments in a three-storey block, many with views of the open countryside. All apartments have access to both a lift and staircase. Half the properties are available for outright purchase and half for rent. There are some parking spaces and a communal garden area. There is a resident warden on site 24 hours and a small team of support workers.

Twilight Housing offers one-bedroom or two-bedroom apartments. Each apartment has a small kitchen and bathroom with easy grip levers on the taps and built-in appliances. All windows and doors have security devices fitted. There are raised height electrical sockets, telephone points and TV aerial sockets to reduce bending.

Each apartment has an intercom system linked to the resident warden. The warden does not undertake cleaning, cooking, other domestic work or nursing. Residents are expected to be sufficiently able-bodied to undertake this work for themselves or if not, with the assistance of family. Residents requiring greater care and support can purchase additional services on site.

There is a communal lounge with a south-facing conservatory. A laundry room with conveniently raised washing machines and dryers is available for use. On site there is a doctor's surgery and treatment room. A resident warden and a small care team offer night cover on site. A GP, chiropodists and a community nurse frequently visit. Guest suites are available for overnight visitors at a small charge.

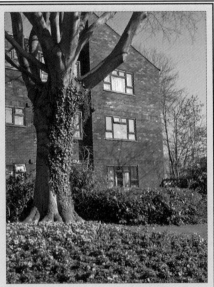

The sale price for a two-bedroom apartment is between **£180,000** and **£215,000**, and for a one-bedroom apartment between **£155,000** and **£170,000**. The service charge includes communal heating and maintenance of gardens and communal areas and is **£35** a week.

The basic rent for a two-bedroom apartment is **£140** per week and **£80** for a one-bedroom apartment, including the service charge.

The ground rent (**£80** per year), council tax, telephone bill, electricity and insurance must also be paid by all residents. In addition, residents are charged for any individual care and services they require.

'Housing design must support independent living for all people – irrespective of disability or circumstance.'

Scottish Office, Breaking Down Barriers in Housing, 06/08/1998

It was the Joseph Rowntree Foundation who developed the concept of 'Lifetime Homes' in 1991. **Lifetime Homes** have 16 design features that ensure a home will be flexible enough to meet the existing and changing needs of households. The design features make the home flexible enough to cope with a variety of potential situations, such as the need for wheelchair or pushchair access.

The Lifetime Homes standards

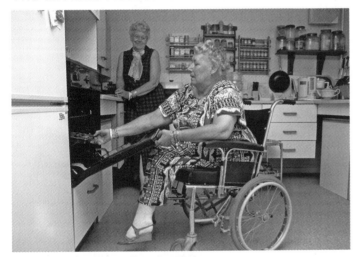

Figure 3.16 *Design for a flexible home*

These standards are set out in *Designing Lifetime Homes*, published by the Joseph Rowntree Foundation in 1999. The key requirements cover car parking, entrances, services and the layout of the home.

The standard width for a car parking space is 2400 mm. Where there is car parking next to the home, it should be capable of enlargement to a width of 3300 mm to accommodate a wheelchair-friendly path. The distance from the car parking space to the home should be kept to a minimum and should be level or gently sloping. The entrance to the housing should be level or gently sloping and should be well lit. Communal stairs should offer easy access. Lifts should be accessible to a wheelchair.

In the home the width of the doorways and hallways should accommodate a wheelchair. The home design should incorporate the provision for a future stair lift and identify space for a through-the-floor lift. There

should be space for turning a wheelchair in the key rooms in the property.

Living room windows should be low and be easy to operate. There should be a toilet at entrance level and drainage provision enabling a shower to be fitted, if required. Walls in bathrooms and toilets should be capable of taking adaptations such as handrails and hoists. The bathroom should be designed to incorporate ease of access to the bath, toilet and wash basin. Switches, sockets, ventilation and service controls should be at a practical height for everybody.

The design standards should not be considered in isolation. The layout of the housing in the community should include an area for parking and green space for recreation. Pedestrians and cyclists need safe routes to access schools, shops and leisure activities.

Roads in the community should have low speed limits which are safer for young children. Road junctions and crossings should be well lit and clearly marked, making it easier for residents to find and follow a route. Appropriate community facilities and services, such as public transport, schools and health services, should be accessible from the housing.

Housing design for individuals and households

Families with dependent young children

Small children have many needs. Their home should be safe and well maintained. They need a safe space to play, possibly a garden. A home should provide adequate bedrooms for the number of children. Ideally, children over ten of the opposite sex should not have to share a bedroom.

There needs to be a space for the family to eat together, prepare food and laundry. Many homes have a large family area where a range of social activities can take place.

The home should include storage space for toys, bicycles and clothes. Older children require a quiet area for homework and study. Good sound insulation between homes is important, especially where there are lots of homes close together.

Students

Student accommodation needs to be inexpensive as students live on a relatively low income. Students usually rent from private landlords at some point during their studies. The quality of the rented accommodation should be considered. The landlord has a responsibility to ensure the housing is safe and appliances are serviced. There should be adequate heating and no damp. Students need a place to sleep, wash, study and prepare meals. Their accommodation must be secure as they often have valuable, portable electrical equipment. Access to transport systems or a location close to their place of study is also important.

Families with dependent older members

Increasingly, grandparents are choosing to live with their children and grandchildren. Many larger new homes are built with a 'granny flat' or the potential for extension. The main consideration is adaptability of the home and the flexibility of room use. A downstairs room may need converting into a bedroom. The relative may require some privacy from the other family members. The design could accommodate a downstairs toilet, wider doorways, handrails, alarm systems, level entrances and allow for a stair lift to be fitted in the future.

The home should be warm and well insulated. It needs to be draught-free. Good lighting is important as older people are more vulnerable to accidents and falls.

The community facilities are important when living with elderly relatives. In a rural community individuals can feel isolated so a good transport system is important. There needs to be easy access to social and health services.

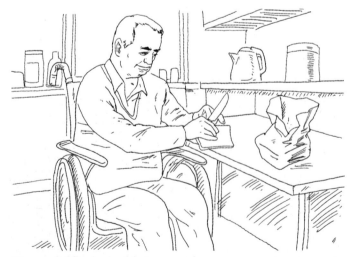

Figure 3.17 *A wheelchair user at home*

Physically disabled individuals

Individuals with physical disabilities, whether young or

old, have special housing needs. Some disabilities only require slight modifications to the home, while others are more significant. Those living in modern housing may be fortunate enough to benefit from the Lifetime Homes Standards mentioned above. However, many people with disabilities live in older property and their needs must be considered.

Security is an issue for the disabled, particularly if they live alone. Windows and doors opening on to a street or road can provide greater security. Bay and corner windows can provide views in different directions, as well as bringing more light into homes.

Access in and out of the home by ramps to front and rear doors is important so the individual does not feel isolated and can easily leave the home and return. A parking area at the front with a dropped kerb may be required. Proximity to good public transport is important.

The installation of toughened glass or guards to fires and stairs contribute to home safety. The individual should be able to access the main rooms in a wheelchair. This may require the widening of doors or installation of a stair lift or a through floor lift. The bath or shower room should be accessible. Downstairs facilities may be required. The housing should include modified kitchen appliances, units for wheelchair use and a work surface with an adjustable height.

To meet comfort needs, switches for lighting and heating controls may need lowering and plug sockets moving up. A heating system that is easy to manage rather than an open fire is preferable. The home should be easy to clean and maintain.

Single person households

Low maintenance costs are important with only one income. Older properties are more likely to require repairs and have higher maintenance costs. A large garden can be time-consuming to maintain and rooms, which are seldom used are expensive to heat. The size of the property is significant and a one-bedroomed property may be sufficient.

Secure parking or access to public transport, possibly a railway station, tram route or bus service would be important. The location of the home is important as it can offer social and leisure opportunities.

Some people who live alone can feel particularly vulnerable and need to feel safe and secure in their own homes.

Effective management of resources

There are three factors to consider in the management of resources in the home: energy, time and money.

The management of energy

Most houses were designed and built before the need to save energy was recognised. Modern houses waste less energy, but many are not very energy-efficient. Wasting energy is not only expensive, but it can also damage the environment. The main use of energy in the home is to heat space and water.

Heat generated in the home is lost through the windows, floor, loft, draughts and walls.

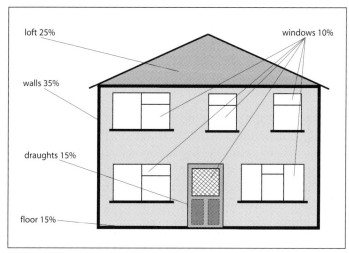

Figure 3.18 *Heat lost from the house*

Simple insulation can eliminate this loss almost completely. The following forms of insulation can be used:

- Cavity wall insulation
  About 35 per cent of the heat lost in a house is through the walls. Cavity wall insulation can reduce heating costs by 15 per cent. In houses built after the 1920s the external walls should consist of two layers with the potential to fill the small gap inbetween. **Cavity wall insulation** involves insulating the walls of the home. A material foam, polystyrene beads or mineral fibre is injected into the outer wall cavity through small bore holes which are subsequently filled back up on completion of the work. It usually costs around £500 and will pay for itself in around five years.

- External wall insulation
  Most homes have solid walls which may have a decorative weatherproof treatment applied to the outside walls. This will act as an insulator. The ideal

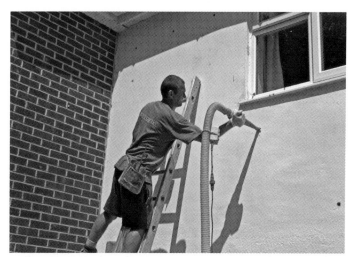

Figure 3.19 *Insulating a cavity wall*

thickness for external wall insulation is between 50 and 100 mm. External wall insulation is more expensive than cavity wall insulation, but it can save around £300 a year. It could pay for itself in around six years.

- Floor insulation
  The floor can allow 15 per cent of heat to escape. Gaps and draughts around skirting and floorboards are simple to fix with silicon sealants available in many DIY stores. This will save around £15 a year on fuel bills.

- Loft insulation
  Insulating the loft is one of the most effective ways to save energy. About 25 per cent of heat is lost through the roof. Loft insulation acts as a blanket, trapping heat rising from the house below. Insulation with mineral wool, fibreglass or recycled paper products can save around £110 a year on heating bills. There is loose-fill insulation including foam, polystyrene beads or mineral fibres which may be

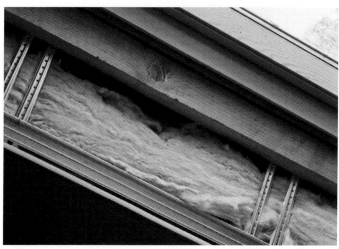

Figure 3.20 *Loft insulation*

more suitable for areas with restricted access. The insulating product should be a minimum thickness of 270 mm for maximum effect.

- **Draught proofing**
  Typically, 15 per cent of all heat loss in the home is through draughts. Draughts are caused by cold air forcing its way through gaps around windows or doors. **Draught proofing** is blocking the gaps to stop the draught entering the home. It will decrease the amount of cold air entering the home and save around £20 a year on heating bills. Draught proofing is a simple and effective way to reduce heating bills. Foam or rubber compressible strips can be used to fill gaps in window and door frames. They are widely available from DIY stores. Nylon brush seals or a spring flap for the letterbox can help reduce draughts, as can a cover on the keyhole.

  Draught strips should not be added to a room with an open fire or a gas fire that does not have a balanced flue or an airbrick near the fire. Fires need a good flow of air to burn safely and there is a danger of being poisoned by carbon monoxide fumes if a room is too tightly sealed.

- **Tanks and pipes insulation**
  Placing a jacket on a hot water cylinder is one of the simplest and easiest ways to save energy. It will cut heat loss by over 75 per cent and save about £20 a year. The jacket should be at least 75 mm thick. They cost around £20. The insulation of hot water pipes will cost about £10 and save around £10 a year.

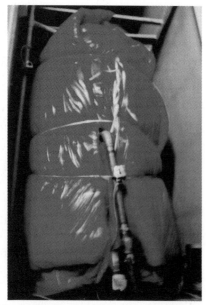

Figure 3.21 *A hot water cylinder with a jacket*

- **Glazing**
  Double glazing is a very popular energy saving measure, but it actually saves less from a typical fuel bill than cavity wall insulation. Only 10 per cent of heat is lost through windows. Double glazing works by trapping air between two panes of glass. It creates an insulating barrier that reduces heat loss, noise and condensation. **Argon gas** can be used to fill the gap as it transmits heat much less readily than the other gases in air, saving even more money.

  Low emissivity or **low e** glass has a special heat-reflective coating between the two panes of glass that will reduce heat loss through the glass by nearly half. The air gap between the panes should ideally be 12 mm to 20 mm to stop heat loss.

  Double glazing cuts heat loss through windows by 50 per cent and can cut a heating bill by around £90 a year. Double glazing can be very expensive to install and can cost several thousand pounds in a modest property.

  Secondary glazing involves the installation of a new fully independent window frame on the room side of the existing window. Secondary glazing is used in older houses that wish to retain their original windows but need to improve their thermal insulation. Secondary glazing is widely used in listed buildings and homes in conservation areas that are subject to planning approval.

- **Heating and hot water**
  The boiler used to heat the home can be inefficient. A boiler over 15 years old probably needs replacing. By law, new gas boilers in England and Wales must now be the high-efficiency condensing type, which can help save up to a third on fuel bills. A condensing boiler will have a better operating efficiency than a conventional non-condensing boiler due to its larger and more efficient heat exchanger.

Whatever forms of insulation are chosen, ventilation is important. Too little ventilation can cause condensation, damp and increase the risk of carbon monoxide being produced.

The following table gives a summary of approximate costs of installation, savings and paybacks.

Energy saving measure	Annual saving each year	Installation/materials cost	Installed payback
Cavity wall insulation	£90	£500	5 years
External wall insulation	£300	£1900	6 years
Floor insulation	£45	£90	2 years
Filling gaps between floor and skirting board	£15	£20 DIY	1 year
Hot water tank jacket	£20	£12 DIY	6 months
Primary pipe insulation	£10	£10 DIY	
Loft insulation (0–270 mm)	£110	£500	4 years
Loft insulation (50–270 mm)	£30	£500	16 years
Draught proofing	£20	£90 DIY	5 years
Double glazing	£80–100	Can be very expensive	10 to 20 years depending on initial cost

Data from www.energysavingtrust.org.uk

Activity 23

Review

Read the following descriptions of different homes. For each property suggest ways in which the occupants could save energy.

Property 1

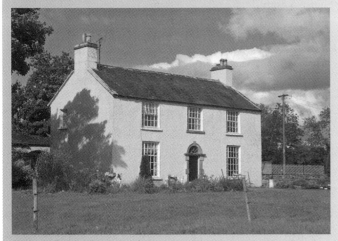

Figure 3.22 *Property 1*

Built during the eighteenth century, the detached house is a listed building. The walls are solid brick and the floors are stone. There are open fires in each room and a few radiators. A very old coal boiler is used to heat the radiators. A copper immersion heater was installed forty years ago and supplies hot water. There is an enormous loft area but many wooden joists support the slate roof, making access difficult.

Property 2

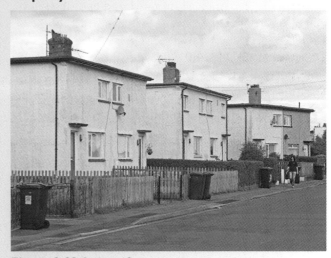

Figure 3.23 *Property 2*

Built in 1955, the small, semi-detached house has three rooms downstairs – a kitchen, lounge and cloakroom. There is no hall and the front door opens into the lounge. Originally the property had an open fire but this was replaced ten years ago by a gas fire and central heating system. The windows are wood with evidence of rot. There is hot water tank and extensive bare copper piping in the airing cupboard. The family has a limited income.

Property 3

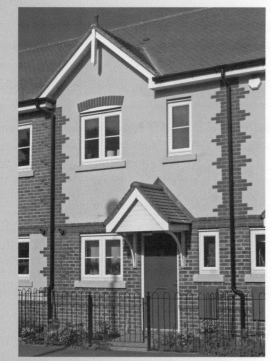

Figure 3.24 *Property 3*

Built in 1990, this mid-terrace mews house is situated on a busy road. It has direct access to the street. The windows are the original double glazed units installed during the construction of the terrace. The loft has been converted to a music room. Tongue and groove wooden flooring was installed throughout the property a few years ago. The staircase, kitchen area and living area are all open plan.

The management of time

The amount of time spent in the home is influenced by whether an individual works or not. Unemployed individuals and the retired may have more available time in the home to complete domestic tasks. Individuals who work full time have less time to complete domestic tasks. In the UK today, many households depend upon the individual members working full or part time. This can make the management of the home environment more challenging, especially if the household contains small children.

Time management in the home is influenced by the number of individuals in the household and their level of dependency. Young children, the elderly, the ill or disabled depend on others to a greater or lesser extent for their care and welfare. Depending on their age, children should be expected to take some responsibility for tasks, such as tidying their bedroom. The parent of

a small child may find it easier to manage work and childcare if they establish a routine. Planned into any routine should be the opportunity for leisure and recreational activities for individual and family groups.

Domestic tasks are time-consuming. Some households are able to 'buy in' services when time is limited and financial resources plentiful such as household cleaning, ironing and oven cleaning. Electrical appliances, such as dishwashers, microwaves and food processors, can help save time completing domestic tasks. By choosing easy-to-clean floor coverings and work surfaces more time can be saved cleaning.

In a household where both adults work full time domestic tasks could be shared.

Activity 24

Review

Below is a list of time-consuming activities completed in the home.

meal preparation	**washing clothes**
changing bedding	**vacuuming the home**
gardening	**cleaning the oven**
food shopping	**ironing clothes**
washing a car	**paying household bills**
cleaning windows	**washing up**
helping children with homework	**household repairs**

Construct a table like the one below, listing the household tasks above and any others you wish to include.

Assign each task to the individual who you think most frequently completes it. Also indicate which tasks could be completed by children.

Household task	Mainly female	Mainly male	Could involve children
Meal preparation			

Group discussion

Is there an equal distribution of tasks between male and females?

In your opinion, are there any tasks that are exclusively female or male?

What impact could both adults working full time have on the completion of tasks?

How could a grandparent living with the family influence the management of tasks?

The management of money

Effective management of money should involve the careful consideration of the household income and outgoings. The development of a budget plan may help to organise the financial resources. A budget should include all the necessary household expenditure. Most households have a monthly mortgage or rent payment to make. All households need to pay for the services they use – gas, electricity, property insurance and a water supply. Money should also be set aside for unforeseen emergencies and ideally saved for significant purchases.

Technology can be used to help manage financial resources. The use of a home computer and specialist software programs can help with budgeting. In addition, technology in the home can help save money. The use of timers to control central heating systems, thermostats to monitor room temperature and shopping online can reduce household expenditure.

Activity 25

Group discussion

Below is a list of the items that make up the household expenditure for a family with one pre-school child and one school-age child.

mortgage payment	credit card
window cleaner	life insurance
household insurance	telephone bill
council tax	food and clothing
toiletries	water bill
television licence	car tax
electricity bill	satellite/cable TV
fuel to run car	gas bill
car insurance	car breakdown cover
swimming lessons (child)	mobile phone
broadband service	
gym membership subscription	
magazine subscription	child pocket money
meals out with family	holiday savings
DIY/repairs to home	nursery fees
insurance on appliances	

What advice could you offer to reduce expenditure and make savings when buying some of these services?

Community facilities and amenities

The provision of different opportunities in the community is very important. Many communities offer a good range of facilities and amenities for individuals and households. Community facilities and amenities are important to consider when looking for suitable housing.

The range of facilities and amenities in a community can affect the cost of renting or purchasing a home. In areas where the opportunities are wide and varied, the price of property may be expensive. If the facilities and amenities are limited, it may be a less desirable area and property may be less expensive.

The facilities and amenities important to consider are those concerned with access to work, schools, services necessary for living and leisure opportunities.

Transport

Access to efficient transport facilities may need to be considered. A regular and reliable public transport system is valuable for getting to work, as well as for access to other local services and facilities. If the housing to be considered is in a rural area, there may not be efficient transport facilities available. In an urban area there is more likely to be efficient transport facilities.

Medical services

Medical services for primary healthcare are necessary and a local health centre not too far away from the housing would be both valuable and convenient. Access to an NHS dentist who has room to accept new patients on their list may also need to be considered. The nearest hospital with an accident and emergency service should ideally be situated within reasonable travelling distance from the home.

Shopping

Access to shops and supermarkets needs to be taken into consideration. Some individuals may need shops and supermarkets for necessary regular shopping to be within walking distance or at least a short bus ride away. Individuals who have a car may be happy to drive to the nearest shops and supermarkets.

Schools

For families with school-age children, the schools in the area are an important consideration. Successful schools may be oversubscribed so moving into the necessary catchment area may need to be considered.

Leisure

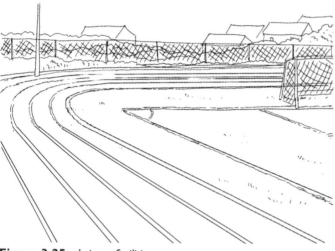

Figure 3.25 *Leisure facilities*

The leisure facilities available may be affected by a number of factors, including the age profile, location, cultural groups and the health, aspirations and socio-economic background of the individuals and households in the community.

Leisure services can be provided by local government, charities, trusts and private businesses. Demand for services will drive the market and the choices available.

Evidence suggests that interest in leisure activities is increasing. The 'Taking Part: the National Survey of Culture, Leisure and Sport' commissioned by the Department for Culture, Media and Sport reported in May 2007 that nine out of ten adults in England had engaged in at least one form of cultural or sporting activity during the past twelve months.

The table below shows a list of leisure opportunities available in a community divided into four broad categories.

Social facilities and clubs	Cultural, history and arts	Sport and recreational facilities	Education and training
Restaurants	Historical houses	Courts for tennis, basket ball, etc	Art and craft courses
Public houses	Museum	Zoo or safari park	Adult education
Cafes and internet cafes	Nature reserve	Winter sports (skiing)	Private tuition (dance, music)
Night clubs	National/country parks	Water sports (fishing, sailing)	Community schools
Village hall/community centre	Historic sites and monuments	Playgrounds	Libraries
Leisure centre/gym/health clubs	Churches and cathedrals	Skateboarding park	Community college
Gambling (bingo, race tracks)	Town parks	Athletic tracks/ football pitches	Communal ICT facilities
Voluntary work	Art gallery	Cycle routes/bridle ways	
Hotels/bed and breakfast	Theatres/amateur drama society	Bowling greens/alleys	
Sport club (golf, tennis, cricket)	Footpaths/walking	Theme park	
Lunch clubs/day centres	Specialist markets/craft fairs	Swimming pool	
Crèches/playgroups	Venues for live music	Allotments	
Youth club/scouts/guides	Cinemas	Open farms	

Activity 26

Group discussion

Review the list of facilities and amenities above for leisure pursuits.

Which of these are available in your area?

Which facilities would appeal to the following groups?:

• families with young children • teenagers • retired people • professional people living alone.

CHECK YOUR UNDERSTANDING

1 Check your understanding of the meaning of the following key terms:

maisonette
owner-occupier
registered social landlord
tenure
assured short-hold tenancy
social housing
private landlord

mortgage
New Build HomeBuy
key worker
Social HomeBuy Scheme
Open Market HomeBuy
tenant
flat

sheltered accommodation
very sheltered accommodation
lifetime homes
cavity wall insulation
draught proofing
repossessed

2 Copy and complete using some of the words above.

Nurses, teachers and social workers are _____. The government introduced _____ to help these groups buy housing in high demand areas.

A person buying a house is called an _____. They will most likely have a _____. If they fail to pay their monthly mortgage repayments their home may be _____. Homeless families can apply for _____. This is usually provided by a _____. Eventually families living in social housing can buy their home in the _____.

A student may choose to rent their housing from a _____. They will have an _____ during the rental period, which protects their rights. The elderly may live in _____ and if they become very frail this could become _____.

The emphasis nowadays is to produce _____ which include design features that ensure a home is flexible enough to meet the changing needs of households.

Exam-style questions

1 Describe the effects of poverty on families. (15 marks)

2 Explain how patterns of employment have changed since the 1990s. (10 marks)

3 Explain the factors which affect the leisure patterns of individuals and families. (10 marks)

4 Discuss the possible effects of homelessness on a secondary school-age child. (15 marks)

5 Describe how the design of a house can ensure energy resources are managed effectively. (15 marks)

6 Explain the housing options available to a young professional. (15 marks)

(Total of 80 marks)

ASSESSMENT HINT!

Describe means write out the main features.

ASSESSMENT HINT!

Explain means set out the facts and reasons for them, make known in detail and make plain or clear.

Environmental issues

Learning objectives

By the end of this chapter you will be able to:

- explain how and why we need to sustain our environment
- identify the range of recycling processes available and how they can be used to sustain our environment
- describe how to manage and conserve energy resources in the home.

Introduction

We all need to be aware and concerned about the need to sustain our environment. A definition of **environment** is the combination of external and physical conditions that affect and influence the growth, development and survival of organisms, circumstances and conditions that surround us.

We need to **sustain** our environment; sustain means to keep in existence, and to maintain. The ever-increasing demand for raw materials is depleting the world's natural resources and supplies of non-renewable energy. The management of waste (rubbish) is a huge issue, and it is important to think carefully about the way we shop, consume and live in order to mimimise the amount of waste we produce. Living in a wasteful way costs the consumer money and harms the environment.

In this chapter you will learn how to reduce waste and the amount of energy used, which in turn will help sustain our environment.

Waste

Waste or rubbish is what people throw away because they no longer need it or want it. Unfortunately we are all producing more waste than ever before. It is said that we live in a 'throwaway society' where everything we do creates some form of waste which we literally throw away.

Here are some facts and figures (taken from www.wasteonline.org.uk):

- The UK produces more than 434 million tonnes of waste every year. This rate of rubbish generation would fill the Albert Hall in London in less than two hours.
- Every year UK households throw away almost 30 million tonnes of waste.
- On average, each person in the UK throws away seven times their body weight (about 500 kg) in rubbish every year.
- Every year an estimated 17.5 billion plastic bags are given away by supermarkets. This is equivalent to over 290 bags for every person in the UK.
- Waste oil from nearly 3 million car oil changes in Britain is not collected. If collected properly, this could meet the annual energy needs of 1.5 million people. (Scottish Oil Care Campaign)
- About one fifth of the contents of household dustbins consists of paper and card, of which half is newspapers and magazines. This is equivalent to over 4 kg of waste paper per household in the UK each week.

● Babies' nappies make up about 2 per cent of average household rubbish.

The fact that we produce waste, and get rid of it, makes a difference to the sustainability of our environment. When we throw something away we have lost the natural resource used to make the product. We do not have a finite supply of these natural resources. It also puts pressure on our environment's ability to cope – obtaining the new resources to make another product, manufacturing and distributing it and then getting rid of our rubbish. When something is thrown away by someone, it is waste to them, and yet another person may not view it as waste – they may be able to use it. A good example of this is scrap metal which has been recycled for many years.

It is also important to consider the future and whether the next generations will have enough of the earth's natural resources. The way in which we use materials will affect whether we have a sustainable society that leaves resources available for future generations to use. We essentially need to:
● use fewer resources
● make products last for longer
● use waste as a resource.

Activity 1

Research opportunity
Look at some websites, such as www.wasteonline.org.uk, and come up with at least five more statistics on UK household waste.

The 'waste hierarchy'

The best way of managing our waste is not to produce it in the first place. This is called 'waste prevention'. After that we can think about reducing the amount of waste we do produce. Then there may be an option to reuse the material. The UK government has developed this approach to derive a hierarchy of options for managing waste, known as 'the waste hierarchy'.

The **waste hierarchy** (Figure 4.1) specifies the order of preference for dealing with our wastes, with those towards the top of the list more desirable than those towards the bottom.

The hierarchy is intended as a guide. In most cases a combination of the options for managing the different wastes produced at home and at work will work best.

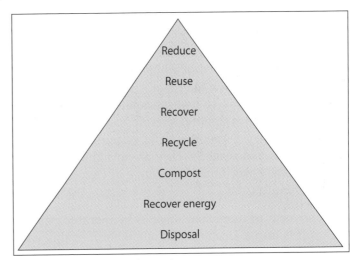

Figure 4.1 *The waste hierarchy*

The basic problem we have today is that more of our rubbish is dealt with towards the bottom end of the hierarchy than the top. The challenge is to change our attitudes and our practices so that much more of our waste is dealt with by options towards the top of the hierarchy.

There are three main ways in which a household can help the environment by adopting positive recycling strategies:
● reduce
● reuse
● recycle.

Activity 2

Review
Produce an information sheet or leaflet which lists and explains ways in which a household can adopt positive recycling practices.

Where does our waste go?

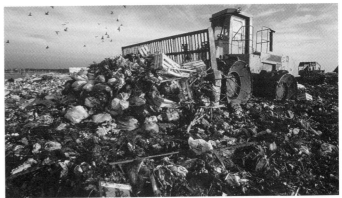

Figure 4.2 *A landfill site*

The vast majority of Britain's waste is disposed of in landfill sites. In the UK 72 per cent of municipal waste (waste collected by local authorities) is **landfilled**, which means it is buried in a hole in the ground. It is actually more complex than that – waste is compacted and covered in 'cells' to prevent pollution. Although carefully controlled, landfill sites do contribute towards pollution as they attract pests and vermin such as rats, flies, pigeons and seagulls. They are unsightly, take up valuable land space and are a source of concern to conservationists.

Nine per cent of municipal waste is **incinerated**, which means it is burnt. Dealing with our rubbish in this way is not ideal.

When we bury or burn our rubbish we are losing valuable natural resources and wasting the energy, water and transport costs used in its production. Landfilling and incineration can harm the environment if not properly managed. Many landfill sites are nearly full and we are rapidly running out of suitable new sites close to where the rubbish is produced. The other issue is that no one wants to live near a landfill site.

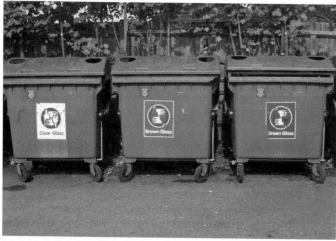

Figure 4.3 *Recycling facilities*

The answer is that we need to use a range of recycling processes and follow the three Rs:

- **Reduce** your rubbish – using less means there is less to throw away.
- **Reuse** bags, card, bottles, jars, paper and other materials rather than throwing them away.
- **Recycle** glass, cans, metal, textiles, batteries, oil, furniture, books, magazines, food and electrical goods.

Reducing

As consumers, we can reduce what we use by:

- Buying only the right quantity of what we really need.
- Choosing products with less packaging – supermarkets need to be lobbied regularly to use less 'double wrapping' on products. We can make a choice not to buy excessively packaged products.
- Buying from producers employing sustainable practices such as Fairtrade.
- Reducing the amount of junk mail received by registering with the mailing preference service. This should reduce the amount of unsolicited post that is produced and therefore the amount of paper which needs to be disposed of.
- Making green choices – buying 'refill packs' to avoid buying containers over and over again and using concentrated washing powders and fabric conditioners.

Reusing

As consumers, we can reuse what we purchase by:

- Giving unwanted items to a charity or charity shop where someone else can reuse them. This can be clothes, furniture, duvet covers, shoes and books. We can also buy our own clothes from a charity shop.
- Selling goods through free local newspapers or the internet.
- Supporting local initiatives to give away rather than throw away – Freecycle operates as a website where unwanted products can be given away.
- Setting the computer printer to print on both sides of the paper.
- Repairing appliances such as a broken washing machine.
- Buying products that have been designed for a longer life. IBM is now making the outer casings of its PCs reusable with upgraded components.
- Refurbishing or recovering old furniture.
- Obtaining milk locally in glass bottles which are then collected (a milk bottle can be reused 20 times).
- Reusing packaging materials for other purposes and making use of jars, boxes, paper and cardboard. Many local schools and nurseries welcome packaging materials which can be used for design and art work.
- Passing PCs to someone else – charities, schools and other groups can all benefit from donations of computers.

- Buying remanufactured items such as retread tyres – car tyres can be retreaded once while truck tyres can be retreaded up to three times.
- Buying products which can be reused easily such as rechargeable batteries, long-lasting light bulbs and concentrated products that all reduce waste and last longer.
- Taking your own shopping bags to a supermarket – some supermarkets offer green loyalty points if you use your own bags.
- Buying real nappies – it is estimated that 8 million nappies are thrown away in the UK each day. Real nappies are not only cheaper in the long run but also much kinder to the environment. Disposable nappies can take up to 500 years to rot down when buried in landfill sites. Families should consider the benefits of using cotton nappies and many local authorities are promoting low-cost starter nappy packs and washing schemes to make it more attractive for families.
- Reusing aluminum foil – recycling 1 kg of aluminum can save up to 8 kg of bauxite, the mineral used to make it.

Food wastage

The average family wastes £430 a year on food. It is inevitable that there will be food left over from many meals. Recycling food is very important because it not only saves money but it also saves on waste. Years ago this was called 'rechauffé' cookery, where the leftovers from one meal were used to create a new dish.

Here are some recycling ideas:
- Leftover cake can be used to make a trifle.
- Leftover meat can be made into a shepherd's pie.
- Leftover chicken can be used to make a curry.
- Leftover potato can be mashed and used in fish cakes.
- Fallen apples can be used to make pies, crumbles and preserves.

Activity 3

Practical opportunity

Create a range of dishes, both sweet and savoury, that use recycled food.

Indicate clearly in each dish what the recycled food is.

Choose your most interesting one to make in a practical session.

The recycling processes available

Only after reducing and reusing waste can we consider recycling. Almost half of the contents of our dustbin could be potentially recycled. Recycling is crucial to sustain our environment because it stops our rubbish going to landfill, saving resources and energy.

Recycling is the processing of waste products to provide the raw material to make new ones. Recycling reduces the demand for raw materials, lessening the impact of extraction and transportation created at the point where the raw material is extracted. Recycling uses less energy than producing goods from raw material and also results in fewer emissions.

Part of the recycling process is buying or using products made from recycled materials. Buying recycled products creates a demand for the collected material, aiding the development of new recycling industries and helping the environment. The symbol in Figure 4.4 (the mobius loop) means that the product has both recycled content and that the product is recyclable.

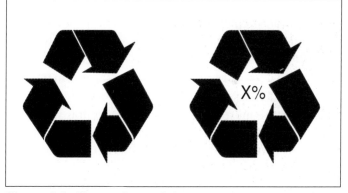

Figure 4.4 *The recycling symbol*

It does not necessarily mean that it is made from 100 per cent recycled material, but can contain any proportion of recycled and raw material. Buying recycled products is an individual action that can make a real difference. Most high street stores, local health food shops, charity shops and supermarkets sell recycled products in some form. Consumers should also look out for the eco labels which indicate that a product has met a specific set of environmental or social standards.

Examples of this are the FAIRTRADE Mark and organic food labels, biodegradable and phosphate-free for cleaning materials and low emissions for cars.

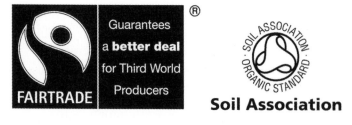

Figure 4.5 *The FAIRTRADE Mark and the Soil Association organic food symbol*

Extended producer responsibility (EPR) laws are now in place that require companies to take back and assume responsibility for disposal of products they sell – from TVs to toasters. Manufacturers have to consider the full impact of their products. It is hoped that they will then get rid of any unnecessary parts, do without excess packaging and design products that can easily be disassembled, recycled, remanufactured or reused. EPR laws also typically ban the landfilling and incineration of these products and establish how the product should be reused and recycled.

In addition, we as consumers can recycle by:

- Saving plastic bottles so that they can be converted into fleeces and garden furniture – many local authorities have a kerbside collection.
- Saving paper, card and magazines – again, many local authorities have a kerbside collection.
- Making the most of any kerbside collection schemes that are in place – it takes little time to sort waste and all members of the family should try and take responsibility.
- Taking waste materials to local recycling banks if kerbside collections are not available – there are recycling facilities in places such as supermarket car parks and local leisure centres.
- Saving aluminium cans – by doing this you can save 95 per cent of the energy used in making a new can, and many local authorities have a kerbside collection.
- Buying goods which use recycled materials.
- Finding out where and how we can recycle goods through our local authority (the website www.recyclenow.com can help).
- Composting kitchen and garden waste as it results in compost that can be used as fertilizer on plants. We could recycle or compost around 68 per cent of our waste, yet we are currently only recycling or composting 15 per cent. Food digesters are also available which enable families to compost cooked food, meat and bones. Many local authorities offer

compost bins, wormeries and food digesters at subsided rates.

- Using recycling facilities such as bottle, can, paper and clothing banks which can be found in supermarket car parks.

Research and development of new technologies to deal with waste, and recycling processes are constantly developing.

Activity 4

Research opportunity

Visit the website www.wasteonline.org.uk and other related websites to find out what the following new technologies are:

- pyrolysis
- gasification
- anaerobic digestion
- mechanical biological treatments.

Write a short guide explaining each technology.

Find out what recycling processes are available in your locality and produce a short information sheet.

Sustaining our environment

Recycling has many positive effects on the environment because it saves valuable resources used to manufacture products.

It prolongs the life of landfill sites which are in short supply. It can boost the economy – recycling creates jobs, reduces imports of raw materials and saves money spent on landfills. It can protect plant and wildlife habitats because fewer raw materials such as bauxite (used to make aluminium) are extracted from huge quarries. Recycling can generate money and many fundraising groups generate cash from collecting products such as cans, stamps, silver foil, mobile phones and ink cartridges. Recycling paper is very good news for the economy. It reduces the import of pulp and water usage, increases jobs in this country, saves landfill space and can protect old growth forests.

The need to sustain the environment is now universally acknowledged and recycling is just one small step to help the bigger problem. The lifestyle we have today is possible because we use energy from fossil fuels such as coal, oil and gas. These are not finite resources – there is not an unlimited supply. Fossil fuels are the main fuels used to generate electricity.

In our homes this energy is used for warmth, light, cooking, refrigeration, freezing and to power a range of electrical appliances to make our life more convenient. The only problem is that as we demand and use more fuel, we are pumping more pollution into our environment. Burning fossil fuels for energy produces carbon dioxide, a greenhouse gas which contributes to global warming. So using less energy is vital. This and a number of other factors contribute to the decline in the quality of our environment.

Activity 5

ICT opportunity

Produce a word-processed information sheet or leaflet on how to be an environmentally friendly consumer.

Factors in the quality of our environment

The factors that influence the quality of our environment include:

- global warming
- ozone depletion
- acid rain
- deforestation
- fisheries depletion.

Global warming

Global warming is an increase in the average temperature of the earth's atmosphere, especially a sustained increase sufficient to cause climatic change.

The atmosphere that surrounds the earth is made up of different gases. One of these is the ozone layer. **The ozone layer** is a layer in the stratosphere (at approximately 20 km) that contains a concentration of ozone sufficient to form a protective shield against most ultraviolet radiation from the sun. Other layers insulate the earth, producing the 'Greenhouse effect'. Both are critical to preserving the balance of life and are affected by the gases produced by man, in particular chlorofluorocarbons (CFCs). The other main greenhouse gas produced by man's activities is carbon dioxide.

There are also several environmental problems associated with refuse disposal which contribute towards the production of greenhouse gases. Methane gas and a toxic liquid called leachate are a by-product of landfill sites. **Methane gas** is created when organic waste breaks down. This has the potential to be explosive and it is also a significant greenhouse gas which can contribute towards global warming.

Since the industrial revolution, we have been upsetting the world's balance by producing more carbon dioxide by burning fossil fuels. Global warming is the result and this leads to changes in the world's climate. These changes could mean rises in sea levels, changes in rainfall patterns and pests and diseases becoming more widespread. Agriculture could see major changes occurring.

There are two main ways to reduce global warming: to remove CFCs and reduce our energy consumption. The government has taken steps to ban certain products containing CFCs. Historically, CFCs were used as coolants in refrigeration and we have not yet found a really good alternative. Some use R22, a CFC with only 5 per cent of the ozone depleting potential of standard CFC. All new air-conditioning systems use R22. All CFCs are drained from old refrigerators before recycling. Polystyrene trays used for packaging meat, fruit and vegetables are now made without CFCs.

The World Meteorological Office and the United Nations have set up panels to monitor climate change carefully over the next few years.

Ozone depletion

The ozone layer is found about 20 km above the earth. In 1984 holes in the ozone layer were found by British scientists. In reality, they are areas that are thinner or depleted. CFCs break down after reaching the upper atmosphere and release chlorine that turns the ozone into oxygen. This cannot protect against UV radiation. CFC gases are used as propellants in aerosols and coolants in refrigerators which have contributed to the depletion of the ozone layer.

Acid rain

Acid rain is rain containing acids that form in the atmosphere when industrial gas emissions (especially sulphur dioxide and nitrogen oxides) combine with water. Acid rain was first identified over 125 years ago. At that time it was suggested that pollutants in the air were dissolving in rainwater, making it acidic and causing damage to buildings and monuments.

It was in the 1970s that the long-range air transport of acidity and its widespread effects on nature were identified. Trees in Europe have been dying or losing foliage due to drought, storms and insects. Sulphur and nitrogen oxide gases from industries are mostly to blame as they dissolve in rain. Lakes have also become acidified and soil has been affected.

One of the main effects of acid rain is that cereal yields have decreased, causing a drop in food production. Metals such as aluminium are leached out of the soil and cause pollution of drinking water. Fish are affected by the acidic water in lakes and rivers. Wildlife declines as a result of lack of food and the toxic effect of acidification. Buildings weather more quickly (blacken) and many famous buildings, such as St Paul's Cathedral, have experienced more damage in more recent years than ever before.

Deforestation

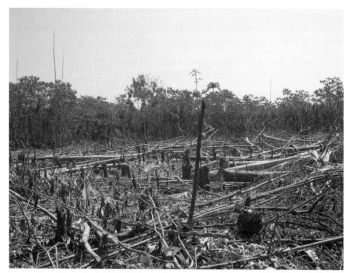

Figure 4.6 *A deforested area*

Deforestation is to cut down and clear away the trees or forests. The gradual loss of trees worldwide has been a major cause of global warming. Tropical forests cover only 7 per cent of the earth's surface but are home to between 50 and 80 per cent of the planet's species. Tropical forests shrink annually by an estimated 80,000 square miles (1 per cent per year), intensifying the greenhouse effect because tropical forests take in carbon dioxide and give out oxygen. When trees are chopped down, the soil no longer has the roots to hold it in place. Rainwater washes the soil away and trees and plants cannot grow back. With the destruction of habitat there is a threat to some plants and animals which may in time become extinct.

Fisheries depletion

Fish stocks have been threatened by continued overfishing. The limit to sustainable fishing has been exceeded – too few fish have been left to maintain stocks. Therefore, measures have been put in place to allow fish stocks to build up again. There are specific areas where fishermen are allowed to fish and there are restrictions on the size of the nets used, to allow the young fish to escape to continue to grow and breed.

Activity 6

Practical opportunity

List and explain as many food-related ways of protecting the environment as you can. Here are two examples:

- buy dolphin-friendly tuna because the tuna is caught in nets which do not trap and injure or even kill dolphins
- buy products with the FAIRTRADE Mark which will guarantee farmers a fair and stable price for their products and ensure that products meet some environmental standards.

Create two dishes, one sweet and one savoury, which include food produced in an environmentally friendly way.

Indicate clearly on each dish the food which is environmentally friendly.

Make your chosen dish in a practical session.

Air, water and noise pollution

Air pollution is a major cause of concern to individuals and the government. Cars, which are driven on petrol, contribute about 20 per cent to total carbon dioxide emissions. Historically, smog has caused major health problems. This forms when nitrogen oxides combine with organic compounds from factories and exhaust fumes.

Transport and air pollution affects the air that we breathe. Measures are being taken to address this. By reducing speed limits and introducing traffic-calming methods, carbon dioxide emissions can be reduced. Road tax is cheaper for less powerful (polluting) cars. A reduction in the use of motor vehicles would help to improve the air we breathe. Relatively small changes in behaviour all add up. For example, walking and cycling rather than taking the car, or sharing a car journey. Traffic-calming measures and congestion charges in cities would reduce the level of traffic.

Air pollution can also result from both incinerated and dumped refuse. Most modern incinerators use state-of-the-art emission control measures, but some fumes do escape into the environment which can contribute towards acid rain and ozone depletion. There is also legislation in place to control when, where and what can be burned.

Activity 7

Practical opportunity

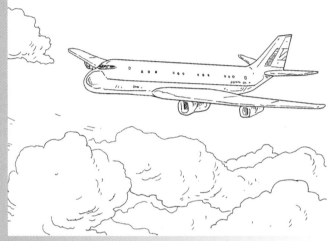

Figure 4.7 *Food is flown around the world*

There has been a significant amount of media coverage about air miles – how far our food travels from around the world to our local supermarket.

Create a display that promotes the fact that your local area has excellent local produce which can be easily purchased and used to create interesting food dishes. The display should include:

- information about your local area
- details of sources of local food within a 30 mile radius of where you live
- a selection of sweet and savoury recipe ideas
- full details of the recipe choice you are going to make – aim, justification of choice, ingredients list, where each ingredient will be sourced, a photo of the final product.

Make your chosen recipe in a practical session.

Water pollution can be caused by a variety of sources. Flooding, sewage, industrial waste, agricultural chemicals and dirty water from landfill sites can pollute watercourses killing fish and wildlife.

Leachate occurs when it rains on a landfill site and the water trickles through the rubbish, carrying with it some of the decomposing substances. This dirty water is highly toxic and can pollute underground water, ground level water courses and rivers. This can result in pollution and the loss of fish and other wildlife. A more responsible approach by individuals and industry would also help to reduce water pollution levels.

Noise pollution from machinery, aircraft, traffic and individuals can make our environment unpleasant to live in. Repetitive noise can lead to stress and make lifestyles miserable especially for the household. It is really important to be a considerate neighbour. People should think about noise emissions and should consider the following:

- turning down stereos and noisy electrical equipment
- preventing dogs from constantly barking
- leaving a house key with a neighbour when you are away from home for long periods if you have a house alarm.

Local authorities employ staff who will investigate complaints about the environment such as chimney smoke, dog noise, bonfires, litter and vandalism.

Activity 8

Research opportunity

The three main factors which influence the quality of our local environment are:

- noise pollution
- water pollution
- air pollution.

Choose one of the above and produce a fact sheet which must include information on what it is, why it is harmful and strategies and solutions to mimimise it.

Agencies for the environment

Agencies have developed over the years to assist in sustaining the environment. They each have a specific and valid role.

The Department of Environmental Health

One of the functions of environmental health officers is that they monitor levels of pollution, including noise, water and air pollution. They will follow up on complaints and ensure that relevant legislation is enforced, including that in the Environmental Protection Act 1990. They will give advice and help to eradicate vermin and pests within the community, helping to reduce the spread of disease.

The Environment Agency

The Environment Agency took over responsibility for waste regulation in April 1996. It is responsible for putting the government's environmental policies into practice. Along with waste management, the Agency took over responsibility for controlling industrial pollution and water management (formerly managed by the National Rivers Authority).

The Department of Environment, Transport and Regions (DETR)

One of DETR's main initiatives is to work in partnership with local and national agencies to improve air quality. It aims to reduce the eight main pollutants that are known to harm human health and which occur widely throughout the UK. These are caused mainly by vehicles and industry. Carbon monoxide, lead and sulphur dioxide are among some of the most harmful pollutants. DETR also monitors concerns about excessive noise pollution especially from air traffic including military aircraft and traffic and road construction noise. It has a specific responsibility for traffic and transport issues. It publishes free literature and offers a consumer helpline.

The Department for Environment, Food and Rural Affairs (DEFRA)

An important function carried out by DEFRA is the air pollution information service. This is a free and easy to understand information service about levels of air pollution in urban and rural communities. The service is available 24 hours a day. It gives forecasts and alert messages when air pollution is likely to be high.

It also offers valuable health advice for people whose health may be affected by air pollution.

Friends of the Earth

Friends of the Earth has local groups all around the country and its major concern is the state of the environment and the threats to it. It raises awareness of what individuals can do to protect it.

Greenpeace

Greenpeace is an independent, non-profit-making, global campaigning organisation that uses non-violent measures to highlight global environmental problems and their causes. It also lobbies for nuclear disarmament and the end of nuclear contamination. Greenpeace does not receive any funding from the government or any political parties. It relies on voluntary donations from its members and other grants from its founders. It is probably most recognised for its initiatives to save dolphins and for campaigning to end high sea, large driftnet fishing.

Environmental Protection UK

Environmental Protection UK (formerly the NSCA) aims to bring together organisations across the public, private and voluntary sectors to promote a balanced and innovative approach to understanding and solving environmental problems. It publishes a number of fact sheets concerned with all aspects of pollution and has a website that offers advice.

The Soil Association

The Soil Association aims to promote organic farming and reduce the use of pesticides and insecticides in the production of food. It carries out research and offers solutions to help provide a more green and peaceful future. It is particularly concerned about the protection of the oceans and forests. It would like to eliminate the use of toxic chemicals and is against the release of genetically modified organisms into nature and the food chain.

To conclude this section, a united approach is required from individuals, local and national government, industry and commerce and international partners in order to bring about significant changes which will sustain our environment. Both a rising world population and rising expectations of higher living standards all threaten to damage the environment. The clear answer is sustainability. We need to meet the needs of the current generation as well as those of future generations.

Activity 9

Review

Consider the most significant ways in which the quality of our environment can be improved and maintained.

Put that information into a table with the following as the two headings:

- Individual responses
- Central and local government responses.

Management and conservation of energy in the home

The British public wastes around £5 billion worth of energy a year. In 20 years' time we could be importing up to 80 per cent of our gas.

In Chapter 3 in the section on housing you learnt how a house can be designed and adapted to reduce energy consumption. In this section you will learn how to make the most efficient use of the energy we consume so that we reduce our energy bills without compromising comfort.

It is easy to bring energy-saving into every aspect of life – work, travel and day-to-day living – and it can make a real difference. The average household could save up to £300 a year on energy bills by being more energy-efficient. About 55 per cent of the total energy used is spent on space heating and 20 per cent is spent on heating water for domestic use. The other main uses are for cooking, lighting and electrical appliances. Advantages of reducing energy expenditure include lower fuel bills, conservation of limited fuel resources, less damage to the environment and reducing condensation in the home.

Purchasing and using electricity

As consumers we can do the following:

- Buy electricity from the greenest energy supplier – check out tariffs on the internet.
- Keep up pressure on the government by writing to your MP demanding more support for renewable energy and energy efficiency.
- Look into an electricity tariff which offers cheaper electricity at night for seven hours. Appliances such as dishwashers, tumble dryers and washing machines can then be used overnight on the cheaper rate.
- Switch off lights.

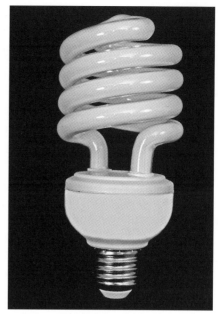

Figure 4.8 *An energy-saving light bulb*

- Boil only the amount of water needed in a kettle or pan.
- Use cooler washing loads – washing clothes at 40 degrees uses a third less electricity. Always ensure that the machine operates with a full load, or if there is not a full load, use the half load facility.
- If buying a new tumble dryer, choose the most energy-efficient model, and avoid drying really wet clothes – hang them outside wherever possible.
- Replace ordinary light bulbs with energy-efficient ones. Just one can save you £100 over the lifetime of the bulb – and they last up to 12 times longer than ordinary light bulbs. If this is not possible, use lower wattage directional bulbs (good for reading) and dimmer switches which help to reduce the amount of electricity used.
- When buying new electrical equipment look out for the energy efficiency label. 'A' rated appliances are the most energy-efficient.
- Try to purchase electrical equipment that has energy saving features, for example washing machines and dishwashers.
- Use electrical equipment sensibly and only when really necessary.
- Do not leave TVs and other electrical items on standby but switch off when not in use. External lighting should be used selectively, be on a timer and be sensor-driven.

Preparing, making and cooking food

As consumers we can do the following:

- Shop online to cut down on traffic pollution. Shopping locally also saves on fuel costs and buying locally supports your local economy.
- Become a 'greener' cook. Recycle food to make new dishes. If you do have any leftovers then compost them. Save energy when cooking by filling the oven or if only cooking one item, use a microwave instead.
- Choose the right pan size for cooking so it fits the ring, cut food into smaller chunks and put lids on pans. The food will cook quicker and use less fuel.
- Make your own meals which can be doubled up on quantities and freeze the other half for a later date.

Water

As consumers we can do the following:

- Shower instead of having a bath. A five-minute shower uses about one third as much water as an average bath.
- When cleaning your teeth do not leave the tap running. Make sure all taps are turned fully off. A dripping tap can waste as much as ten litres a day.
- Toilets account for 35 per cent of domestic water usage. Fitting a water 'hippo' bag saves up to three litres of water with every flush. The eco flush is a flush with high and low settings and can reduce the water used to flush a toilet by a third.
- Hot water tanks should always be lagged. The lagging should be 75 mm thick and will save around £20 a year. These are easy and cheap to fit and the initial outlay is recouped very quickly through energy savings. Most modern houses have water heating tanks that are already insulated. Hot water pipes can also be lagged which will reduce energy use. Check the temperature of your water; the cylinder thermostat should not need to be set higher than 60°C/140°F.

Heating

As consumers we can do the following:

- Use a timer and only heat the home when there.
- Reduce the heating temperature by 1°C. This will knock 10 per cent off the bill, an average saving of £40 per year.
- Use thermostatic controls on radiator valves as they considerably reduce heating bills. Check the layout of rooms to ensure that there are no large pieces of furniture in front of a radiator. Boilers need to be regularly serviced in order to maintain their efficiency.
- Use easy insulation methods – thick-lined curtains are a much less expensive way to reduce draughts around unglazed windows. Make sure that any draughts are prevented. Plastic, foam or metal brush strips should be fitted to doors and windows. Draughts waste heat and they can easily be solved by DIY measures.
- Thick carpets and underlay will also reduce draughts through floorboards, and unused chimneys should be blocked to eliminate drafts.

Activity 10

Review
List ten ways in which a householder can reduce their energy bills without outlaying any money.

Activity 11

Check your understanding
Check your understanding of the meaning of the following key terms:

environment	waste
waste hierarchy	land filled
incinerated	sustain
recycling	global warming
ozone layer	acid rain
methane gas	

Exam-style question

Explain the advice that could be offered to families who wish to reduce their household energy expenditure.

ASSESSMENT HINT!

Each point you make must be well explained.
Remember PEGEX – make the point, explain it and give an example.

Here is an example:

If the family wishes to buy a new dishwasher and chooses one which is A rated on the energy efficiency scale, it will be more energy-efficient. This means it will use less electricity and therefore cost less to run.

Point = energy efficiency labelling
Explanation = A rated means more energy-efficient
Example = a dishwasher which will cost less electricity to run.

Social issues

Learning objectives

By the end of this chapter you will be able to:

- explain what is meant by the term 'welfare state'
- identify some of the issues in providing welfare services
- describe how health and social services can be provided by statutory, voluntary and private organisations.

Introduction

In this chapter you will investigate the development of the welfare state and the concept of the state providing a comprehensive system of health and social care for individuals. Services provided by the state are referred to as **statutory** services. Statutory services are provided after law has been passed in parliament. They are funded from taxation and include the National Health Service and local social services. To supplement statutory services, voluntary and private organisations can provide services for individuals. Voluntary organisations are non-statutory and independent. Some are set up to help and support individuals who need help meeting their health and social needs, such as Age Concern. Private organisations are run by businesses to make a profit and are increasingly involved in delivering health and personal social care services to individuals.

We explore in detail how the state, voluntary and private organisations contribute to providing both health and social care in the UK.

The welfare state

The **welfare state** is a system supported by the government that attempts to provide economic security

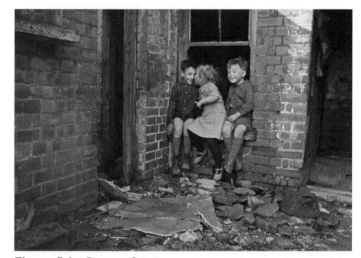

Figure 5.1 *Post-war Britain*

for people when they are unemployed, ill or elderly. Examples are the National Health Service (NHS) and state benefits.

The idea of a welfare state was developed by the economist and social reformer William Beveridge during the Second World War. He produced a report which pulled together many different ideas about social reform. It became known as the Beveridge Report. Implementing the Beveridge Report was immediately seen as part of winning the peace after the war and gave the government a major role in providing decent health care, housing and employment opportunities for the nation. The report offered security 'from the cradle to the grave'. It was established to fight the five 'evil giants' that faced post-war Britain.

These five giants were:

- **Want**: Many people were very poor. Being unable to work was the key cause of poverty. The report created National Insurance, a tax paid by workers to provide sickness and unemployment benefit, retirement pensions and a widows and maternity benefit for those unable to work.
- **Disease**: Everyone had to pay for medical treatment. The health of the nation was poor and the poorest could not afford health care. With new legislation the NHS was formed and every British citizen received free medical, dental and optical services.
- **Ignorance**: Most children left school at 14 or before. Welfare reform made education free and compulsory from 5 to 15 years. It provided meals, milk and medical services at every school.
- **Squalor**: Many people lived in poor housing. The war had devastated many towns and cities. Social housing was introduced and decent homes were available for all. During the post-war period large numbers of council houses were built and new towns created.
- **Idleness**: After the war there was a very high employment rate. Industries were nationalised (taken over by the government) to help keep full employment.

Activity 1

Group discussion and review

What are the advantages and disadvantages of a state funded welfare system?

Discuss this in a group and then make your own notes on what you learn from the discussion. You can present your notes as two sets of bulleted lists (advantages and disadvantages).

Welfare reform

Many of the good intentions of the welfare reforms introduced after the war did meet problems.
The cost of running the NHS continued to rise, driven by a combination of rising expectations about personal health and health services, by advances in

medical technology and by a rapid growth in life expectancy.

Charges were introduced for some health services. When the NHS was introduced in 1948, it was expected that it would cost £400 million. In its first year it actually cost £700 million. It was predicted in the 2007 budget that the NHS would cost nearly £90 billion in 2007/8.

The NHS now

Here is a snapshot from the Department of Heath NHS Plan 2005.

On a typical day in the NHS:

- Almost one million people visit their family doctor.
- 130,000 go to the dentist for a check-up.
- 33,000 people get the care they need in accident and emergency.
- 8000 people are carried in an NHS ambulance.
- 1.5 million prescriptions are dispensed.
- 2000 babies are delivered.
- 25,000 operations are carried out including 320 heart and 125 kidney operations.
- 30,000 people receive a free eye test.
- District nurses make 100,000 visits.

In addition to the expenditure on the NHS, the cost of welfare benefits is rising. Welfare benefits were not paid at a high enough level to prevent many people from living in poverty. By the 1970s unemployment began to rise and the goal of full employment was abandoned. The cost of providing welfare benefits is an increasing burden and a new approach was required.

The emphasis is now on 'welfare to work' and not 'welfare to live on' to tackle poverty. **Welfare to work** is a range of strategies to help the unemployed into work and off benefits. Living on welfare benefits as a way of life is no longer acceptable. The early welfare state did recognise the importance of work in creating a decent society. But the new debate concentrates on how long-term employment opportunities and training can be provided. Individuals are to have a much greater responsibility in supporting themselves and their families. Personal responsibility is now seen as key in tackling poverty and building aspirations for everyone in our society.

There will always be those who cannot work and the state will support them. But increasingly welfare is restricted to a system of safety nets for the most vulnerable in society.

The delivery of welfare services has also changed and now a combination of state, voluntary and private organisations provide care.

Statutory, private and voluntary provision

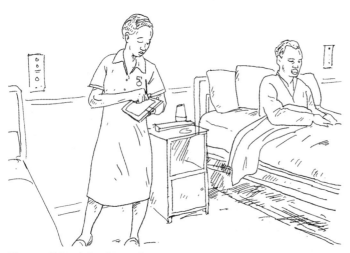

Figure 5.2 *A health worker*

In the UK the state provides free health care as a right for every individual. This has been traditionally provided by the NHS. The NHS is a government-run service which provides doctors (GPs), hospitals and community health services which meet the health care needs of individuals.

The main sources of health and social services providers are:

- statutory health and social services provided by law which are free of charge
- private sector health and social services which need to be paid for by the individual
- voluntary health and social services which is provided by charities and voluntary organisations
- informal health care which is provided by an individual's family, friends or neighbours.

Statutory provision

The NHS core principles are as follows:

- It meets the needs of everyone.
- It is free at the point of need.

- It is based on a patient's clinical need and not their ability to pay.

The NHS provides a comprehensive range of services throughout primary and secondary care. The NHS will also provide information services and support to individuals in relation to health promotion, disease prevention, self-care, rehabilitation and after-care. The NHS works in partnership with:

- patients, their carers, families and NHS staff
- the health and social care sector and social services
- various government departments
- the public sector, voluntary organisations and private providers.

Figure 5.3 shows how the NHS structure works in England.

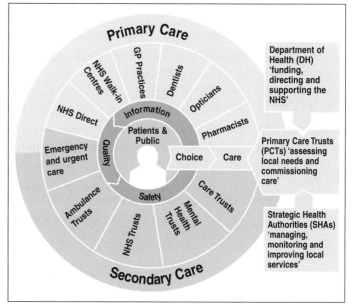

Figure 5.3 *The structure of the NHS*   *Source: NHS Choices*

- **Department of Health**
  This government department funds, directs and supports the NHS.

- **Primary Care Trusts (PCTs)**
  Primary Care Trusts are local health organisations which manage the health services in a local area – hospitals, doctors, dentists and mental health services. They are now at the centre of the NHS and control 80 per cent of the budget.

- **Strategic health authorities (SHAs)**
  Strategic health authorities have overall responsibility for improving the health services in their local area. They make sure local health services are of a high quality and are performing well.

Strategic health authorities manage the NHS locally and are a key link between the Department of Health and the NHS.

The care that is offered to us by the NHS is divided into two areas: primary care and secondary care.

Primary care

Primary care is provided by health professionals at the first or primary stage of health care. Much of the health care provided remains in the primary care stage. It is the health care provided by the people you normally see when you have a health problem. It consists of:

- GPs
- NHS walk-in centres
- NHS direct
- dentists
- opticians
- pharmacists.

Primary health care aims to prevent the illness or problems getting worse. It will refer individuals to secondary health care when necessary.

The statutory services provided by primary care include:

- **NHS direct:** This provides a telephone service to offer advice and support, particularly out of hours.
- **NHS walk-in centres:** If you become ill out of hours and phone your GP and need medical help, you can be referred to an NHS walk-in centre where you can be seen by a health professional.
- **GP practices:** Your local **GP** provides a wide range of family health services including:
  - advice on health problems
  - vaccinations
  - examinations and treatment
  - prescriptions for medicines
  - referrals to other health services and social services
  - medical tests.
- **Dentist:** NHS dentists provide dentistry for urgent and out-of-hours care in your area.
- **Opticians:** They look for signs of eye disease which may need treatment from a doctor or eye surgeon and prescribe and fit glasses and contact lenses.
- **Pharmacists:** Also known as chemists, they are experts in medicines and how they work. They play a key role in providing quality health care to patients. They dispense prescriptions and are often willing to give advice.

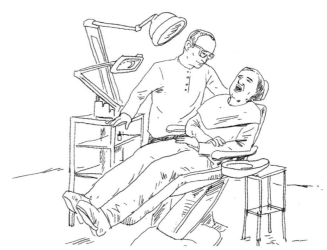

Figure 5.4 *A dentist*

Secondary care

Secondary care is provided if a health condition requires further treatment. As this is not possible in primary care, a referral is made to secondary health care, which is provided in hospitals. It consists of:

- emergency and urgent care
- acute trusts
- NHS trusts and foundation trusts
- ambulance trusts
- care trusts
- mental health trusts.

When treatment has been received and the condition is dealt with, or at least improved sufficiently, the patient is returned again to primary care.

The statutory services provided by secondary care are:

- **Emergency and urgent care:** This is provided by the 999 emergency care system and accident and emergency departments of hospitals.

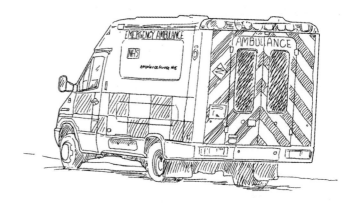

Figure 5.5 *An ambulance*

- **Acute trusts:** Hospitals are managed by acute trusts. Acute trusts employ a large part of the NHS workforce – nurses, doctors, pharmacists, midwives and health visitors. It also includes people doing jobs related to medicine – physiotherapists, radiographers, speech and language therapists, counsellors and psychologists.
- **NHS trusts and foundation trusts:** These are new types of NHS hospitals run by local managers, staff and members of the public, which are tailored to the needs of the local population.
- **Ambulance trusts:** These provide emergency access to health care. The NHS is also responsible for providing transport to get patients to hospital for treatment. In many areas it is the ambulance trust that provides this service.
- **Care trusts and mental health trusts:** These will be considered later in this chapter because they are mainly concerned with social care provision.

Activity 2

Group discussion

Carry out some research – in the media, on the internet – on what you consider are the problems within the NHS today.

Discuss your findings with your group.

Some starting points for your discussion are given at the back of the book.

Statutory provision of social services

Social services are a wide range of support and care services which look after our health and welfare. They are also referred to as social care services. Many of us are likely to become clients of social care services at some point in our lives. The people most likely to need social care services are the following:

- children or families under stress
- people with disabilities
- people with emotional or psychological difficulties
- people with financial or housing problems
- the elderly who need help with daily living activities.

Social care services are provided by local councils, voluntary (not-for-profit) organisations and private agencies. Councils with social services responsibilities have a statutory responsibility to ensure that the social care needs of people are met. These are sometimes met

in conjunction with local NHS providers and other organisations. Many councils often work together to run social care services.

In England the responsibility to provide social care services rests primarily with local councils. At any one time, up to 1.5 million of the most vulnerable people in society are relying on social workers and support staff for help. Social care services also make a major contribution to tackling social exclusion.

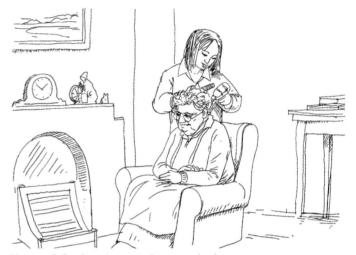

Figure 5.6 *Providing social care in the home*

There is a huge variety of social care available:

- **Personal care** is offered in the individual's home for help with bathing, toileting, dressing, companionship, hairdressing, manicure and feeding.
- **Domestic care** is offered in the individual's home for help with garden maintenance, equipment repairs, laundry, cooking, shopping, cooking and cleaning.
- **Auxiliary care** is offered in the individual's home for help with gardening, transport and odd jobs.
- **Social support and surveillance** is offered in some communities. It may include visiting, companionship, social events, trips out and pet care. These services can be supplied by voluntary organisations.
- **Community nursing care** is carried out by community nurses. They provide medical care in people's homes, GP surgeries and health centres. They work with the most vulnerable groups including older people, children or adults with learning disabilities. Community nurses visit people at home to change dressings, give injections and offer advice on home nursing aids and equipment.
- **Day services,** in the form of residential or nursing home care, can be provided. Day centres are where

elderly people or mentally ill people can go to socialise and meet friends or have a hot meal. Transport may be offered to allow the person to travel to and from the day centre.

- **Respite care** where an individual goes into short-term residential care to give their carer a break. A carer is anyone who provides care for another person or people.
- **Residential care** is given in a care home. It is available to individuals who are unable to live independently. These can be run by local councils or as private businesses.
- **Palliative and supportive care** is for individuals and families where there is serious long-term illness or the advanced stages of a terminal disease. Supportive care is given with diagnosis and treatment and includes advice and counselling. Palliative care helps control symptoms of disease and provides emotional support usually by specialist nursing (Macmillan nurses). Care can be provided in the community to help individuals live their lives as actively as possible or in specialist care settings.

Social workers

Social workers work with adults and children within the community, giving support and advice to help solve problems. They work closely with organisations such as the police, the local authority, NHS, schools and the probation service. They provide two services:

- **Adult services**: working with people with mental health problems or learning difficulties. They work with offenders in the community and support them to find work. They assist people with HIV/AIDS and work with older people in their homes to help to solve problems with their care package, health, housing or benefits.
- **Children and young people services**: providing help and advice to keep families together. Social workers manage the adoption and foster care processes. They provide support to young people leaving care and help young offenders. They help children who have problems at school or are facing difficulties due to issues at home.

Trusts

Care trusts are set up when the NHS and local authorities agree to work together. They are organisations that work in both health and social care. They may carry out a range of services, including social care, mental health services or primary care services.

Mental health trusts provide health and social care services for people with mental health problems. This might include counselling, community and family support or general health screening. For example, people suffering bereavement, depression, stress or anxiety can get help.

Children's trusts bring together all services for children and young people in an area. Children's trusts aim to listen to children and focus on improving child health care provisions. In 2008 every area should have a children's trust.

Access to social care services

Self-referral is where a person chooses to ask for help. They may visit their GP as a starting point who may refer them to the social services department as part of their treatment. They will be assigned to a social worker who will take responsibility for managing their care.

The social worker assesses the individual and their home circumstances to decide what is needed. Visits will be made to the individual's home to assess any particular needs. Decisions can then be made on the level of care needed.

Professional referral is where you are referred on to someone offering more specialist care. For example, a GP may refer an individual to a physiotherapist for help with mobility.

Third-party referral is where an individual is put in contact with a service by a friend, family or neighbour.

Under the National Health Service and Community Care Act 1990, anyone who needs social care services is entitled to have their needs assessed. Needs are assessed by social workers and other professional staff to assess what services are needed for the individual.

Assessment results in a **care plan**. This is a written document that outlines how the needs of an individual are to be met. Many people have complex needs that may result in **multidisciplinary care**. This is where care is provided by a range of different agencies and professional carers. For example, an older person in their own home may be unable to do housework or shopping because they are recovering from a broken leg. They may receive occupational therapy to help with daily living activities, home care to assist with the shopping and nursing care to assist with their leg.

Activity 3

Review

To help you understand the differences between primary and secondary care, outline the services provided by primary and secondary care within the NHS.

ASSESSMENT HINT!

If you are asked to outline something you should write out the main points or a general plan, but omit the minor details.

Private provision of health and social services

Some aspects of the health service are not free. Individuals may have to pay for some services or they may just prefer to do so.

Private medical insurance

With private insurance, health care is provided by private companies. An individual pays medical insurance to a health care company, and if they need treatment the costs are met by the company. Some people receive this insurance as part of their job. Private medical insurance covers the costs of private treatment for acute conditions. These are diseases, illnesses or injuries that are likely to respond quickly to treatment. In general, the insurance does not cover the treatment of long-term and incurable illnesses.

Having private medical insurance can mean quicker consultations and treatment. A private patient can often choose when treatment will take place, the specialist they will see and where the treatment will be given.

Private medical insurance is not designed to replace the services offered by the NHS. Accident and emergency treatment are beyond the scope of most private hospitals. Alternatively, some people prefer to pay for treatment as they require it. If their GP refers them to a local hospital for treatment, rather than be placed on a waiting list, they prefer to book to see a consultant privately. Any subsequent treatment could be paid for in the private system or they could return to the NHS.

Dental services

In April 2006 NHS dental services changed. Some people still receive free treatment – those aged under 18, those aged 18 and in full-time education, pregnant women and women who have had a baby in the last 12 months, an NHS dental hospital patient, or someone receiving income support or income-based jobseeker's allowance. Everyone else who is registered with an NHS dentist is charged using three standard price bands for all NHS dental treatments. The maximum charge for the most complex treatment is £194.

These charges help to meet some of the treatment cost. Dentists are obliged to give NHS registered patients the treatment they need to meet all their clinical needs under the NHS. But advances in dentistry have led to many people demanding treatment which is more than clinical need. Private dentists offer treatments which are not available on the NHS, such as cosmetic dentistry including tooth whitening, porcelain dental veneers and dental implants. This treatment can be very expensive. Many dental surgeries provide a mixture of NHS and private care.

Optical services

Some people are entitled to a free NHS sight test. They include those who are:

- under 16 or under 19 and in full-time education
- aged 60 and over
- registered blind or partially sighted
- suffering from diabetes or glaucoma or are at risk of glaucoma
- receiving income support or income-based jobseeker's allowance.

For those on a low income, NHS optical vouchers are available to meet the cost of a prescription. Opticians will charge everyone else for sight tests, contact lenses and spectacles.

Fertility treatment

In vitro fertilisation (IVF) is the most well-known fertility treatment. Women under the age of 40 are offered one free IVF cycle. The average cost of an IVF cycle was estimated to be about £2800 in February 2004. Any subsequent treatment, and those already with children, have to pay privately for treatment.

Chiropodists

Chiropodists (now often called podiatrists) treat conditions of the foot and lower limb such as verrucas, ingrown toenails and arthritis. They work with all ages, but are very important in helping older or disabled people to stay mobile and independent. Podiatry or chiropody is available on the NHS free of charge, but free treatment usually requires a GP referral. Many people who require treatment pay for the service privately.

Cosmetic surgery

Cosmetic surgery is usually provided by private health care. The term is used to describe operations that change the appearance, structure or position of features to produce a result that patients perceive to be more desirable. Cosmetic surgery procedures include face lifts, nose reshaping, breast enlargements and liposuction. These operations can be very expensive. Generally, the NHS will not provide surgery just for cosmetic reasons. However, reconstructive surgery and cosmetic surgery to correct or improve birth defects and injuries due to accidents are usually carried out free of charge.

Health screening

The NHS provides some free health screening services for men and women including bowel cancer, breast cancer and cervical cancer. However, there is no national NHS screening programme for prostate and testicular cancer, osteoporosis and glaucoma. The private sector fills the gap and provides a wide range of health screening services.

Care homes

If social services are involved in providing a nursing and residential home, they expect a contribution towards the fees. If social services consider there is a need for residential or nursing home care, the amount the individual pays depends upon a national set of rules. This involves looking at income, benefits, pensions, savings, investments and the value of any property owned. Generally most of the income goes towards the cost of the care. Private applications to nursing and residential homes can be made directly without the involvement of social services.

There are two main types of care home:

- **Residential care homes**
  Residential care homes provide personal care. The staff in a residential home can help with personal care such as washing, going to the toilet, taking a bath, getting up or dressing. All meals are provided and there are activities and outings. All residential homes have to be registered with the Department of Health's Commission for Social Care Inspection. Its inspectors visit residential homes to make sure that they meet the standards that have been set by the government.

- **Nursing homes**
  Many nursing homes are privately owned and managed. Nursing homes care for people who are more dependent. They provide expert nursing care. All nursing homes are required by law to have a qualified nurse on duty 24 hours a day. They have to be registered and are inspected by the National Care Standards Commission.

Some care homes are dual registered. This means that the home will take people needing either residential or nursing care. Some people may wish to choose a dual-registered home so that if their condition deteriorates they do not have to move to a different home. Or a couple with differing needs may wish to go into the same home.

Social care

There are several services which come under the heading of social care:

- **Home care services**
  Home care services provide help in an individual's home with personal tasks including bathing and washing, getting up and going to bed and shopping. Providing home care may involve a carer visiting the home daily. There are charges for this service.

- **Home helps**
  Home helps are people who help with domestic tasks including cleaning and cooking. There are charges for this service.

- **Adaptations to the home**
  Adaptations to the home are important in allowing independence and improving quality of life. Major adaptations could include the installation of a stair lift, downstairs toilet or the lowering of worktops in the kitchen. Minor adaptations include installing

hand rails and hoists. The cost of these adaptations may be met by social services or privately by the individuals.

● Meals
The provision of meals as a community care service could mean a daily delivery of a meal or, in some areas, the delivery of a weekly or monthly supply of frozen food. It could also mean providing meals at a day centre or lunch club. The cost of these meals varies considerably in different parts of the UK.

● Recreational and occupational activities
Many local authority social services departments provide a range of recreational, educational and cultural activities. These may be held in a day centre. Activities include lectures, games, outings, and help with living skills and budgeting. The local authority's social services department may provide transport to enable use of the facilities. The cost of transport and refreshments may be met privately.

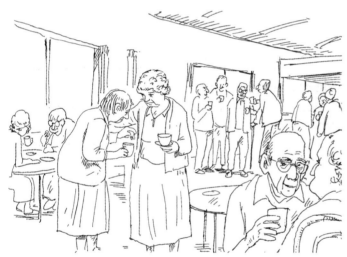

Figure 5.7 *Socialising at a day centre*

Voluntary provision of health and social services

Voluntary organisations are non-statutory bodies, set up and run by their members rather than by government. They are accountable to their members rather than to the public through democratic procedures. Most such organisations operating in the health field are registered charities and therefore enjoy financial benefits of tax relief on funds donated.

Essentially, voluntary bodies are private organisations operating on non-commercial or social principles. They make extensive but not exclusive use of

volunteers. Substantial numbers of paid employees work within the voluntary sector. Some voluntary bodies in the field of health and personal social services receive funding from the government and local authorities

They play a crucial role by complementing state provision, in that they make a major contribution to health care and social welfare. They can be flexible and act quickly to help those who have a particular problem and in immediate need. They are useful in befriending individuals who may need to re-establish themselves within the community if they have been in an institution or are recently bereaved. They are an outlet for religious feeling, social care, goodwill and generosity. They are useful as a pressure group for reform by being critical of service shortcomings and alerting the authorities to any gaps. They may use their own provision to fill an official gap, such as the organisation Women's Aid, which provides shelters for women and children who have been subjected to abuse from a violent partner. They also provide an interest and work for those who are otherwise unemployed.

The activities undertaken by voluntary organisations include:
● providing a service for individuals in need
● identifying unmet needs
● meeting minority needs
● educating the public
● raising funds
● acting as a pressure group.

Types of voluntary organisations

Voluntary organisations vary enormously in size and scope of activities, from international groups such as the Red Cross, to national concerns such as Relate, Age Concern and Mind, down to district and local groups, for example, a club for the unemployed who are suffering from stress caused by debt or low self-esteem.

Here are some examples of voluntary organisations:

● **The Samaritans** offer a free counselling service to those in need. They have experienced and trained counsellors available 24 hours every day. Counsellors deal with any topic of concern and cope with every level of concern from mild worries to those contemplating suicide. The service is confidential and help is usually give over the telephone so that anonymity can be maintained. Appointments are not necessary.

- **Women's shelters** offer help and refuge support to stressed women and their children who have aggressive or abusive partners.
- **Gingerbread groups** are for single parents offering mutual support in dealing with the stress involved in single parenting.
- **Help the Aged** and **Age Concern** target help to the elderly who may need support if they are to remain living in their own homes. They also provide day care centres where specific help, such as hairdressing, may be available as well as social contact.

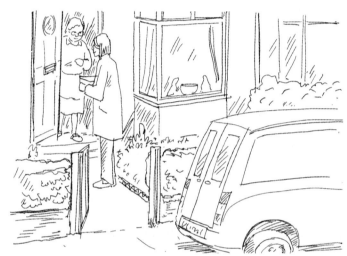

Figure 5.8 A 'Meals on Wheels' delivery

- The **Women's Royal Voluntary Service (WRVS)** provide 'Meals on Wheels' for elderly and disabled people who are housebound. They also respond in times of crisis in the event of flood or fire, by setting up emergency shelters and feeding centres.

Activity 4

Practical opportunity

Suggest a selection of hot main meals and hot puddings which would be suitable for an elderly, housebound person.

Make one of them in your practical session.

- The **Salvation Army** supports the homeless as well as providing care for the elderly or people in poverty.
- **Shelter** provides support to those who are homeless or are having difficulties with housing and poverty.
- **Alcoholics Anonymous** provides support to individuals who have alcohol problems.

- **Drug dependency groups** provide support to individuals who have drug problems.
- **Relate** provides support to people with relationship problems.
- **The Citizens Advice Bureau (CAB)** can offer information and specific advice on legal or financial matters. It can also help individuals with practical problems. For example, if debt is causing someone stress and ill-health, the CAB can offer practical help to remove the cause. It is usually necessary to make an appointment.

Activity 5

Review

Summarise the information on voluntary organisations, making sure you include information on:

- what they are
- what they do
- some examples.

Activity 6

Research opportunity

Choose a voluntary organisation and find out what services they offer and to whom.

Present your work in the form of an information sheet of no more than one side of A4.

Compare your information sheet with other members of your group.

Activity 7

Review

Check your understanding of the meaning of the following terms. Write a sentence using each word.

statutory	GP	social services
informal care	NHS	care plan
primary care	social services	
voluntary organisations	multidisciplinary care	
personal care	secondary care	
primary care	pharmacists	
residential care	home helps	welfare state
welfare to work		

Exam-style questions

Read the case study on the right.

Gerry is 85 years old and lives alone. He can be a bit forgetful. Sometimes he forgets to eat lunch. Gerry has a close friendship with a neighbour who will do some shopping and gardening for him. Gerry has arthritis and finds it difficult to use the cooker and washing machine. Gerry has two grandchildren but he only sees them at the weekends.

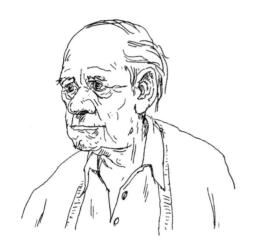

Figure 5.9 *Gerry*

Answer these questions:

1 Identify two problems Gerry may experience. (2 marks)

2 Describe three ways social services could support Gerry at home. (6 marks)

3 Describe three adaptations that could be made to a home to help the elderly? (6 marks)

4 Define the term 'welfare state'. (2 marks)

5 Explain the term 'from cradle to grave'. (2 marks)

6 Explain why we need to change the welfare state. (4 marks)

7 Complete the table below, giving examples of different organisations which provide health and social services. (8 marks)

Provider	Description of service	Example
Statutory		
Private		
Voluntary		
Informal		

8 Describe the range of social care provision today. (15 marks)

(Total of 45 marks)

Health

Learning objectives

By the end of this chapter you will be able to:

- explain the factors which may cause ill health
- understand the incidence and causes of major health problems in the UK
- describe the conditions diabetes, coeliac disease and osteoporosis
- describe the condition, incidence and risk factors associated with coronary heart disease
- explain how diet influences health and interpret data relevant to dietary-related health issues
- identify reports and advice relating to health and consider the value of current health education policies.

Introduction

This chapter will focus on the incidence and causes of health problems in the UK today. You will learn about diet-related conditions and how they can be addressed by changing the diet. The current government advice regarding healthy eating and the role of health education will also be investigated.

You will begin with an attempt to define health. This is not simple as health is linked to a range of individual, lifestyle, social and environmental factors. The impact of these factors has a significant effect on the individuals' opportunity and choice to remain healthy.

What is health?

Health was defined by the World Health Organization (WHO) in 1948 as:

'A state of complete physical, social and mental well-being and not merely the absence of disease or infirmity.'

Activity 1

Group discussion

What is physical, social and mental health?
List the key words you associate with each type of health.

The WHO definition is considered to be an ideal rather than a practical goal. It is often criticised as inadequate and having limitations. People with mental illness and physical disabilities may feel offended by the definition. What do you think? If the individual is well supported and feels content with their condition should they be regarded as healthy?

It is also disputed that health cannot be defined as a state, but as a resource that can adapt to the changing demands and expectations of life. In 1986 WHO broadened its definition:

'Health is therefore seen as a resource for everyday life, not the objective of living. It is a positive concept emphasising social and personal resources as well as physical capabilities.'

Ottawa Charter for Health Promotion, 1986

Health promoters have now come to regard health in broader terms. They link health to much wider physical, social, lifestyle and societal factors. These factors may include family values, aspirations, housing, employment, self-esteem and the environment. It is now believed that to reduce ill health, the impact of these factors should be addressed.

You will now investigate how these factors can influence health.

Factors affecting health

In recent years the approach to health policy in the UK has included more focus on social and lifestyle issues as causes of ill health. It is now recognised that an individual's health is controlled by a range of factors which are related to each other.

These layers of influence are represented in Figure 6.1.

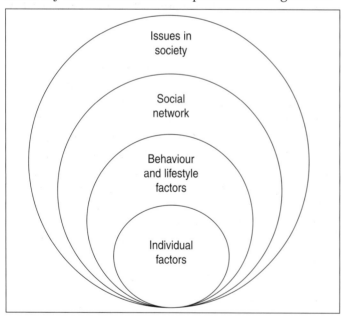

Figure 6.1 *Layers of influence on health*

Individual factors

These are fixed factors which can cause ill health. The fixed factors are difficult to change. They include our genetic make-up, gender and age, over which we have no control. Growing older increases the risk of developing problems with vision or movement. Some people are born with genetic diseases which affect their health. Research suggests that males are more likely to develop coronary heart disease than females. There is little doubt that future generations will have more control in this area thanks to developments in genetic science and drug treatments.

Behaviour and lifestyle factors

Behaviour and lifestyle factors have an important impact on health and can be modified. These may include cigarette smoking, alcohol consumption, taking drugs, exercising, diet and sexual activity. All these factors could influence the health and life expectancy of an individual. The contribution of behaviour and lifestyle factors to the incidence of disease will be explored later in this chapter.

However, it should be remembered that healthy choices are not always straightforward. Some individuals find it difficult to make healthy choices because of their personal circumstances. Their priorities may focus on more immediate problems and coping with their present situation. For example, an unemployed man who feels depressed may drink more alcohol to escape his situation.

Social network

A social network is the support and care given by friends and family. This will influence our behaviour and lifestyle. Individuals with strong social ties are more likely to be healthier than those who feel socially isolated. Research suggests that unemployment, drug and alcohol misuse and living alone can all contribute to the incidence of suicide. The Department of Health reported in 2002 that suicide is the commonest cause of death in men under 35 years and that young men from the poorest groups in society are at the greatest risk.

Issues in society

The final area of influence on health is the wider society. These are sometimes referred to as **societal factors**. Within this area there are some factors we have less control over. In the UK social and economic factors can contribute to the incidence of ill health. Where we live and work, our access to health services, as well as food, knowledge and education are all important. When social problems, such as poverty, poor housing, unemployment and limited access to health care, are combined, an individual's health can suffer disproportionately.

The values and expectations in society can also impact on our health, such as not smoking in enclosed public places. This makes the environment smoke-free and reduces the risk of diseases associated with smoking.

This multilayered approach to studying health supports the view that intervention is more effective when aimed at the wider issues in society. Targeted campaigns which just concentrate on individual or lifestyle factors appear to be less successful. When trying to improve health a co-ordinated approach is important as it recognises the links and influences of all the layers.

Activity 2

Group discussion

Discuss how the following situations may influence the ability of an individual to make healthy choices:

- living in temporary accommodation
- being unemployed
- being unable to read and write English.

Incidence and causes of major health problems

There has been a shift over the last century in the causes of ill health. In the 1900s, 25 per cent of deaths were caused by infectious diseases. This compares to only 1 per cent of deaths in 2000. Improvements in housing, health care and sanitation have contributed to a lower incidence of infectious disease. However, the relative proportion of deaths caused by cancer, coronary heart disease and stroke has increased. These diseases account for around two-thirds of all deaths and are a major source of ill health for many in the UK.

Diet and lifestyle

A balanced diet is an important way of protecting health. Poor diet is associated with some cancers, heart disease and stroke as well as tooth decay. Research from the British Nutrition Foundation in 2006 suggested that a third of all cancers were the result of a poor diet.

Families and households on low incomes spend proportionally more money on food but do not always make healthy choices. Limited transport means they are less likely to be able to reach supermarkets and take advantage of special offers and discounts. Research suggests that they are more likely to consume a diet low in fresh fruit and vegetables and large quantities of foods rich in fat, sugar and salt.

Incidence of obesity

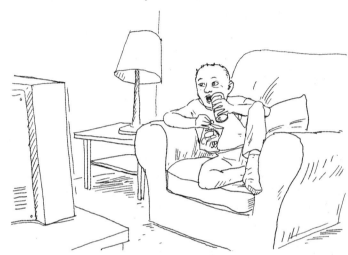

Figure 6.2 *An imbalance between calories consumed and energy used*

Obesity results from an imbalance between energy intake and energy needs. It has been suggested that children today are less active than previous generations. Too many children spend too much time travelling by car instead of walking or cycling. They watch TV or play computer games instead of playing sport. The increase in obesity suggests that the number of calories consumed is too high for the inactive child. King-sized portions, the increased consumption of sugary drinks and the popularity of fast food outlets serving energy-dense foods may have also contributed to the rise in obesity.

Doctors calculate obesity using a formula known as the body mass index (BMI). A BMI of 25 to 29.9 is considered overweight. **Obesity** is a BMI of 30 or above.

'If current trends continue, at least one fifth of boys and one third of girls will be obese by 2020'.
British Medical Journal, January 2007

Activity 3

Research opportunity

Investigate the consequences of childhood obesity. Describe the methods used to reduce the incidence.

ASSESSMENT HINT!

Investigate means you will need to consult a wide range of information sources and draw some conclusions.

Activity 4

Practical opportunity

1. Some children are eating meals which contain too much energy. Investigate the energy intake of children.

   Identify which foods or dishes eaten by children are high in energy.

   Take the recipe of a high-energy dish or meal (pizza) and adapt the ingredients to produce a low-energy version.

   Plan and prepare the dish in a practical session.

2. Investigate why the consumption of fruit and vegetables is important.

   Explain how fruit can be used to produce a low-energy dessert for children.

   Plan and prepare a dish in a practical session.

3. Red meat has an important place in the diet but can be high in fat. Investigate how the fat content of red meat dishes can be reduced.

The Department of Health suggests that obesity is responsible for more than 9000 premature deaths per year in England. In addition, it is a risk factor associated with heart disease, stroke, some cancers and type 2 diabetes.

Obese people are more likely to suffer from low self-image and confidence, social stigma and reduced mobility.

The National Audit Office predicts that by reducing the number of obese people in the UK by one million it could reduce the number of people with coronary heart disease by around 15,000. The number with type 2 diabetes would fall by 34,000 and 99,000 fewer people would develop high blood pressure.

The incidence of obesity is not evenly spread in the population. The graph below shows the proportions of obese men and women over 25 years but under retirement age related to their income.

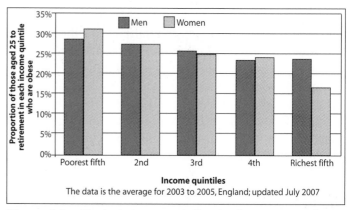

Figure 6.3 *Obesity in income quintiles; the data is average for 2003–2005, England, updated July 2007*

Activity 5

Review

1. With reference to the graph above, what proportion of women from the poorest fifth of households is likely to be obese?

2. What proportion of women from the richest fifth of households is likely to be obese?

3. Describe the data on obese men across all households.

4. What are the risk factors associated with obesity?

Dental decay

Internationally tooth decay is a significant health problem. In the UK the dental health of children has improved in recent years, but there are still some concerns. The Children's Dental Health Survey in 2003 suggested that children attending deprived primary schools were found to have more tooth decay than children in non-deprived schools. In deprived schools 60 per cent of five-year-olds had obvious decay experience in their milk teeth, compared with 40 per cent of five-year-olds from non-deprived schools.

Tooth decay is caused by sticky deposits called dental plaque collecting around the gum line and in crevices between teeth. The dental plaque consists of food remains and bacteria in the saliva. It is acidic and will

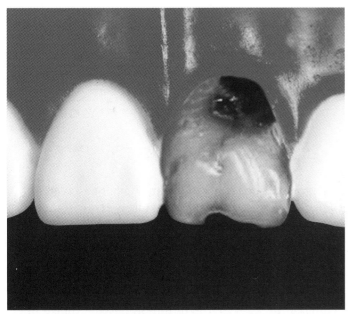

Figure 6.4 *A decayed tooth*

start to dissolve the tooth enamel. If the dental plaque is not removed by careful brushing, it may cause tooth decay. The dental plaque will harden into a substance called tartar. Both tartar and dental plaque are acidic and will dissolve away the protective enamel coating of the tooth, creating cavities if left unchecked.

This process can take months but eventually the softer, inner structure called dentine in the tooth and the blood supply will be damaged. This damage is permanent and if left untreated could result in tooth loss.

The link between tooth decay and sugar is well documented. A diet rich in sugar and starch will increase the risk of tooth decay. Frequent snacking increases the amount of time that acids are in contact with the teeth. Establishing a routine of brushing teeth with young children is important to reduce the incidence.

Activity 6

Research and ICT opportunity

Investigate the ways of avoiding tooth decay.

Design and produce a leaflet for primary school children to help them understand how to prevent tooth decay.

Activity 7

Practical opportunity

1. 'My five-year-old daughter loves very sweet, sticky snacks in her school lunchbox.' Identify products that could be offered as an alternative to a sweet, sticky snack.

   Plan and prepare a savoury snack and a low sugar snack suitable for a child's lunchbox.

2. Investigate the range of lower calorie sugars and sweeteners.

   Prepare biscuits using a low-calorie sugar product and standard sugar.

   Complete a sensory profile of the outcomes.

Physical activity

Physical activity is important in preventing heart disease, building healthy bones and helping to maintain good mental health. The Department of Health suggests that physical inactivity is a risk factor for a number of diseases including coronary heart disease, stroke, type 2 diabetes, high blood pressure and mental health problems.

Not everyone exercises. Research has shown that individuals from high socio-economic groups do more physical activity as a leisure pursuit than individuals from low socio-economic groups. Affordable leisure services make it easier for individuals to be more physically active. In communities where leisure facilities and services are not widely available the choice to participate is also limited.

Smoking

Smoking is the most significant cause of diseases which lead to early deaths in England. A study for the Health Development Agency in 2006 found more than 1600 people in England die each week because of smoking. The greatest number of deaths occur in the most deprived areas. It also showed that 85 per cent of lung cancer deaths were estimated to be caused by smoking. Smoking is the main cause of lung cancer and is linked to heart disease, chronic bronchitis and asthma. It may also contribute to cancer of the mouth, bladder, kidney, stomach and pancreas. Evidence suggests that mothers who smoke significantly increase the risk of cot deaths in their babies.

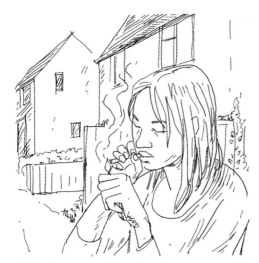

Figure 6.5 *A teenage girl smoking*

In 2004 a survey of school pupils found the proportion of regular smokers increases with age. The Office of National Statistics reported in 2006 that 26 per cent of girls and 16 per cent of boys smoked regularly by the age of 15. Overall, the number of adult smokers is declining, but young smokers are not giving up cigarettes at the same rate as other age groups. In the UK smoking remains a significant health issue.

The graph below shows the percentage of adults in different age groups who smoked in Great Britain in 2004.

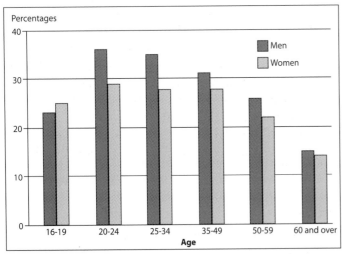

Figure 6.6 *Percentage of adults who smoke cigarettes, by age and sex, 2004, Great Britain*

Activity 8

Review

1. With reference to the graph above, which age group contains the largest number of smokers?
2. At which age is the number of women who smoke greater than men?
3. What health risks are associated with smoking?

Passive smoking is breathing in someone's cigarette smoke. This 'second-hand' smoke is a major source of indoor air pollution and contributes to the development of disease. Research evidence suggests that non-smokers, who are exposed to passive smoking at home, have a 25 per cent increased risk of developing heart disease and lung cancer. The British Medical Journal estimated in 2005 that exposure to passive smoke in the home caused around 2700 deaths in people aged 20 to 64 years and a further 8000 deaths a year among people aged 65 years or older.

Alcohol

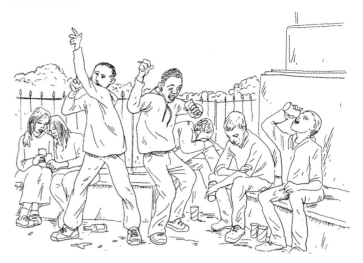

Figure 6.7 *Binge drinking*

Drinking alcohol is socially accepted behaviour which for the majority of people has few long-term effects on their health. However, some people do not drink sensibly. The Department of Health advises that adult women should not regularly drink more than two to three units of alcohol a day and adult men should not regularly drink more than three to four units of alcohol a day. Pregnant women or women trying to conceive should avoid drinking alcohol. If they do choose to drink, to protect their baby they should not drink more than one to two units of alcohol once or twice a week and should not get drunk.

The alcohol-related death rate has more than doubled, increasing from 6.9 per 100,000 populations in 1991 to 12.9 in 2005. Alcohol consumption is associated with cancer of the mouth, liver and breast, heart disease and stroke, and cirrhosis of the liver.

Alcohol has also been linked to domestic violence, car accidents, drownings, falls and alcohol poisonings. Young people who drink are potentially at greatest risk to the harmful physical and social consequences of excessive alcohol consumption.

Figure 6.8 shows the number of units of alcohol consumed weekly by young people aged 11 to 15 years in England.

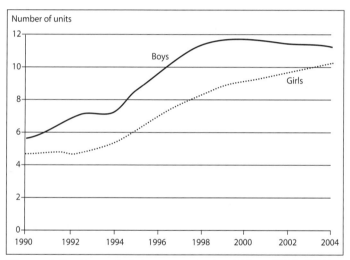

Figure 6.8 *Mean alcohol consumption by children, 1990–2004 (ONS, 2006)*

Activity 9

Group discussion

With reference to the graph above, what does the trend suggest?

What measures could reduce alcohol consumption?

Sexual health

Teenage girls living in deprived areas are four times more likely to fall pregnant than those living in more affluent areas (ONS, 2006). Young teenage girls who become pregnant increase their own health risks and their baby's health. Infant mortality rates for babies born to mothers under the age of 18 are twice the average rate (DOH, 2006).

Teenage pregnancy is often associated with a lack of educational achievement which is tied to limited employment prospects and poor living conditions which can result in health problems in the long term.

Sexually transmitted diseases are increasing. As many as one in ten sexually active young women may be infected with chlamydia. This may cause infertility if untreated (DOH, 2004).

Drugs

The use of illegal drugs threatens both individuals and communities. Research evidence has suggested a relationship between social deprivation and rates of drug-related deaths. Young men from deprived areas are six times more likely to die from drug-related conditions than their counterparts living in less deprived areas. Recent data from the Department of Health and the National Treatment Agency for Substance Misuse suggests the number of overdoses is increasing and incidence of blood-borne viruses has started to rise again.

The inequalities in health

There are health inequalities in the UK. Not everyone has the same chance to be healthy. Inequality is to some extent embedded in our social structure and difficult to change. The Acheson Report (Independent Inquiry into Inequalities in Health, 1998) clearly showed some inequalities in health. It has since directed the approach to managing public health in the UK. Acheson stressed the importance of tackling the wider causes of health inequalities, such as tax and benefits, education and employment, housing, environment and transport. A discussion of these factors will highlight the considerable inequality that still exists.

Poverty

Poverty can affect health in a number of ways. Households living in poverty are more likely to suffer ill health due to lifestyle habits including smoking, drinking, too much alcohol and not exercising. Diseases of the respiratory system, some cancers and heart disease are more frequent. A report by the charity Diabetes UK 2006 found that Britain's poorest communities are 2.5 times more likely to develop type 2 diabetes than the general population. They were also

3.5 times more likely to develop serious complications of diabetes including heart disease.

In addition, poverty can bring mental health problems, babies with a low birth weight. Road accidents involving pedestrians are more common in poorer communities.

Poverty can affect life expectancy and health. The gap in life expectancy is large and growing in some areas. The 2003 report 'Tackling Health Inequalities: A Programme for Action' suggests that the gap in death rates between professional and unskilled manual workers (male) since the 1930s has increased almost two and a half times. There are significant regional differences in life expectancy. In 1999/2001 newborn boys in North Devon could expect to live 9.5 years longer than boys born in Manchester in the same year.

Employment

Work is better for health than unemployment. Unemployment has been clearly linked to poor physical and mental health. The employed live longer than the unemployed. The unemployed are more likely than people in work to die from cancer, heart disease, accidents and suicide. Research has suggested that unemployment is associated with changes in health-related behaviour, such as an increased likelihood of smoking. Evidence suggests that unemployment amongst the middle aged is harmful on mental and physical health. The stress associated with factory closure has been shown to have a strong link with a decline in health among many older workers.

Housing

Housing has an impact on health. People who live in poor housing are almost twice as likely to suffer from poor health as those who do not. Data from the charity Shelter in 2007 has shown that children living in unfit or overcrowded homes are almost a third more likely to suffer from respiratory problems, such as asthma and bronchitis, than other children. Overcrowded conditions can lead to accidents, sleeplessness, stress and the rapid spread of infections.

A lack of heating contributes towards many deaths each winter. The elderly and the very young are vulnerable to cold weather. In the UK about a million homes have inadequate standards of energy efficiency, putting the health of those who live in them at risk when it's cold.

Access to health services

Health services must be accessible to all and meet the needs of the community. Equal access to services is not a reality everywhere. Research evidence suggests that deprived communities are in greatest need, but are the least likely to access the health services that they require. Many deprived communities are also less likely than affluent ones to receive heart surgery, hip replacements and other services such as health screening. There is a lower uptake of health checks, breast and cervical cancer screening and immunisation among some disadvantaged groups. There are concerns about the range and quality of GP services available in some deprived areas.

Activity

Research opportunity

'Health and life expectancy are still linked to social circumstances and childhood poverty. Despite improvements, the gap in health outcomes between those at the top and bottom ends of the social scale remains large and in some areas continues to widen.'

Tackling Health Inequalities: A Programme for Action, 2003

Investigate the government response to inequalities in life expectancy and infant mortality in the UK.
Write up your findings in a format of your choice.

Diets for diabetes, coeliac disease and osteoporosis

You will now look at these three conditions and see how important a role diet has in their management.

Diabetes

The full name for **diabetes** is Diabetes Mellitus. It is a condition in which the amount of glucose in the blood is too high. The reason why it becomes too high is because the body's method of converting glucose into energy does not work properly and allows the level of glucose to rise. Glucose is converted into energy by a hormone called insulin. **Insulin** is made by the **pancreas**, a gland lying just behind the stomach. Insulin controls the level of blood sugar and glucose and helps glucose to enter the cells in parts of the body such as the muscles, liver and adipose (fat) tissue. It is important that insulin works properly because both low and high levels of blood sugar are harmful to the body.

Type 1 diabetes

Type 1 diabetes, also known as insulin-dependent diabetes (IDDM), usually develops in childhood and is treated by a combination of diet and drugs. It develops if the body becomes unable to produce insulin. The main symptoms of type 1 diabetes include:

- increased thirst
- need to pass urine much more often, especially at night
- weight loss
- tiredness
- itching of the genital organs
- blurred vision.

It is important to maintain blood glucose level in order to eradicate the symptoms and prevent any problems which may occur in the long term, particularly poor circulation and damage to nerves, kidneys and eyes. Type 1 diabetes is treated by injections of insulin coupled with a healthy diet.

Type 2 diabetes

Type 2 diabetes is also known as non-insulin-dependent diabetes (NIDDM). It develops when the body produces some but not enough of the insulin it needs, or when the body is not able to use the insulin properly. It is often found in people who are overweight. Type 2 diabetes is usually managed by diet on its own or by diet and drugs in the form of insulin. It is increasing rapidly in the UK. This is thought to be linked with the fact that there are more overweight and obese people. The worldwide prevalence of type 2 diabetes has been predicted to be 215 million people by 2010 (according to the British Nutrition Foundation).

The role of diet in diabetes

The dietary advice for people with diabetes has changed considerably over the years. People with diabetes used to be told to eliminate all sugar and sugary foods from their diet. This resulted in people with diabetes buying special diabetic foods to replace everyday sugar-containing food products. Special diabetic jams, cakes, biscuits or pastries are of no particular benefit and they usually contain too much fat and are often expensive. Sound nutritional knowledge means that diabetics should not have to buy 'specialist' food at all if they choose to follow the healthy eating advice.

The most important message for people with diabetes is to eat healthily, in exactly the same way that is recommended for everyone – a balanced diet based on starchy foods and plenty of fruit and vegetables, and low in fat, salt and sugar. Eating more starchy foods such as bread, potatoes, rice and pasta will help reduce the amount of fat and increase the amount of fibre in the diet. A diet high in saturated fat and low in fibre can be harmful because it may cause weight gain and also impair insulin action.

A small amount of sugar and sugar-containing foods can be eaten, preferably as part of a healthy meal. Diabetics do need to be able to understand food labels, particularly when different forms of sugar are listed (fructose, invert sugar). A glucose carbohydrate snack may be carried at all times to prevent blood sugar levels falling below normal.

Diabetics should always plan their diet. They need to take care that portions are controlled and there are no leftovers for second helpings. All fat should be trimmed from meat, oil skimmed off dishes and methods of cooking should include baking or grilling rather than frying or roasting. They should use butter and margarine sparingly. Packet and bottled sauces are often high in sugar and calories and should be avoided.

Alcohol is a source of calories and care should be taken over quantity. Low sugar and sugar-free drinks are useful for diabetics.

Smoking should be avoided because it accelerates arterial disease and can affect the eyes and kidneys. Exercise is a useful activity in maintaining a healthy weight, particularly for people with type 2 diabetes. Exercise and sport can lower blood glucose levels so is a good idea. But type 1 diabetics do need to monitor their glucose levels if participating in intensive sporting activities regularly.

To conclude, the basic recommendations for people with diabetes is to:
- maintain a healthy body weight
- exercise regularly
- eat a healthy, balanced diet.

Activity 11

Review

1. Explain the difference between the two types of diabetes.
2. Discuss the implications of diabetes for an individual.

Activity 12

Practical opportunity

Design a leaflet which gives advice on diet for a diabetic. Include in your leaflet a range of healthy main meals which are low in fat, high in fibre and starch. Choose a dish to make in your next practical session.

Activity 13

Check your understanding

Check your understanding of the meaning of the following terms:

diabetes	glucose	insulin
pancreas	type 1 diabetes	type 2 diabetes

Coeliac disease

Coeliac disease is the main form of wheat intolerance. It is a bowel disease and it is an intolerance of gluten. Gluten is a protein present in a number of cereals: wheat, rye, oats and barley. When wheat flour is combined with water, the proteins in flour called gliadin and glutenin form another protein – **gluten**.

It is a permanent condition and may present at any age. A person suffering from coeliac disease is called a **coeliac**. The lining of the small intestine consists of villi. **Villi** are tiny finger-like projections which normally provide the very large absorptive surface of the small intestine. Characteristic of coeliac disease is that the villi are stunted. This stunting means that the body is less effective at taking up nutrients provided by foods. If a coeliac eats a product containing gluten it causes the villi to flatten and nutrients are no longer absorbed by the body and are passed out of the body in the faeces.

There are two important factors necessary for the disease to occur:

- It can be genetic and run in families.
- There is gluten in the diet to trigger the condition. It is estimated to have a prevalence of about 1 person in 100 although this is reduced to 1 in 10 in families where coeliac disease exists.

Possible symptoms of the disease are:

- diarrhoea
- irritability
- malabsorption which may also leave people tired and weak or it may be because of anaemia caused by iron or folate deficiency
- abdominal swelling
- loss of appetite and vomiting
- children may not gain weight or grow properly
- problems with bone development because of reduced calcium absorption
- possible long-term problems include infertility and osteoporosis
- a skin condition known as dermatitis herpetoformis which results in a red blistery rash.

Figure 6.9 *This logo shows that food is gluten-free*

The role of diet in coeliac disease

People with coeliac disease can still follow a tasty, healthy, balanced diet. But in order to avoid the long-term complications of the disease, people with coeliac disease must follow a strict gluten-free diet.

To have to follow a diet which does not contain wheat is very difficult but it can be done with careful thought and planning. Wheat is an important and nutritious staple in the UK diet and is found in a number of foods. It is found in flour, baked products, bread, cakes, pasta and breakfast cereals and is used as a thickener or extender in soups, sauces, sausages and pâté.

To omit wheat from the diet would mean the loss of valuable nutrients. Flour contains iron, vitamin B and some flours are fortified with calcium. Wholegrain products are also high in fibre and starchy carbohydrates. The nutrients that a coeliac would be unable to gain from wheat need to be sourced elsewhere:

- Iron can come from meat.
- The vitamin B group can come from offal, milk, eggs and green vegetables.
- Calcium can come from dairy products and nuts.
- Fibre can come from the skin of fruit and vegetables, nuts and pulses.

Socially a coeliac can find eating out more difficult in terms of food choice. As they become more knowledgeable and aware of their own condition, they usually gain more confidence about eating out and are more able to select the most appropriate foods from a given menu.

Coelaics must take care when choosing processed foods because of the likelihood of wheat being present.

Many foods are naturally gluten-free such as fresh meat, fish, cheese, eggs, milk, fruit, vegetables, rice, maize, potatoes, all kinds of vegetables and fruit, nuts, seeds, pulses and beans, as long as they are not cooked with wheat flour, batter, breadcrumbs or sauces.

There is now gluten-free flour which is readily available in health food shops and in most supermarkets. It is possible to bake cakes, biscuits and bread using gluten-free flour. There are also gluten-free baked products available to buy readymade. The foods are made gluten-free by the removal of gluten from wheat flour to produce wheat starch. The taste tends to be better, but often the texture is sometimes not as good as products baked with gluten-containing flour.

Regular tests are recommended to check for osteoporosis, so appropriate treatment can be given if necessary. A diet rich in calcium and vitamin D is therefore very important.

Sound nutritional knowledge is very useful because it can mean that coeliacs do not have to buy specialist food all the time. It may sometimes be necessary to prepare separate meals if flour is being used, but there are many occasions where everyone can eat the same meal – a roast dinner where the coeliac might just avoid gravy thickened with flour.

During pregnancy coeliac disease should be well controlled at all times and the baby should be fine.

Activity 14

Practical opportunity
Try some recipes using gluten-free flour in a practical session.

Write up your results on a computer using the title 'Does gluten-free flour produce acceptable results?'

Here are two examples of recipes you could use.

Gluten-free fairy cakes

75 g margarine

75 g caster sugar

2 eggs

$1/2$ teaspoon vanilla essence

75 g gluten-free flour

1 tablespoon milk

$1/2$ teaspoon baking powder

Preheat oven to gas 6/200°C

Beat all ingredients together until smooth and creamy

Divide into 12 cases

Bake for 10 to 12 minutes

Chocolate brownies

100 g margarine

75 g chocolate chips

100 g gluten-free flour

3 eggs

200 g caster sugar

1 teaspoon baking powder

Preheat oven to gas 4/180°C

Gently melt the butter

In a separate bowl mix flour, baking powder and sugar

Beat in eggs, butter and chocolate chips

Pour into a greased and lined tin 15 cm by 20 cm

Bake for 30 minutes

Activity 15

Check your understanding
Check your understanding of the meaning of the following terms:

coeliac disease   **gluten**   **villi**

ASSESSMENT HINT!

Never ever waste time writing out the question.

Osteoporosis

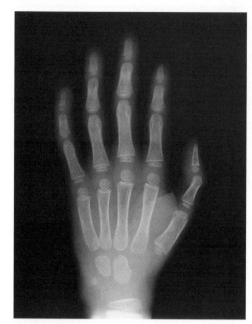

Figure 6.10 *Bone structure*

Osteoporosis is a diet-related condition which involves the thinning of the bone, involving loss of organic matter and bone mineral. It is a **multifactorial disease** which means that many factors increase the risk of osteoporosis. However, most of the contributing factors can be modified to reduce the risk in later life. The most significant factor contributing to the disease is diet.

We are all potentially at risk of osteoporosis because of the bone loss that occurs as we get older, particularly as we are living longer as a population. People can modify their diet and lifestyle when younger to reduce the risk of osteoporosis in later life.

You cannot see or feel your bone getting thinner so osteoporosis is often called a silent disease. For most people, the first sign that something is wrong is when they break a bone. You can find out if you have osteoporosis by having a bone density scan, called a dual energy x-ray absorptiometry (DXA) scan. This scan measures the **density** (thickness) of bones and compares this to a normal range. This test is currently the most accurate and reliable means of assessing the strength of bones and the risk of fracture.

Hormones play a part in osteoporosis. Women can get osteoporosis due to a lack of oestrogen. Lack of oestrogen is caused by an early **menopause** (before age 45), early **hysterectomy** (before the age of 45), particularly when both ovaries are removed, and by

missing periods for six months or more (excluding pregnancy) as a result of over-exercising or over-dieting. Men can get osteoporosis if they have low levels of the male hormone testosterone.

Men and women can be more at risk from osteoporosis for the following reasons:

- If they use high dose tablets for conditions such as arthritis and asthma long term.
- If there is a family history of osteoporosis.
- If they have other medical conditions such as liver and thyroid problems.
- If they have **malabsorption** problems such as coeliac disease, Crohn's disease and gastric surgery.
- If there is long-term immobility.
- If they drink heavily.
- If they smoke.

Your genetic make-up determines the potential height and strength of your skeleton, but lifestyle factors and diet will contribute to the thickness and strength of your bones. What you do when you are young in terms of strengthening your bones has a huge impact on the quality of your bones in later life.

The role of diet in osteoporosis

Healthy bones need a well balanced diet. A well balanced diet should consist of an adequate supply of minerals and vitamins, particularly calcium and vitamin D.

The material that gives hardness to bone is calcium phosphate. Bones are cartilage, but as calcium phosphate becomes enmeshed in the cartilage, the bones become stronger. This is known as calcification. More than 1500 mg of calcium phosphate per day for children can contribute to an increase in bone mass that can hinder the onset of osteoporosis in later life. For women, calcium consumption after menopause has little or no effect on the rate of bone loss so it is essential that calcium consumption is high when young.

The best sources of calcium are milk and dairy products such as cheese and yoghurt. Non-dairy sources of calcium include green leafy vegetables, baked beans, bony fish, nuts and dried fruit. Vitamin D which aids the absorption of calcium can be derived from UV light in the summer and margarine and oily fish in the winter. Calcium is hormone-controlled so with the onset of menopause it can be lost more readily.

The role of lifestyle factors in osteoporosis

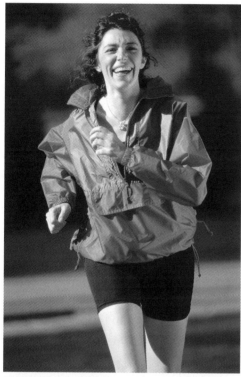

Figure 6.11 *Weight-bearing exercise will strengthen bones*

Taking regular, weight-bearing exercise will help strengthen bones. The best forms of exercise are running, skipping, aerobics, tennis and even brisk walking. Government recommendations are to try to exercise at least three times a week for a minimum of 20 minutes.

Smoking has a toxic effect on bone in men and women. It can cause women to have an early menopause and may increase the risk of hip fracture in later life. Stopping smoking will benefit bones, health and fitness.

Drinking too much alcohol is damaging to bones. The Department of Health advises that men should limit their alcohol intake to a maximum of 21 units per week and women to 14 units.

Activity 16

Review

1. Outline the condition of osteoporosis.
2. Explain who is most at risk and why.
3. What advice would you give to young people on diet and lifestyle to help reduce the risk of osteoporosis in later life?

Activity 17

Review

Devise a fact sheet on how the diet can be modified for the following people:

- a diabetic
- a coeliac
- a young person wishing to ensure they do not suffer from osteoporosis in later life.

Activity 18

Practical opportunity

Make two lists:

- As many foods as possible which are rich sources of calcium.
- As many foods as possible which are rich sources of Vitamin D.

Using a computer program such as Food in Focus or Food Tables, create a table showing the foods with the most calcium per 100 g of the food.

Choose a dish which incorporates a calcium-rich food and make it in a practical session.

Activity 19

Check your understanding

Check your understanding of the meaning of the following terms:

osteoporosis   multifactorial disease

density   hormone   menopause

hysterectomy   malabsorption

Coronary heart disease

Coronary heart disease (CHD) is a disease of the heart caused by the narrowing of the arteries that supply the heart with oxygen. This narrowing is caused by **arterial plaque,** consisting of fat globules and cholesterol, being deposited on the walls of the arteries. This process is known as **atherosclerosis.**

This restricts the supply of blood and oxygen to the heart, particularly during exertion when there are more demands on the heart muscle. At the same time the blood becomes more prone to clotting. Arterial plaque may block the delivery of nutrients to the artery walls, causing the arteries to lose their elasticity. In turn, this can lead to high blood pressure. It can result in chest pain known as **angina.**

A heart attack, also known as **myocardial infarction,** occurs when one of the coronary arteries blocks completely. This usually happens when arterial plaque splits open causing a blood clot to form on its surface that obstructs the flow of blood.

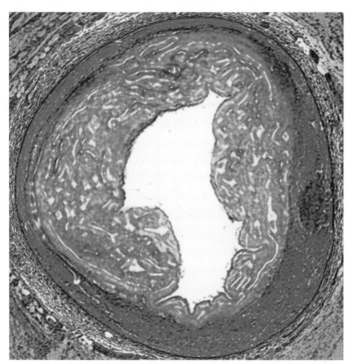

Figure 6.12 *A diseased artery*

The incidence of coronary heart disease

Figure 6.13 shows the four main causes of death between 1911 and 2003 in men and women in England and Wales. Circulatory diseases include heart disease and strokes.

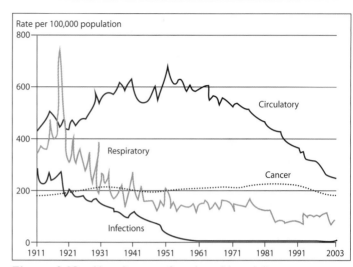

Figure 6.13 *Mortality rates for selected broad disease groups, 1911–2003, England and Wales*

Activity 20

Review

1. With reference to the graph above, which three types of diseases were the main causes of death in 2003?
2. Suggest a reason why the number of deaths from infections and respiratory diseases has fallen.
3. Which type of disease since 1921 has been the major cause of death?

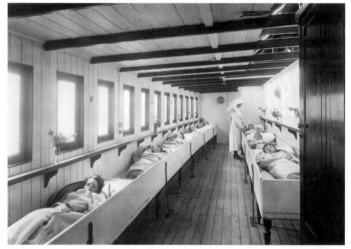

Figure 6.14 *A TB ward in a hospital, when TB was much more significant than it is today*

There has been considerable debate about the potential risk factors in the development of CHD. Some are more significant than others and some combinations of risk factors are more serious than others. For example, high blood cholesterol levels, smoking and high blood pressure together are significant risk factors. However, having one or two risk factors does not mean you will definitely develop the disease.

Health, social and environmental factors

Family history

Those with a family history of CHD could be at an increased risk of developing the disease. The risk is higher if there is a family history of early coronary heart disease, including a heart attack or sudden death before age 55 in the father or before age 65 in the mother.

Increasing age

Old age increases the risk as the disease develops over time. The peak age for men to develop the disease is between 55 to 64 years and women between 75 to 84 years.

Ethnic background

If you are black or Asian you have a higher risk of developing heart disease. If you are Asian, this is due to your increased risk of type 2 diabetes, which is a risk factor for CHD. If you are of black origin, you are more at risk of high blood pressure and in turn CHD.

Gender

Men are at greater risk of developing the disease than women. Women before menopause rarely suffer from heart disease. It has been suggested the hormone oestrogen appears to protect them.

Socio-economic disadvantage

The highest incidence of the disease is amongst the unskilled groups. Individuals from a higher social class have less risk of developing the disease. Research suggests the gap between the rich and the poor is still evident in the incidence of disease.

Low birth weight

Studies have shown that babies with a low birth weight have a greater risk of developing CHD in later life. They also have an increased risk of high blood pressure and raised blood cholesterol levels.

Smoking

Smoking contributes significantly to the incidence of CHD. The Department of Health suggests ten million people smoke in England, and approximately 20 per cent of heart disease deaths in men and 17 per cent in women are linked to smoking. The risk of thrombosis (blood clots) also increases. The heart and circulatory system has to work harder in a smoker to supply the body with oxygen.

High blood pressure

Raised blood pressure is an important risk factor. High blood pressure damages blood vessels and increases the risk of arterial plaque deposits which contribute to the development of the disease. It increases the heart's workload, causing the heart to enlarge and weaken over time.

Obesity

The risk of heart disease significantly increases in individuals with a body mass index above 30. The distribution of body fat is also significant as those people carrying abdominal fat, known as 'apples', are at greater risk than those carrying peripheral fat deposits on the hips, known as 'pears'. Approximately 22 per cent of men and 23 per cent of women in England were obese in 2004 according to the Department of Health.

Stress

Stress can be caused by work, unemployment, debt, lack of sleep, health or relationship problems. Too much stress and tension can raise the blood pressure and may make relaxation and sleep difficult. This can increase the risk of coronary heart disease.

Lack of exercise

Lack of exercise and fresh air will reduce the efficiency of the heart and the whole circulatory system. A sedentary lifestyle also contributes to this as a significant proportion of people only do minimal exercise.

High blood cholesterol

Cholesterol is a waxy substance found in the bloodstream and all body cells. Cholesterol is an essential part of a healthy body because it is used for producing cell membranes and some hormones. But high levels of cholesterol have a strong association with coronary heart disease. The amount of cholesterol in the blood depends on diet but genetic factors are also important.

When we eat cholesterol-rich foods some cholesterol may enter our bloodstream. In the bloodstream it combines with proteins called **lipoproteins**. There are two types of lipoproteins formed: **low-density lipoproteins** (LDL) and **high-density lipoproteins** (HDL). The cholesterol that combines with low-density lipoproteins is the LDL cholesterol or 'bad' cholesterol. It forms arterial plaque in the blood vessels. High levels of LDL cholesterol in the blood are associated with an increased risk of heart attack. The cholesterol that combines with high-density lipoproteins is the 'good' cholesterol or HDL cholesterol. It can remove arterial plaque from blood vessels. This is the type of cholesterol we want in the blood. Low levels of HDL cholesterol have been associated with an increased risk of heart attacks.

Type 2 diabetes

Research has suggested that individuals with type 2 diabetes have an increased risk of developing heart disease. Diabetics can have problems with the flow of blood around the body. They are more prone to higher blood pressure and higher LDL cholesterol levels than the general population. Poorly controlled diabetes can result in high levels of sugar in the blood, which can make the blood 'sticky' and likely to clump. Diabetes also magnifies the other risk factors for CHD such as raised cholesterol levels, raised blood pressure and obesity.

Diet and lifestyle factors

Type and quantity of fats consumed

LDL cholesterol has already been suggested as a risk factor. But the consumption of food rich in saturated fat can be more significant than dietary cholesterol. A high saturated fat intake can significantly increase the amount of cholesterol in the blood. Saturated fats are found in a range of foods including cooking fats, dairy and meat products, pastries, biscuits and cakes.

In recent years there has been concern over the processing of fats to produce convenience foods. Processing changes the structure of fatty acids and can result in the formation of **trans fatty acids**. Trans fatty acids can be produced during the processing of oils to make spreads and margarines. Trans fatty acids can

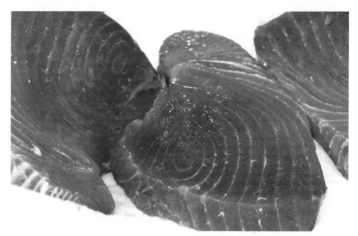

Figure 6.15 *Tuna, an oily fish*

raise blood LDL cholesterol levels and have been associated with increasing the risk of heart disease.

There are three types of fat: saturated; mono-unsaturated and polyunsaturated. Polyunsaturates are the healthiest type of fat and they can be divided into two groups of essential fatty acids (EFAs): omega 3 and omega 6.

Omega 3 fats are polyunsaturated fatty acids which are believed to be beneficial to health. They have to be consumed in the diet as the body cannot manufacture them. Food sources include oily fish, nuts and seeds. Research has suggested that the consumption of omega 3 fatty acids may cut the risk of heart disease – but the evidence is not conclusive. Many food manufacturers still add omega 3 to fruit juices, breads, margarines, spreads and children's drinks. Eggs can be produced which are high in omega 3 if hens are fed omega 3-rich diets.

Levels of salt

There are possible links between salt intake and high blood pressure. High blood pressure is recognised as a significant risk factor in the development of coronary heart disease. There could be some benefit for those susceptible to coronary heart disease in reducing their salt intake.

Levels of calcium

The minerals found in drinking water vary around the country. In some areas the water is described as hard water. This means that the water contains more minerals such as calcium and magnesium. A high calcium intake has been associated in some studies with a reduced incidence of coronary heart disease.

Alcohol consumption

A high alcohol intake can contribute to CHD in a number of ways. Research has found that a regular high alcohol intake increases the risk of high blood pressure and damage to heart muscles. Alcoholic drinks are high in calories and regular alcohol consumption is likely to contribute to excessive weight gain. Obesity brings several associated health problems including increased risk of developing coronary heart disease.

Fruit and vegetable consumption

Recent research has associated high rates of CHD with low body levels of **antioxidant vitamins and minerals**.

Antioxidant vitamins are vitamin E, C and beta carotene (a form of vitamin A). It has been suggested that vitamin C, beta carotene and vitamin E may offer some protection against coronary heart disease by preventing the development of fatty deposits in the arteries.

Antioxidants stop the build up of free radicals which damage cells in the body. **Free radicals** are unstable molecules produced as by-products of normal body metabolism. They can damage healthy cells and research has suggested that they may trigger conditions such as heart disease and cancers.

Activity 21

Review

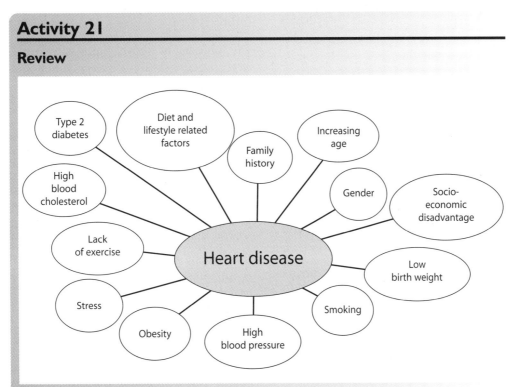

Figure 6.16 *Summary of risk factors for CHD*

Choose four risk factors from the diagram above and explain how they may contribute to CHD.

Activity 22

Check your understanding

Write a sentence to explain each of the following terms:

angina	salt	antioxidant vitamins and minerals	alcohol
myocardial infarction	fruit and vegetables	lipoproteins	cholesterol
high-density lipoproteins	trans fatty acids	free radicals	omega 3
calcium	arterial plaque	atherosclerosis	

Activity 23

Practical opportunity

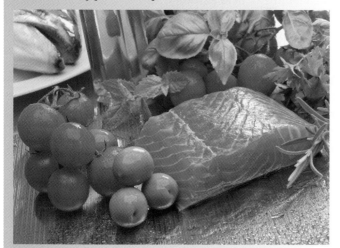

Figure 6.17 *The 'Mediterranean' diet*

The **'Mediterranean' diet** is a diet rich in fruit, vegetables, oily fish, lean meat and olive oil. Find some recipes containing the typical Mediterranean diet ingredients.

Plan and prepare a dish in a practical session.

Health of the nation

Data is constantly being collected in order to establish current dietary habits and how they influence our health. This information is obtained from many sources such as expenditure and food surveys, health surveys and social trends surveys.

It is well known that diet has an important influence on weight and general health. Today, many of the most common causes of death and **premature** death in the UK are linked to our diet, levels of physical activity, smoking and drinking.

You are now going to examine data which indicates the current trends of dietary-related health conditions, how they influence the health of our society and investigate how current policies are aiming to address these issues.

Life expectancy

Life expectancy is a widely used indicator of the state of the nation's health. Large improvements in life expectancy have occurred over the years. In 1901 the life expectancy for males born in the UK was 45 years and for females 49 years.

By 2005 life expectancy for males born in the UK was 77 years and for females 81 years. The gap between males and females has been steadily narrowing, with this trend projected to continue until around 2014, when the difference is expected to level off at around 3.7 years. Life expectancy is projected to continue rising for both sexes, to reach over 80 years for males and almost 84 years for females by 2021.

It is really important to note that life expectancy takes no account of the quality of life and whether it is lived in good health or with a disability or dependency. What is happening today is that although people have been living longer, the number of years spent in poor health has been increasing. This will also have an impact on health and social care services in the future.

The table below shows figures for Great Britain for life expectancy, healthy life expectancy and disability-free expectancy at birth by sex.

	Males		Females	
	1981	2002	1981	2002
Life expectancy	70.9	76.0	76.8	80.5
Healthy life expectancy	6.4	67.2	66.7	69.9
Years spent in poor health	6.4	8.8	10.1	10.6
Disability-free expectancy	58.1	60.9	60.8	63.0
Years spent with disability	12.8	15.0	16.0	17.5

(Adapted from Government's Actuary Department and Office for National Statistics)

Current dietary trends

Diet has an important influence on weight and general health. Diets which are high in fat (particularly **saturated fat**), sodium and sugar and low in fresh fruit and vegetables can contribute to a person being overweight or obese. This increases the risk of **chronic** diseases such as cardiovascular disease and cancer.

Obesity is linked to heart disease, diabetes and premature death. In recent years the proportion of the adult population and children in England who are obese has been rising. This is a worrying trend for the future health of the UK. Current dietary habits suggest that many people are consuming more food than they need for the energy they are expending and they may also not be eating foods in the right proportion to maintain health.

Government reports have highlighted the need for dietary changes to improve the health of society. Previous reports, such as the 1994 report of the Government's Committee on the Medical Aspects of Food and Nutrition Policy (COMA), recommended a reduction in fat intake, particularly saturated fat intake, and sodium intake (salt) and an increase in fruit and vegetable and complex carbohydrate intake. In the 2003 report 'Salt and Health', the Scientific Advisory Committee on Nutrition repeated COMA's guidance on salt intake in adults and introduced additional guidance on reducing salt intake in children.

In 2005 the government's dietary objectives were reiterated, reviewed and updated in 'Choosing a better diet: a food and health action plan'. The table below illustrates these dietary targets for England.

	Target
Total fat	To maintain the average total intake of fat at 35 per cent of food energy
Saturated fat	To reduce the average total intake of saturated fat to 11 per cent of food energy
Fruit and vegetables	To increase the average consumption of a variety of fruit and vegetables to at least five portions per day
Fibre	To increase the average intake of dietary fibre to 18 grams per day
Sugar	To reduce the average intake of added sugar to 11 per cent of food energy
Salt	To reduce the average intake of salt to 6 grams per day by 2010

Fat consumption

It is pleasing to note that the percentage of total energy derived from total fat in the British diet is decreasing, but only gradually, from around 40 per cent in 1975 to just less than 37 per cent in 2004/05.

However, the type of fat eaten has changed more significantly. There has been a decrease in the consumption of many different types of foods with a relatively high total fat and saturated fat content, including whole milk and butter. There have also been increases in the consumption of foods which are relatively lower in total fat and/or saturated fat such as reduced fat milks and spreads.

Fruit and vegetables

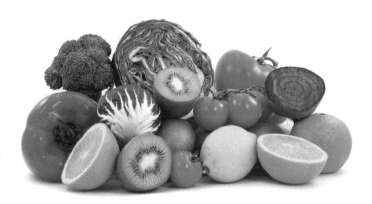

Figure 6.18 *Fruit and vegetables are essential in a healthy diet*

The Department of Health recommends that a healthy diet should include at least five portions a day of a variety of fruit and vegetables (excluding potatoes).

Current statistics tell us that the combined consumption of fruit and vegetables has risen but only slightly. In 2005 only 26 per cent of men and 30 per cent of women aged 16 and over in England met this target on a daily basis. Although children aged 5 to 15 tend to eat less fruit and vegetables than adults, their consumption has increased over the past year. In 2005 both boys and girls ate an average of 3.1 portions a day compared with an average of between 2.4 and 2.7 portions for boys and 2.6 to 2.7 portions for girls between 2001 and 2005.

The relatively high price of fruit and vegetables compared to processed foods or confectionery has long been considered a potential barrier to a healthy diet. Looking at social trends, people from the highest income group spent nearly 20 per cent more on fruit and vegetables than those from the lowest income group.

Some supermarkets use fruit and vegetables in regular promotions, which may encourage increased consumption. Research from the World Health Organization has highlighted the specific importance of low fruit and vegetable consumption as a cause of CHD. The World Health Report 2002 estimated that around 4 per cent of diseases in developed countries were caused by low fruit and vegetable consumption, and that just under 30 per cent of CHD and almost 20 per cent of strokes in developed countries were due to fruit and vegetable consumption levels below 600 grams a day.

Salt consumption

Data from the National Food Survey suggests that the consumption of salt added to cooking and at the table has declined considerably over the last half century. However, this does not mean that total salt intake has declined. This is because we obtain approximately 75 per cent of our salt from manufactured foods. Salt consumption in the National Diet and Nutrition Surveys shows an increase in both men (up by 9 per cent from 10.1 to 11.0 grams) and in women (up by 5 per cent from 7.7 to 8.1 grams) over a period of 15 years.

Lifestyle and food choices

One of the trends in society today is that because many people have busy lifestyles they claim to not have enough time to prepare fresh food. The consequence of this is that we have become more reliant on convenience foods, particularly ready meals which are often high in salt and fat.

The Food Standards Agency (FSA) found that around 20 per cent of people believed they had time to prepare a meal from raw ingredients at most once a week. So there has been a decline in home-cooked meals as fewer people have the skills or the time to cook, and more pre-prepared and convenience foods are consumed.

Snack foods, which are very widely consumed, tend to be high in sodium content and fat and sugar. This means that the national intake of these is too high.

More foods are eaten away from the home in work or school canteens, cafes, pubs and restaurants, as well as takeaway foods consumed at home, in cars or in the immediate environment where they are bought. These foods frequently have a high fat and salt content.

Many people choose not to eat breakfast at all or have a very light, quick breakfast rather than the previously traditional high protein breakfast of fried egg and bacon. Breakfast for those who still regularly eat it is often a drink and a piece of toast or a bowl of cereal with milk.

Food choice is affected by many factors which are explored in Chapter 8.

Activity 24

Review and group discussion

Find out the health implications of a diet that is:
- too high in salt
- too high in saturated fat
- too high in sugar
- too low in fibre.

Discuss your findings with the other members of your group.

Write up your findings as notes.

Activity 25

Group discussion

Study this survey on household food and drink expenditure in 2004–5.

United Kingdom	Pence per person per week
Milk and cream	156
Cheese	60
Meat and meat products	494
Fish	99
Eggs	18
Fats and oils	37
Sugars and preserves	17
Potatoes	102
Vegetables (excluding potatoes)	182
Fruit	167
Bread	93
Cereals (excluding bread)	283
Beverages	42
Soft drinks (excluding pure fruit juices)	80
Confectionery	84
Takeaways	159
Alcoholic drinks (average for the whole preparation)	266

Source: Family Food, DEFRA, 2004–5

Using the data, discuss the patterns of expenditure on food in relation to the guidelines for healthy eating.

People need to be aware of how they can achieve the government's dietary targets. Information has been produced to inform individuals on how they can achieve a healthy diet. One source of information is the Eatwell plate.

The Eatwell plate

The Eatwell plate has recently replaced the 'Balance of good health' as a visual representation of how to eat healthily. You should choose a variety of foods from each of these four food groups every day:

- bread, other cereals and potatoes
- fruit and vegetables
- milk and dairy foods
- meat, fish and alternatives.

Foods in the fifth group – foods containing fat and foods containing sugar – should be eaten in moderation.

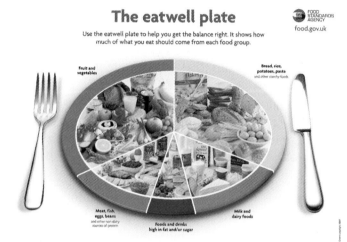

Figure 6.19 *The Eatwell plate*
Source: Crown copyright material is reproduced with permission of the Controller of HMSO and Queen's Printer for Scotland.

The Eatwell plate is consistent with the government's eight tips for eating well, published in October 2005, which are:

- Base your meals on starchy foods.
- Eat lots of fruit and vegetables.
- Eat more fish.
- Cut down on saturated fat and sugar.
- Try to eat less salt – no more than 6 grams a day.
- Get active and try to be a healthy weight.
- Drink plenty of water.
- Don't skip breakfast.

The advice continues as follows:

- Base your meals on starchy foods such as bread, potatoes, rice and pasta. This will help reduce the amount of fat and increase the amount of fibre in the diet.
- Cut down on saturated fat by trimming all visible fat and skin from meat and poultry.
- Choose cooking methods that do not add fat, for example, grill instead of fry.
- Take care with your consumption of milk and its products, fatty meat, biscuits, cakes, pastries, butter and lard which contain saturated fat.
- Eat lots of fruits and vegetables because all fruits and vegetables count towards the target of at least five portions per day, except for potatoes (which are classed as a starchy food). The fruits and vegetables do not need to be fresh or raw; canned, dried, frozen and juiced are just as good. Fruit juice counts as one portion which is particularly useful for children, as do beans and pulses.

Activity 26

Research opportunity

Visit the following websites:

- www.nutrition.org.uk – British Nutrition Foundation
- www.dh.gov.uk – Department of Health
- www.food.gov.uk – Food Standards Agency

Using the information you find, produce an informative, easy-to-understand information sheet or leaflet designed for families to encourage them to eat healthier. The aim of the leaflet is to show how easy it is to make your eating habits healthier.

Activity 27

Practical opportunity

Gordon Ramsay's campaign in his 2007 television series 'The F Word' was 'To redefine the concept of fast food and prove that anyone can prepare speedy meals in less time than it takes to get a pizza delivered.'

Create seven recipe ideas for a week's worth of evening meals for a busy couple. Each dish should be created from start to finish in 30 minutes. Use as many fresh ingredients as you can.

Justify your choice of recipe – explain why you have chosen certain ingredients and methods.

Then create three desserts that are also quick to make that could be used for a special occasion.

In your next practical session make one of your chosen dishes. This could be either a main dish or a dessert.

Physical exercise

Here are some interesting statistics:

- In 2004 in England 35 per cent of men and 24 per cent of women reported achieving the physical activity recommendations for adults (at least 30 minutes of at least moderate intensity activity at least five times a week).
- In 2005 the main reasons for adults not participating in active sports was that their health was not good enough (50 per cent) followed by difficulty in finding the time (18 per cent) and not being interested (15 per cent).
- In 2002, 70 per cent of boys and 61 per cent of girls met current physical activity guidelines for children (achieving 60 minutes or more on seven days a week).
- During 2005/06, 80 per cent of pupils took part in at least two hours of high quality PE and sport a week.

Choosing health

The government has attempted to address some of the causes of ill health by introducing legislation, strategies and policies to change our behaviour. One of these ways was to publish a white paper in 2004 called 'Choosing Health: Making healthy choices easier'.

It outlined the fact that there has been a sharp rise in obesity, a slow decline of smoking rates, growing problems with alcohol, teenage pregnancy and sexually transmitted diseases. It also identified key health priorities which were to:

- reduce the number of people who smoke
- reduce obesity and improve diet and nutrition
- increase exercise
- encourage and support sensible drinking
- improve sexual and mental health.

The document sets out ways in which the government can make it easier for people to choose healthy lives:

- Make it easier for people to choose healthy lives by giving them information about their health, help poorer people make good choices about health, and try to stop so many people buying unhealthy food, cigarettes and alcohol, especially children and young people.
- Help children and young people to be healthy by giving better information about health to parents, children and young people and working with schools to help children to be healthier. This includes providing children with healthy food to eat, making

sure children see a school nurse, encouraging children to do sport and exercise and reinforcing the message that the sale of cigarettes to children under 18 years is an offence.

- Help local communities to help people be healthier by making sure the NHS and local authorities work with groups and organisations. Initiatives have led to the support of sports clubs to help people do more sport, making it easier to cycle and walk and stopping smoking in public places.
- Make health a way of life by issuing health guides to anyone who wants one, and giving everyone the opportunity to get advice about healthier living.
- Support the NHS to help people be healthier by training NHS staff so they can teach people about being healthy, to help everyone get the health services they need, work with people who have been ill and to make sure that services are good and easy to use.
- Help people be healthier at work by helping more people get a job, making working conditions better, giving more support to employers to help their staff be healthy and to make sure the NHS is a healthy place to work.

The emphasis was put on people making informed choices, personalising health care to meet individual needs, and encouraging a range of organisations to work together.

People need to make informed choices about what they need to do to be healthy. The government cannot dictate what people can and cannot consume, but what they can do is provide access to information that shows the advantages of adopting a healthy lifestyle – and the dangers of excess drinking, smoking, taking illegal drugs or having unsafe sex. They can also put strategies and initiatives in place to support these choices.

Here are the strategies and initiatives which have been put in place to enable us to make healthier choices easier.

The 'Five a Day' programme

The government's 'Five a Day' programme encourages people to eat at least five portions of fruit and vegetables every day to promote a healthy diet.

The '5 a Day' logo was developed in consultation with industry, health professionals, the voluntary sector, consumers and other government departments to spread the health message that we should all eat five

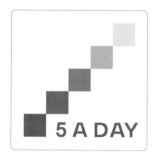

Just Eat More
(fruit & veg)

Figure 6.20 *The 5 a Day logo*

portions of fruit and vegetables each day. Only products without any added sugar, fat or salt may carry the logo or portion indicator.

All major supermarkets have agreed to support the government policies and campaigns aimed at improving healthy eating. They advertise and promote healthy eating messages on food packaging, in the stores and on their websites. Many supermarkets have developed their own range of 'healthy' food products. These food products often attract premium prices. This may prevent some consumers from making purchases and taking advantage of the health benefits these products may offer.

The school fruit and vegetable scheme

This scheme is part of the Five a Day programme to increase fruit and vegetable consumption. Under the scheme all four to six-year-old children in local authority infant, primary and special schools are entitled to a free piece of fruit or vegetable each school day. The scheme was extended when carrots and tomatoes were added to apples, pears, bananas and easy-peel citrus fruit.

Activity 28

Practical opportunity

List all the methods of cooking fruit and vegetables giving examples.

Then find two recipes which use cooked fruit and cooked vegetables.

Personal advice

Personal support has been promised to people who want to live more healthily. NHS accredited trainers will be available to provide advice and support on healthy eating. Since 2007 a new telephone, online and digital service has provided confidential advice on improving lifestyles and support for those who wish to take responsibility for their own health.

Interventions

The Choosing Health consultation showed that people are in favour of the idea that the government should act to make less healthy foods less appealing to children. Children are not old enough to be able to make informed decisions about what they eat. Yet a great deal of food and drink advertising is aimed at them. The government is working with the food industry to improve food labelling and restrict advertisements for foods high in sugar and fat during children's programmes to improve the food choices they make.

Healthy Start

Healthy Start replaces the Welfare Food Scheme. It is now available throughout Great Britain and Northern Ireland. It enables people who claim benefits, are pregnant or under 18 to claim free vouchers every week which can be swapped for fresh fruit and vegetables, as well as milk and infant formula milk. It also includes free vitamin supplements for children from six months until their fourth birthday. Many retailers accept these vouchers throughout the UK. In addition, the scheme also supports breastfeeding and encourages earlier and closer contact between health professionals and families from disadvantaged groups.

The School Food Trust

The School Food Trust was established by the Department for Education and Skills in September 2005. Its aim was to transform school food and food skills, promote the education and health of children and young people and improve the quality of food in schools.

Research was carried out that showed that children were not making healthy food choices at lunchtime and that school meals did not meet their nutritional needs. As a consequence, new standards were developed to increase the intake of healthier foods, restrict junk foods high in fat, sugar and salt, improve the quality of food and set minimum levels for the nutritional content of school meals.

The food-based standards for school food other than lunch were introduced in all schools in September 2007 and many schools adopted these standards before the deadline date.

A new, full set of food-based standards is to be introduced into primary schools by September 2008 and secondary schools by September 2009 at the latest. These new standards will specify the levels of a number of nutrients that a school lunch should provide. It is hoped that as a consequence children will be able to eat more balanced meals at lunchtime.

The current standards state that school meals should include the following:

- They have to provide more oily fish and bread.
- They have to provide more fruit and vegetables.
- They have to provide only healthy drinks such as water, milk and pure fruit juices.
- Foods that can be sold at mid-morning break are sandwiches and baguettes, fruit, salads, toast, pizza, yoghurt and drinks such as water, milk and fruit juices.
- Foods such as chocolate, sweets and crisps and sugary or sweetened drinks are no longer allowed.
- The serving of deep-fried foods and manufactured meat products is restricted.

There are no standards for packed lunches that are brought from home, but the School Food Trust provides advice for parents on how to provide healthier packed lunches. Some schools choose to set rules on the contents of packed lunches brought from home. One primary school allows the children to bring crisps for a snack on a Friday – it is called crisp Friday. From Monday to Thursday the children are encouraged to bring in healthy snacks.

Activity 29

Practical opportunity

Create a menu for five main meals for a primary school kitchen which address the current dietary guidelines

Choose one of the dishes to make in a practical session.

The National Healthy Schools Programme

Schools can apply for the status of a 'healthy school'. A detailed plan needs to be developed and realised in order to achieve this status. The aim of becoming a healthy school is that it helps young people and their schools to be healthy.

The programme has four themes:

- **Personal, social and health education (PSHE):** This is a subject taught in schools and its scheme of work usually includes sex and relationship education and drug education (including alcohol, tobacco and volatile substance abuse). It contributes significantly to the government's 'Every Child Matters' agenda which states that children should be healthy, stay safe, enjoy and achieve, make a positive contribution and have economic well-being. PSHE can also provide young people with the knowledge, understanding, skills and attitudes to make informed decisions about the choices they make throughout their lives
- **Healthy eating:** This helps young people to develop the confidence, skills, knowledge and understanding to make healthy food choices. The school also has to ensure that healthy and nutritious food and drink are available across the school day.
- **Physical activity:** This contributes significantly to the health of young people. Schools can provide young people with a diverse range of opportunities to take part in physical activity such as sport. Participation in all sports is encouraged, with girls and boys having the same sports available to them. PE is also now a thriving GCSE and A level subject. Many schools offer a wide range of extracurricular sporting activities and provide areas around the school for ball games to be played.
- **Emotional health and well-being:** This contributes again to the Every Child Matters agenda. The promotion of positive emotional health and well-being helps children and young people to understand and express their feelings, build their confidence and emotional resilience, and therefore their ability to learn.

The Walk Once a Week scheme (WoW)

The WoW scheme encourages parents and pupils to walk to school at least once a week. It was developed to promote walking to school and to reduce the number of children who are driven to school. It is also a way of increasing physical activity. The scheme asks schools to pledge to be a 'WoW school'. A WoW school is one that agrees to promote walking to and from school as the preferred travel choice on a regular basis. The individual school can decide when it is going to promote walking and small rewards are available for the children who do it.

Cycling to school

With the worrying rise of childhood obesity and the recognised benefits of exercise as part of a healthy lifestyle, cycling is an enjoyable and affordable way of getting some exercise. It helps develop confidence and independence. Encouraging and developing a school cycling policy, which could be part of a school travel plan, is beneficial to young people. Many primary schools provide the opportunity for the children to undertake basic cycling training by completing a cycling proficiency test.

Extended schools

As part of the extended schools initiative, many schools are considering and setting up before and after school provision. One of the initiatives has been to offer a breakfast club which opens before school aiming to target young people who arrive at school having skipped breakfast.

Schools' own initiatives

Here is an example of one school's own initiatives.

The Chase School in Malvern has Healthy School status and has a number of strategies in place to support the healthy well-being of its students. It has a breakfast club which opens at 8am in the school canteen. It holds tasting sessions to enable children to try new, healthier foods. It has held competitions such as a raffle with the prize of a mountain bike, for which tickets were given every time a piece of fresh fruit was bought. Water fountains are available in school to encourage the drinking of water.

To support the emotional well-being of students, some year 10 and 11 students have received training in counselling skills and become TICS (talking in confidence students). They provide support to younger students, particularly the new year 7 students.

A school nurse is available to provide support for any student who wants it and a trained counsellor is on site for drop-in sessions. The pastoral team can set up a series of counselling sessions for students who would benefit from this support.

Each year the school devotes a week's activity to promote an aspect of healthy living. It has run a sustainability week and a healthy eating week.

Activity 30

Review

Find out what strategies are in place at your school to support the health of the students.

The value of health education policies

The policies and campaigns now running have all been developed since the Health of the Nation Report 1991, which identified the importance of **preventative** health measures. It also emphasised the principle that individuals should take some responsibility for their own health instead of expecting solutions to problems after they have developed. It was at this time too that rising costs and huge demands on the health service meant that there was a need for more people to take positive steps to improve their health to avoid becoming a burden on the NHS.

Health education is therefore important to improve the nation's health which, if successful, would have the potential to reduce health costs. It is difficult to quantify how successful each policy or campaign is, but one measure would be how widely recognised the content of such campaigns is and how memorable a campaign is. A healthy diet is important for everybody so it is important that dietary messages are clear and simple and can be easily interpreted by everybody.

The Eatwell plate campaign involved the use of a clear illustration of how foods should be grouped and eaten in healthy proportions. The merit of this campaign was its emphasis on an illustration that made it accessible to most people, including those with no specialist nutritional knowledge. It is important when assessing any policy or campaign to be aware of who the target market is and if the materials are suitable for the target.

The 5 a Day logo is also well recognised and it may be that it has had an impact because the consumption of fruit and vegetables is slightly higher than it was.

The ultimate measure of the success of any policy or campaign aimed at improving the nation's diet has to be an improvement in health and diet-related health problems. Another indicator of success is a reduction in the average adult body weight that can be detected in statistics achieved after a length of time sufficient to achieve a quantifiable result.

Time will tell as to how successful and valuable 'Choosing Health' and other campaigns are. It is certainly true that they are valuable because they give a large number of the population up-to-date information that is relevant to them. The campaigns are also generally accessible, particularly with many households having access to the internet.

However, it has also to be taken into consideration that they may be ignored or not perceived as being useful or relevant for some people. They may not be as easy to implement by people on a very limited income. The healthy start vouchers are hoping to address this.

Activity 31

Check your understanding
Check your understanding of the meaning of the following terms:

dietary	premature	life expectancy
diet	saturated fat	chronic
preventative	intervention	

Exam-style questions

Coeliac disease

1 Describe the condition known as coeliac disease. (4 marks)

2 Describe the symptoms and explain the dietary implications of this condition. (6 marks)

(Total of 10 marks)

Healthy eating (1)

'We are what we eat' is a common saying. Examine how diet can influence the health of an individual. (15 marks)

ASSESSMENT HINT!

Always read the question carefully and note exactly what you are asked to do. The context (in this case 'We are what we eat' is a common saying) usually sets the scene and can offer some clues.

Examine means to look at or study closely and find out the facts.

Healthy eating (2)

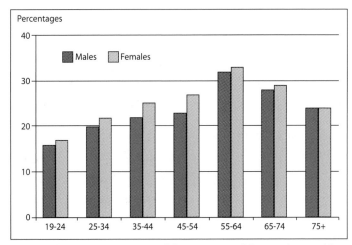

Figure 6.21 *Consumption of five portions of fruit and vegetables per day, by age and sex*

Figure 6.21 shows the consumption of five or more portions of fruit and vegetables by different age groups and sexes.

1 a Which age group is most likely to eat five portions of fruit and vegetables a day? (1 mark)

  b Which age group consumes the least amount of fruit and vegetables? (1 mark)

  c Approximately what percentage of men aged 19 to 24 years eat five fruit and vegetables a day? (1 mark)

  d Approximately what percentage of women aged 55 to 64 years eat five fruit and vegetables a day? (1 mark)

2 Explain why it is important to eat fruit and vegetables. (6 marks)

3 Describe the ways that parents and schools can encourage young children to eat fruit and vegetables. (15 marks)

(Total of 25 marks)

Resource Management

This unit matches AS Unit 2: Resource Management (G002) from your course.

Learning objectives

By the end of this chapter you will be able to:

- identify the factors that affect how time, energy and money are managed
- explain how to manage resources in response to social, economic, cultural and technological change
- describe how to reduce consumption of time, energy and money
- describe how to balance income against expenditure
- maintain a balanced yet cost-effective diet.

Introduction

This chapter will focus on the management of the resources time, money, human and fuel energy in the home environment. Individuals and **households** need to manage these resources as part of everyday life, and the aim essentially is to balance income against expenditure in order to enjoy a balanced diet and good health.

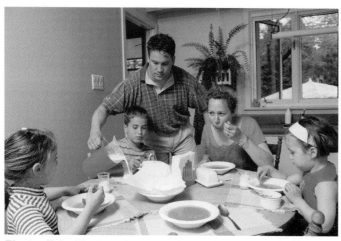

Figure 7.1 *The home environment*

Management of resources

The three primary resources which need to be managed in the home are:

- time
- energy (as in managing **amenities** such as fuel and water)
- money (income, **occupation**, budgeting).

You will see how to manage these resources in response to social, economic, cultural and technological change.

Time management

It is vital when considering time management in the home environment that proper consideration is given not only to necessary routines but to socialising and fun. It is important for every individual to have personal time and space, as well as for the family to have opportunities to socialise and enjoy activities together

As many women now work in paid employment it is important that all able members of the household should take a share of the necessary household **chores** according to their age, physical health and capabilities, as well as what is reasonable with the other demands on their time. Children should be expected to take responsibility for some tasks appropriate to their age and relevant to their own activities.

While children are very young their parents will have to do more for them. But as they grow up, there should be a more **equitable** division of time use in the home so no single member of a household is overburdened while others are failing to take an appropriate share. Parents will need to manage the time the children spend on school work until the children are old enough to take responsibility for themselves. It will also be necessary to manage bed times in order to ensure that children get enough sleep to help them cope effectively with the demands of school and home.

In order to apportion tasks that might be done by different members of a household, consideration should be given to those tasks that must be done daily and weekly, as well as those that need to be done less frequently.

Time and energy-saving techniques

Here are some techniques for saving time and energy in the home.

Timers on household appliances allow householders to set programmes or cycles on washing machines and dishwashers so that they can operate while other activities are completed – so saving time and human energy.

News items and radio and television programmes can be accessed on the internet, which is useful to individuals and households if they cannot be at home to see or hear programmes at the time of the original broadcast. This may be important for the effective management of time.

Corresponding by email can be much quicker than waiting for the normal postal system and can save time and energy as well as reducing frustration caused by possible delays in the post. Savings can be made on the cost of international telephone calls if it is possible to communicate via the web instead.

Labour-saving equipment such as food mixers and processors can be used to mix, knead, chop or grate ingredients quickly and can save both time and energy.

Kettles can be bought which have automatic cut-off mechanisms that operate when the water boils. These allow the individual to get on with other things rather than wasting time waiting for the kettle to boil so that it can be turned off.

The continued use of refrigerators and freezers has enabled individuals and householders to store perishable foods for longer periods and therefore made it unnecessary to shop so frequently. Batch baking or bulk preparation of some food mixtures may be time-saving as the surplus can be frozen and defrosted for use when time is short. This saves both time and energy.

Energy management

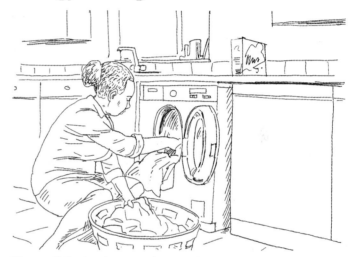

Figure 7.2 *Loading a washing machine*

Energy management in the home includes personal human energy as well as fuel and heat energy. Many of the points concerned with human energy are considered above.

Human energy is involved in running and maintaining a home so any design feature or equipment aimed to make the home easy to clean and manage will save both time and human energy. A well designed house that is a suitable size for the household will save both human and fuel energy. Effort will not be wasted maintaining space that is either not being used or is so cramped that it is difficult to easily maintain.

Smooth easy-to-maintain surfaces will be easy to clean and minimise opportunities for dust and dirt to collect. Plenty of easily accessible storage space ensures that possessions can be properly stored so they do not clutter living space and result in wasted time when things cannot be found. Effective lighting can also save energy in the same way because possessions are less likely to be lost.

Teflon coatings on the surface of household equipment, such as saucepans and kitchen utensils, mean that food does not stick to the coated surface and therefore they are easy to clean – saving both time and energy. The same coating applied to the sole plate of irons makes ironing clothes quicker and more efficient because the surface of the iron is less resistant to friction.

Technological fixtures and fittings can save human energy. Examples are the systems controlling light, heating and ventilation using pre-set controls which operate with the use of sensors and thermostats. These features remove the need to think about or operate equipment to achieve a comfortable living environment.

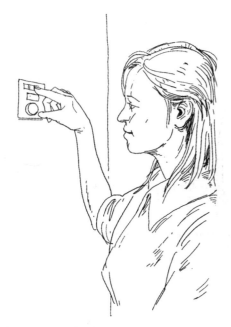

Figure 7.3 *Adjusting a thermostat*

Thermostats on appliances that require temperature control save energy because only the temperature required is achieved and maintained automatically and does not have to be controlled manually by constant attention. Some examples of temperature-controlled appliances are cookers, freezers, refrigerators and toasters.

Microwave ovens cook, defrost or reheat much more quickly than is possible using conventional heating methods. It is clear therefore that a considerable time saving can be achieved.

Dishwashers and washing machines make the necessary and regular household chores of laundry and washing up much less labour-intensive and therefore save both human energy and time. It is only necessary to load the machines and to empty them when the cycle of operation is complete. However, care should be taken because of the amount of electricity and water they use. They should be used responsibly by only using when there is a full load. The temperature setting should be 40 degrees or less, and if possible the machine should be used on a tariff that has cheaper electricity at night.

Reducing fuel energy

The use of fuel energy is a major household cost that can be considerably reduced with effective insulation and the right choice of heating system.

All new housing must comply with new building regulations that stipulate the need for good insulation. Insulation can be added to homes if the standard of insulation was not adequate in the original build. Cavity wall insulation can be added, as can insulation in the roof and double glazing of the windows. The hot water cylinder should also be lagged to save fuel energy. This is very easy to do and extremely cost-effective.

Central heating is the most effective way to heat an entire house and the system can be controlled on a time switch so that it can be programmed to come on when needed. Radiators can be fitted with individual thermostats so that the temperature of each area in the home can be set and controlled according to need and therefore avoid heat being wasted unnecessarily. The temperature setting of both the domestic hot water supply can also be controlled according to the needs of the household. The lower the temperature settings, the easier it is to save money on water and space heating.

Solar powered heating is an effective system, but it can be expensive to install though cheap to maintain.

Money management

Good money management requires an evaluation of total income from all sources and the development of a realistic budget plan. A realistic budget must include all the necessary regular expenses, while allowing some extra money for savings or an emergency such as repairs to a car or washing machine.

If the household has any very young or elderly members there may be the extra cost of increased heating bills, childcare, special medical supplies or special diet.

Online banking can enable people to access banking information outside banking hours as well enabling them to complete some transactions such as paying utility bills over the internet. This can also save time.

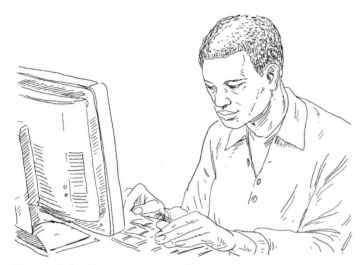

Figure 7.4 *Managing money online*

We can shop online for goods or services. It saves time and money to shop this way as well as the personal energy that would otherwise have to be used to buy goods or services direct. Even quite major purchases can be made on the internet and it is possible to buy items from outside the UK although such items may involve shipping costs.

Regular grocery shopping from most supermarkets can be done online although there is often a delivery charge. But it saves both time and energy and can save money because there are no travelling or parking costs and less 'impulse buying'. So it can save money in the long run.

If planning a major purchase, like a car or major household item, it is possible to access information from a variety of sources to inform decision-making. Some sites offer comparative information about different brands of the same product as well as the likely maintenance costs. This offers an efficient way of conducting initial research that can save both time and energy and possibly also money.

Factors affecting time, energy and money management

There are many factors which affect how we manage the resources of time, energy and money.

The number of people in any household will be an important factor in the home because it has a direct relevance to the amount of resources available.

The ages of the members of the household will be a factor because the very young or the very elderly will inevitably take up time and energy of the other members of the household in looking after them and providing for them. Dependent members of any household also involve additional costs without them being able to contribute a large amount in financial terms to the household resources.

The health of the household is important. Members of a household may suffer periods of ill health or disability. Or there may be a disabled member of the household who, like the very young or the elderly, is a greater consumer of resources than a contributor.

The gender of household members may affect what they are able to do – or at least what they perceive is an acceptable role for a man or woman. This may affect what individuals are willing to do with regard to saving time, money or energy. Men may be prepared to complete quite physically demanding building work required in the home but be unprepared or unable to share daily domestic chores.

The skills and talents of all members of the household will determine the ways in which they are able to contribute to the pool of resources of money, time and energy available. A good cook in the household could save money as they can be creative with the minimum of foods bought.

The geographical location of the home will be a relevant factor – how near it is to work, school or college. Travelling will affect costs, whether it be public transport costs or fuel costs for running a vehicle. There is also the time issue in the amount of time taken travelling to and from work and the energy required to make the necessary journeys.

The location of the home also affects the cost of living. Costs may be higher in the south than in the north and some sought-after regions can be expensive areas in which to live. Heating costs could be higher in colder areas of the far north of England or Scotland. Transport costs are likely to be higher for those living in rural areas than for those living in towns.

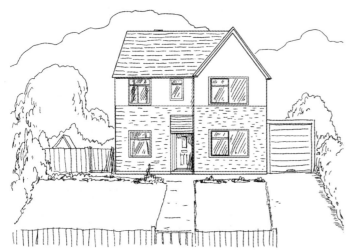

Figure 7.5 *The nature and size of a house affect the cost of its maintenance*

The nature and size of the house will determine the cost of its maintenance, as well as heating costs and the ease or difficulty of keeping it clean and well ordered. Generally, the smaller and more modern the property, the easier it should be to clean and maintain. Terraced properties are usually cheaper to heat than a detached property. A larger house will obviously take more time and effort to look after than a small one.

Not only the house but also the nature and quantity of its content, surfaces, equipment and furnishings will affect how difficult and time-consuming it is to maintain.

Labour-saving appliances and technological aids can save time and energy and therefore will help to determine what time and energy can be saved. There may be cost implications for a household who decide to invest in labour-saving equipment for family members who have little time but who may be more 'cash-rich'.

Leisure hours and the chosen activities of household members can have both cost and time implications as well as the amount of energy expended by each individual in their leisure activities.

Any help available to the household in the form of support from friends, neighbours or extended family may be particularly important if it has dependent members. In addition, some households may be able to employ help with domestic work or gardening, but this will depend on costs and income.

The working hours and the nature of the work done by each household member will affect how cash-rich or time-poor the household is.

Activity 2

Review

Summarise in the form of bullet points the factors affecting time, energy and money management.

Then make notes on their relevance to the needs of the following family types and households:

- Nuclear family – mother working part-time, father working full-time, daughter aged 16 and son aged 17, both at school.
- Extended family – mother at home, father working full-time, three boys aged 14, 11 and 8, very elderly grandmother needing part-time nursing care.
- University student household consisting of two males and two females.
- Single professional person living alone.

The interrelationship between time, money and energy

It is possible to interlink the resources of time, money and energy when managing them as part of everyday life. By doing this it is easier to reduce the consumption of each, maintain a balanced yet affordable diet and ensure we remain healthy.

The following statements illustrate some ways in which each of the resources interlink together.

1. Those with little time will spend more on convenience foods which may not be beneficial to our diet.

2. How much income we have will determine how much money we can spend on food.

3. Time switches can be used to use electricity during the night on a cheaper tariff – appliances such as washing machines, tumble driers and dishwashers can be used overnight to save money on electricity.

4. How much money we have will depend on how well we can look after our health so that our energy levels are maintained.

5. Children can sometimes take responsibility for jobs at home if both parents are working and have less time.

6. If you have time, shopping wisely for food can save money.

7. Our occupation decides what income we have.

8. Thermostats can help save fuel energy

9. Insulating the home – cavity walls, double glazing, carpets, curtains, a well lagged tank – saves on fuel.

10. The lower the disposable income, the fewer choices we have in what we eat, where we spend our leisure time and where we live.

11. Roles within the family between husband and wife are often shared due to the pressures of time and work.

12. Good budgeting is essential to ensure that all bills are accounted for.

13. A well designed home will ensure heating and water costs are kept to a minimum.

14. Income affects our health – those on a low income are less likely to afford a healthy diet.

15. Those on a low income may be less likely to own their own home and may pay a lot of money to rent their homes.

16. Many women are now working, leaving them less time to manage the home.

Activity 3

Review
Create a visual diagram (a spider diagram) using different colours to show the interrelationship between time, money and energy.

Financial planning

Financial planning is very important in order to avoid financial difficulties. Balancing income and expenditure is crucial, the idea being that income and necessary expenditure are calculated, and what is left over is called **disposable income**. This can be used for items such as major purchases, holidays and savings.

It is also possible to analyse data from national statistics which illustrate current income and expenditure patterns.

Sources of income

Activity 4

Group discussion
Identify as many sources of income as you can.

There are many sources of income available to individuals and households.

Source of income	%
Wages and salary	51%
Self-employment and rent	13%
Property development	12%
Benefits and pensions	19%
Grants, transfers from abroad	5%

Source: Adapted from Social Trends 37 Table 5.2

Composition of household income in the UK in 2004

Activity 5

The use of data
With reference to the data above, what does it tell us about the sources of income in 2004?

Wages and salary

A major source of income is likely to be earnings paid as wages or salary. As an employee carrying out work for an employer you would expect to be paid wages (paid weekly) or a salary (paid monthly).

Welfare benefits

If a person is unemployed, on a low income, sick or disabled and therefore unable to work there are **welfare benefits** that can be claimed to supplement or replace income. If a person has children, child benefit can be claimed. It is paid at a slightly higher rate for the eldest child. It is paid to the primary carer (usually the mother) and is payable until each child leaves full-time education.

Working family tax credits are payable to low income-earning families and can be added to earned income and received directly in the pay packet.

Other benefits that may be claimed are:
- old age pension
- jobseeker's allowance
- housing benefit
- incapacity benefit
- disability allowance
- education maintenance allowance
- income support.

Interest on savings and investments

Interest payable on savings and investments is unearned income and therefore may be taxable. However, unless savings are substantial the interest gained is unlikely to be significant.

Individual Savings Accounts (ISAs) offer good rates of interest, but there are limits to the amount of savings that can be put into an ISA in any financial year.

Premium bonds can be bought from National Savings and Investments and then entered into a draw with cash prizes. The capital invested can be withdrawn at any time. Any winnings from either of these sources are not liable to tax.

Allowances

Private medical and dental care may be offered as an employee benefit. A low interest rate mortgage or free banking may be available to some employees of banks and building societies.

The use of a company car, car loan or leasing facility may be supplied by an employer and would be a valuable benefit.

Help with transport to work is sometimes available from employers.

Methods of payment

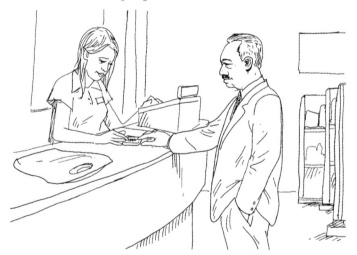

Figure 7.6 *Paying by credit card*

Activity 6

Research opportunity

Visit the Department of Work and Pensions website: www.dwp.gov.uk.

For each of the benefits listed below find out how much they are worth:
- child benefit
- working family tax credits
- old age pension
- jobseeker's allowance
- housing benefit
- incapacity benefit
- disability allowance
- education maintenance allowance
- income support.

Then note who might be eligible for each of these benefits and why.

Activity 7

Group discussion

Identify as many methods of payment as you can.

When an individual buys goods and services they can pay in a variety of ways. In all cases the goods can be taken home immediately. There are many different methods of payment, and the individual needs to choose the best option for them. Often that will depend upon the type of goods or services being purchased.

The different methods of payment to choose from when paying for goods or services are as follows.

Cash

Cash is generally acceptable everywhere. With cash there are no interest charges to pay for and the goods become your own property the moment they have been bought. Cash normally comes in the form of coins and notes. It is easier to keep control of your budget if you pay by cash and overspending is less likely. It has the disadvantage that it reduces your capital which could be earning a higher rate of interest if invested. Cash can also be lost or stolen and is difficult to trace if that occurs.

Direct debit cards

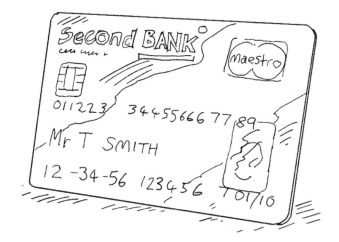

Figure 7.7 *A debit card*

In order to have a direct debit card, a bank or building society account is needed. These cards take the place of both cash and cheques and they speed up the purchasing transaction. The card is swiped at the time of purchase and the money is electronically debited from your account. This has advantages for the retailer as there is less money to process and the transferred funds are cleared quicker. The customer then uses the 'chip and pin' system. This system replaces the need for the customer to sign a slip and is safer to use as there is less chance of fraudulent use.

Customers also have to have enough money in their account. If they do not, the transaction will not go through.

Credit cards

Credit cards can be beneficial as spending can be spread over a period of weeks and when used carefully, interest charges can be avoided. But when monthly balances are not cleared, interest charges can be very high and it is easy for someone to overspend. It is also possible to collect a number of credit cards, as they are readily available, and for large debts to accrue. It is very easy for consumers to lose track of the amounts that have been spent.

Credit card fraud can be a problem, so care needs to be taken when carrying them. Major credit cards can be used worldwide and they reduce the need to carry large sums of money or purchase travellers' cheques.

Store and charge cards

Store and charge cards are available in a large number of chain stores. Interest charges are usually high and the cardholder would need to ensure payments are made on time to avoid further penalties. At the end of each month the customer receives a statement from the store and it is wise to pay the total amount. It is easy to overspend with these cards and to lose track of when they were used.

Hire purchase agreements

Using a hire purchase agreement, goods can be purchased in advance of having the funds available to purchase them. Monthly payments are usually made and interest is applied at a high rate. The goods do not belong to the purchaser until the final payment has been made. Goods can be repossessed if the customer does not keep up with the payments.

Credit agreements

This is where goods can be bought immediately and paid for later. Some credit agreements are offered on an interest free basis and these can be used to the consumer's advantage. Care needs to be taken with some of these because they can involve high interest rates. Mortgages are a long-term form of credit agreement and consumers should shop around to achieve the most attractive rates.

Bank loan

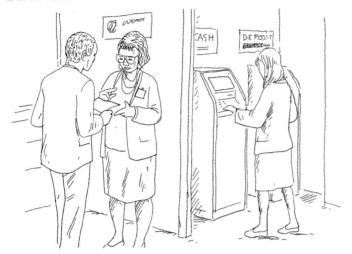

Figure 7.8 *Using banking facilities*

A bank or a building society has the facility to offer a bank loan or overdraft to pay for goods and services. A loan is for a fixed sum which is lent to the customer on condition that it is paid back at regular intervals or at a given time. If the loan is a large one, security may be needed.

Student loans are the accepted way to finance further and higher education. They often have the advantage of low interest charges and repayment is often delayed until the student is earning a decent salary.

Bank overdraft

An overdraft is more flexible and interest is only charged on the overdrawn amount. Overdrafts can be helpful to cover emergency expenditure. Some people operate on semi-permanent overdrafts which may be a costly way to finance expenditure.

Direct debits and standing order payments

Direct debits and standing order payments can be set up through a bank or building society to pay a number of fixed regular payments, such as rent, mortgage, council tax or credit agreement payments. These have many advantages to the consumer, including convenience, and they can help with budgeting.

Activity 8

Review
Make a table to illustrate the advantages and disadvantages of each method of payment.

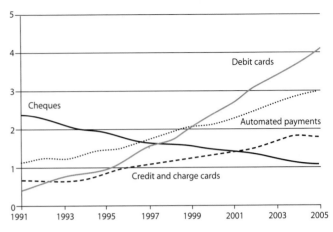

United Kingdom
Billions (£)

Figure 7.9 *Non-cash transactions by method of payment*
Source: Social Trends 37, Table 6.11

Activity 9

Group discussion and the use of data
What does Figure 7.9 above tell us about the trends in methods of payment?
The answer is given at the back of the book.

Debit card	1996	2001	2005
Food and drink	43	29	23
Motoring	12	13	14
Household	6	9	7
Mixed business	10	7	7
Clothing	6	6	5
Travel	5	7	6
Entertainment	3	5	5
Hotels	1	1	1
Other retail	9	10	10
Other services	4	12	21
of which financial	–	–	10

Payment of goods and services by debit card in %

Credit card	1996	2001	2005
Food and drink	13	11	11
Motoring	13	13	12
Household	10	12	11
Mixed business	7	6	7
Clothing	6	5	5
Travel	14	12	11
Entertainment	7	7	7
Hotels	6	5	4
Other retail	14	16	16
Other services	10	14	16
of which financial	–	–	7

Source: Social Trends 37, adapted from Table 6.12

Payment of goods and services by credit card in %

Activity 10

Group discussion

What do the two tables above tell us about the trends in paying by debit and credit cards?

The answer is given at the back of the book.

Activity 11

Review

Find out how the Consumer Credit Act protects the consumer when paying for goods on credit.

Which method of payment would you suggest is the most suitable when buying the following:

- a car
- a house
- a holiday
- a dishwasher
- some new clothes for a new job?

Explain your answers.

Income and expenditure

Income and expenditure vary throughout the various stages of family life:

- single person, student or professional
- couple married or living together
- couple with young children
- couple with school-age children
- couple with children at university or college or who have moved away
- elderly couple
- widowed elderly person.

Activity 12

Group discussion

Discuss the different sources of income for each of the stages of family life, and what would be the main items of expenditure for each stage.

When planning financially it is necessary to calculate the income coming in and the expenditure going out. Expenditure should be less than the income coming in to avoid living beyond your means and getting into debt. In order to budget carefully, households and individuals should write down all the income received and all expenditure to be able to calculate the sum when one is deducted from the other. If families can balance incomings with outgoings in this way financial difficulties should not arise.

Before income and expenditure can be calculated, it is useful to consider the factors affecting income and expenditure:

- **Age:** A person's age will influence their interests and activities and therefore how much they spend.
- **Employment:** The type of employment – self-employment, having short-term contracts, annual bonuses and seasonal work – can affect income and expenditure.
- **Location:** Where you live will affect expenditure due to access to social opportunities and transport costs. Some parts of the UK are more expensive to live in than others.
- **Spending:** How much is regularly spent each week or month so that a pattern can be established.
- **Shopping:** Shopping for food needs to take into account the individual's dietary needs. Convenience may influence some individuals to buy ready meals or takeaways.
- **Eating out:** Where you eat, how frequently and how often takeaways are consumed should be considered.
- **Transport:** The implications of running costs of owning one or more cars need to be considered, as do public transport costs.

- **Clothes:** Clothing for the family, fashion, accessories and cosmetics all need to be considered.
- **Heating costs:** These are often dependent upon who lives in the household. Having an elderly person in the family or a baby will probably increase the costs.
- **Housing costs:** These are crucial to provide somewhere to live which could take the form of a mortgage or rent.
- **Insurances:** There are a number of insurances that are needed or taken on as optional such as house contents, car and life insurance.
- **Recreation:** Leisure activities such as holidays, swimming lessons and gym membership will need to be budgeted for.
- **Technology:** The increased production and availability of appliances and the increased use of internet, mobiles and emails may have an impact on household bills.

Income can come from the following:
- wages and salary
- welfare benefits
- interest on savings and investments
- allowances
- gifts
- lottery wins.

Expenditure and money going out can be spent on the following:
- home/household costs to include rent or mortgage and council tax
- household insurance, buildings and contents
- heating costs, gas, electricity and water
- TV licence, telephone charges, mobiles and internet
- repairs and renewals
- food and groceries, school and work lunches
- clothing – school uniform, work and casual clothing
- travel – car purchase, car tax and insurance, petrol, car servicing, public transport fares
- financial commitments – credit and store card payments, bank charges, pension contributions, loan repayments and other financial obligations
- miscellaneous outgoings – holidays, savings, cigarettes, alcohol, subscriptions, meals out, child/spouse maintenance, university/college fees, Christmas, birthdays, newspapers and savings.

Activity 13

Review
Create a table of your income and expenditure. Do you have any money left over at the end of the month?

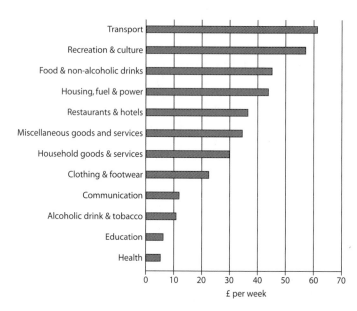

Figure 7.10 *Average weekly household expenditure on main commodities and services in 2005 and 2006 in the UK*
Source: Expenditure and Food Survey, Office for National Statistics

Activity 14

Group discussion and the use of data
Discuss what Figure 7.10 above tells us about trends in expenditure.
The answer is given at the back of the book.

Other data showed that the average weekly expenditure was highest among households consisting of three or more adults and children – £744 a week. The lowest expenditure was reported among one-person retired households who were mainly dependent on the state pension. Households with two adults and two children spent an average of £642 a week.

Expenditure also varies with the age of the household 'reference' person. Those households where the reference person was aged 30 to 49 spent the most – on average £547 a week. Those where the reference person was aged 75 or over had the lowest average household expenditure – £206 a week.

Once the income and expenditure have been calculated, the ideal situation is that there is money left over. If there is not and expenditure is higher than income, then financial strategies will need to be employed. This is called **budgeting**.

Financial strategies

There are several strategies a household can use to balance their income and expenditure. It is possible to budget for food with careful planning.

Households can spread large bills so that they can be paid monthly. Direct debits can be set up so that costs for services are reduced and paid monthly. This should reduce the burden of large bills arriving through the post.

They can shop around for credit deals. When using loans, overdrafts, mortgages or other forms of credit, consumers should shop around for the best deal and consider changing banks or credit provider. Consumers should also be aware of interest charges. If credit is a necessity, they can try to find interest-free credit while being aware of the timing for the payments and any penalty clauses that may apply.

They can plan their food shopping carefully. Food shopping is a large outgoing for most families but expenditure can be reduced with sensible planning. An amount of money to be spent on food must be decided upon, and stuck to. They can use shops with loyalty cards or money back schemes. They can use coupons collected from magazines, newspapers or mail shots to reduce shopping bills. They can buy food resources which are on special offer or are offered in 'buy one, get one free' packages. They can try shopping at discount supermarkets such as Lidl, Netto or Aldi. Markets are also frequently cheaper sources of fresh and locally produced foods, and bargains can sometimes be obtained at the end of the day when fresh food needs to be sold before the sell-by date. They can buy some foods in bulk if funds allow and if the food can be stored properly and used during the time its quality can be maintained. They can buy a supermarket's own economy ranges. Research has shown that these products represent good value for money.

Knowledge of food will equip an individual to make wise choices when purchasing food – to store it correctly to maintain quality, and to prepare and cook it to avoid waste and to maximise food value. Here is some good advice:

- Starchy carbohydrate foods can be the basis of main meals and are cheap, easy to store, prepare and cook. They are also extremely versatile and filling. Good examples are pasta, rice, bread, potatoes and cereals.
- Protein foods do not need to be eaten in large quantities. These are generally more expensive foods. Knowledge of cuts of meat and poultry would enable a consumer to be discerning while saving money.
- Eggs represent very good value for money and can be used in a variety of ways in both sweet and savoury dishes.
- Milk is an excellent source of calcium as well as being a good source of protein and can be bought cheaply in supermarkets.
- Cheese can be served in many different ways, both cooked and 'raw' and is an excellent source of protein.
- Fruits and vegetables can be expensive, but with knowledge of the different varieties available and their seasons, it is possible to buy wisely and to have high quality produce at relatively low cost.
- Baked beans are a cheap and excellent food for health.
- Cooking larger quantities of mixtures or 'batch baking' is also an economical use of food and fuel and products can be frozen.

Activity 15

Review

Complete a table to show how it is possible to manage food resources when feeding a family. Use the following headings:
- Shopping for food
- Choosing food
- Cooking food.

Consider unnecessary expenditure

A household can reduce unnecessary expenditure such as alcohol, cigarettes and going out. A social life is important but a household should have a budget and stick to it. If then at a later date economies have to be made, savings on socialising could be made.

It can review expenditure on luxury goods and holidays or extravagant purchases and make necessary purchases carefully. For example, it can hire DVDs rather than visit the cinema, or join the local library where DVDs can be loaned for free or at a small cost.

Other ways to reduce unnecessary expenditure are as follows:

- **Conserve energy:** Conserving as much water, electricity and gas in the home to reduce bills and help the environment.
- **Skills:** Learning DIY skills so that home maintenance can be done without the need to hire a tradesperson. Repairing items rather than replacing them if at all possible. Avoiding waste and making items that are within personal capability.
- **Savings:** Saving a little money each month so that funds are available in case an emergency arises.
- Transport: Reducing transport costs. Walking, cycling or car sharing as much as possible. Consider the size of car to minimise costs.
- **Clothing:** Only replacing clothes if they wear out. Looking out for items in a genuine sale. Visiting charity shops as they can be an excellent source of good quality clothing.
- **Shop around:** Seeking bargains from charity shops or car boot sales. Using internet shopping sites to find the most competitive prices for major purchases. Selling unwanted goods at car boot sales or on ebay.
- **Increase earning power:** Taking on extra work if possible or additional part-time work.
- **Communication:** Paying bills online can save on postage and may attract discounts. Monitor the use of mobile phones, limit the time of calls and make sure of the best deal if signing a contract. Pay as you go can be better.

There are a number of free and low-cost financial planning services available, including banks and building societies, which offer support if financial help is needed.

The Financial Services Authority (FSA) has a helpline which can answer general enquiries about financial products and services. The Citizens Advice Bureau offers independent advice on financial issues. Its advice will be impartial and free. It also offers debt counselling. It helps families to work out how much money is coming in each week and balance that out against weekly expenditure.

The worst thing families can do if they experience financial problems is to try and borrow to pay off other debts. This course of action, although advertised extensively, can increase problems and make matters worse.

In order to try and prevent financial difficulties in the first place, budgeting is the key.

Activity 20

Review

Obtain as much information from the Citizens Advice Bureau as possible in the form of leaflets or go to its website (www.citizensadvice.org.uk).

Condense the information and produce a helpsheet to help families with their financial planning. Give your helpsheet a catchy title to make it appealing.

Activity 21

Review

Check your understanding of the meaning of the following terms:

amenities	occupation	household
chores	equitable	income
expenditure	disposable income	budgeting
welfare benefits		

Exam-style question

With the ever increasing cost of housing, many people are choosing to live in a shared household. Discuss how resources can be effectively managed in such a household. (15 marks)

Food provision

Learning objectives

By the end of this chapter you will be able to:

- understand the reasons why patterns of eating have changed
- identify the four types of food products which combine to make meals
- describe the food choices available outside the home
- understand how we develop food habits and the different factors which can affect our food choices
- describe the ways you can purchase food resources to meet individual and household needs
- understand the basic principles of meal planning
- explain how the management of resources to provide meals can be applied to different contexts.

Introduction

In this chapter we will explore the patterns of eating and how they have changed. The range and choice of food products available and the issues affecting food choice will be investigated. We will also examine the management of resources when providing meals for individuals and households.

Eating patterns

An **eating pattern** can be described as where, when and how you eat. Traditional eating patterns could be described as eating three meals (breakfast, lunch and dinner) a day and two or three snacks each day. The main meal of the day would be taken in the evening at home with the family.

A **meal** is an eating occasion which usually takes place at a specific time and place. The meal may contain a selection of two or more different food products. The components of a meal vary across cultures, but could include grains, such as rice, pasta or noodles served with meat or fish, beans and vegetables.

A **snack** consists of a small amount of food or beverage taken between meals to relieve hunger. Snacks are usually purchased by the consumer and are ready-to-eat products. The ready-to-eat nature of snack products can make them expensive.

Activity 1

Review and group discussion

Keep a food diary until your next lesson. Write down when, where and what you eat.

Discuss the results with your group.

Changing eating patterns

There is little doubt that the way we eat and what we eat is changing. There are many issues in society which have contributed towards the change in eating patterns.

Eating patterns during the 1950s and 1960s were different from today. Then, the majority of families ate their main meal together five or six times a week in the home around a table. Many people never ate outside the home unless it was a special occasion.

At the turn of this century the situation is different. A survey in 2004 found that 20 per cent of families said they sat down to eat together once a week or less often. Children frequently had meals in their bedrooms while watching TV or playing computer games (www.raisingkids.co.uk, Back to the Table, 2004).

Meal times have become more flexible. The possible reasons for more flexible meal times are that less time is spent in the home by working women, many people work longer hours and more time is spent travelling to and from work.

Snacking or grazing during the day is becoming more common. The term **grazing** is used to describe the practice of eating snacks throughout the day instead of meals.

The distinction between a meal and a snack has become blurred. Meals eaten at work at a desk, travelling on a train or at the roadside in a car could be classified as snacks. Research from market analysts Datamonitor in 2006 found European consumers had on average 242 'on the go' food occasions each year. This is expected to rise each year.

In 2008 it is predicted that snacking will account for 44 per cent of all eating occasions. In 2008 we will spend £10.3 billion on bakery items, bagged snacks, dairy snacks, fruit and vegetables, and confectionery (excluding snacks eaten as part of a meal).

People snack for many reasons including:
- Snack products are widely available.
- Eating snack products is enjoyable.
- They have poor food preparation skills.
- There is a lack of time to eat a meal.
- They are available at certain social occasions – a football match or the cinema.
- They satisfy hunger.
- They relieve boredom.

Activity 2

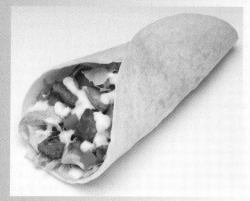

Figure 8.1 *A snack product*

Review
Produce a web diagram of foods eaten as snacks.
Divide these into groups. Note down some general comments that can be made about the products you have identified.

Research from the Office of National Statistics in 2005/6 on family spending demonstrated that the younger generation are bringing changes to the way we all eat. Those under 30 years spend about £14 each week on eating out, compared to an average £7.50 each week spent by those aged 65 to 74 years and just under £5 in those aged 75 years or older.

Activity 3

Practical opportunity
Produce a web diagram showing all the places you can buy snack products.
List all the foods available in school vending machines. Make general comments about their nutritional value.
Plan and prepare a snack product suitable for sale in a school vending machine.

Dashboard dining

Dashboard dining is food eaten in a car. Mintel's 'Dashboard dining' report published in February 2005 showed that 22 per cent of consumers frequently eat or drink in the car on a long journey. It also claimed that typically wealthy socio-economic groups make up nearly one third of dashboard diners. Increased car ownership and busier lifestyles may have contributed to this finding.

Many garage forecourts offer a range of hot and cold snack products. The hand-held savoury bar or slice has been developed by food manufacturers for this market. Many larger establishments offer hot beverage dispensers, in-store bakeries and microwave facilities.

The 'drive thru' fast food restaurant has been in existence for many years. This market is diversifying to meet changing needs with the emerging 'healthier' 'drive thru' sandwich and salad retailers.

The desk breakfast or deskfast

Traditionally in the UK breakfast has been eaten at home. However, in recent years evidence suggests this is changing. The term **deskfast** is used to describe breakfast that is eaten at a desk, usually at work. Research has found that more people are leaving home in the morning and waiting until they reach their destination before eating breakfast. Datamonitor estimated in 2003 that British workers spent over £1 billion on breakfast at work.

Fast food restaurants like McDonald's and Burger King have been catering for the 'no breakfast' at home consumer for some years. The increasing popularity of the portable breakfast has led to more innovations in the food industry. A wide range of 'healthy' products are available including ready-to-eat oats mixed with milk that just require heating, cereal bars, yoghurt-based products, muffins and pastries.

Reasons for the changes in patterns of eating

More disposable income

Patterns of eating and what is eaten are affected by the household income. Households with two wage earners may have more disposable income. Research suggests more money is being spent on ready-to-eat 'premium' food products and some people who have more disposable income want higher quality food with minimal preparation.

Research from an IGM report, 'Brits shun fast-food for healthy home cooking' published in August 2007, found that rather than eat fast food or ready meals, some consumers are indulging their desire to prepare and eat high quality home cooked meals. The food industry refers to this group as the 'foodies'. Foodies are more likely to be adventurous in their choice of food and be inspired by celebrity chefs. They are more likely to buy expensive premium food products. By

contrast, the report refers to 'fuelies' as another group who eat mainly to satisfy hunger and are less adventurous in their food choice. They consume more ready meals and takeaways and eat snacks or graze (IGM 2006 Shopper Trends).

Households and families where there is more money available are also choosing to spend more on non-essential items like meals outside the home.

Working mothers

Patterns of eating have been affected by changes in the labour market. More women are working which could reduce the amount of time and motivation they have to cook meals every evening. Social Trends 2006 estimated that 67 per cent of women with dependent children work. Working mothers can find preparing meals after working all day tiring and for convenience choose to eat outside the home, purchase ready meals or part-prepared food products.

More people live alone

Government statistics suggest that one in three households is now a single person household, compared to one in five at the start of the 1970s. The effect of this change has been significant on the food industry. The number of single portion ready meals purchased and consumed has grown tremendously.

A single-person household could be a retired person. Research suggests that many retired people do not wish to spend more time preparing meals. They want convenience and ease of preparation. The retired are not necessarily an affluent group and the numbers choosing to eat outside the home falls with increasing age.

More places to eat out

Patterns of eating have changed as the number and range of eating out establishments have increased. There is a greater choice of places to eat and prices to suit all budgets. According to the Office of National Statistics, between 1992 and 2004 spending on food and drink products consumed outside the home grew by 102.2 per cent to £87.5 billion.

Eating out has become a family activity. The typical British pub has changed considerably over the last few decades. The pub is no longer regarded as a male dominated environment serving just simple food and cask beers. Today many pubs offer a range of beverages and food choices. They welcome children and family dining with purpose-built play areas and special menus. According to Mintel, in 2005 pub catering accounted for 23 per cent of the eating out market, second only to fast food catering at 27 per cent.

The eating out market is dominated by fast food establishments. In the UK we consume more fast food than any other European country. The number of fast food restaurants in the UK has grown considerably since the first McDonald's opened in Woolwich in 1974 and there are now over 1200 McDonald's in the UK. Other large chains include KFC and Burger King which have become household names and are a common sight on many high streets. Fast food restaurants now appear in entertainment complexes, airports and hospitals.

Limited skill and knowledge of how to cook

Eating patterns have changed because some people lack the basic skills and knowledge to cook. The skills needed to prepare meals may not be passed from mother to daughter or son. The contribution of schools in developing the skills to cook meals has in many cases been reduced. Many young people leave school and home to start higher education with minimal knowledge of food preparation. This may create a dependence on ready-to-eat meals and convenience foods.

The preparation of some food is regarded as complicated and difficult to recreate authentically in the home. The number of speciality restaurants offering ethnic foods has risen. In 2006 DEFRA found the sales of takeaway meat-based meals, rice dishes and pizza rose considerably between 1974 and 2005–6, while sales of takeaway fish fell.

Lack of time

Eating patterns have changed as some people feel they have less leisure time. Compared to other European nations, research suggests that the British work the longest hours. Non-work time is increasingly precious for the workforce and the inconvenience of shopping for food, preparing a meal, cooking and washing up weigh increasingly in favour of the appeal of ready meals.

The perception of eating out has changed

Eating out is no longer regarded as a special treat for many households or families but has become a way of life. More disposable income has contributed to the fact that some people feel wealthier and choose to eat out more frequently.

The food catering market has changed too. Many restaurants offer special 'meal deals' and 'two for one' promotions to attract custom, particularly in the early evening or on week nights. The 'all you can eat' Indian or Chinese buffet is popular as many consumers regard it as good value for money. Eating out is no longer considered to be very expensive and only appropriate for special occasions.

The choice of food inside and outside the home

The range and types of food products available has changed considerably over the past fifty years. Developments in technology and changes in society have contributed to this change. Food retailers and manufacturers now regard separate food products as meal solutions. **Meal solutions** consist of a range of food products that can be combined to make a meal, including some products which are ready to make, ready prepared or ready to eat.

The IGD is a research organisation for the food and grocery industry. It divides the food we purchase to make meals into four categories.

Ready to make

These are raw ingredients bought by the consumer that are made or used in food preparation. These products include minced beef, chicken breasts, vegetables, flour, eggs, butter and milk.

Ready prepared

These fall into two further groups:
- Prepared meal components: These are parts of a meal that have been prepared by the manufacturer. They can be raw or ready to use. Examples include beef burgers, marinated pork chops, sausages, fish fingers, breadcrumb-coated chicken and ready-made pasta sauces.
- Part-prepared light meals: This is a meal that can be prepared quickly by the consumer and is sometimes eaten as a snack. Examples include tinned soup, pot meals, baked beans and dried soups. Some of the preparation is completed by the manufacturer.

Ready to heat

A complete frozen or chilled meal at least part-cooked by the manufacturer. Examples include pizza, pasta-based meals, curries, oriental-style meals and fish pies. Chilled 'freshly' prepared meal components can be sold on a delicatessen counter – samosas, sausage rolls, pasties and pies. These are often referred to as ready meals.

Ready to eat

This category includes hot or cold food ready for immediate consumption and suitable for eating on the move. Examples include sandwiches, wraps, salad tubs and hot food from a rotisserie – chicken pieces and pork ribs.

An example of a meal solution may be:

- **ready prepared** – uncooked chicken breasts in a lemon and garlic marinade
- **ready to make** – fresh carrots
- **ready prepared** – roast potatoes with oil and herbs in a foil tray
- **ready to heat** – chilled gravy
- **ready to eat** – fresh fruit salad.

Activity 4

Review

Take each of the four types of food product and collect some packaging from each.

Investigate the following:

- How is it useful to the consumer?
- Who do you think the product is aimed at?
- Does it make any marketing claims?
- What did the product cost?

There is an enormous selection of food available to purchase. You will explore some of the more significant developments in food choice.

Frozen and cook-chilled food products

The domestic refrigerator has become widely available since the 1960s. This has meant that perishable foods like dairy produce, meat and cooked food can be stored safely for much longer at home. The freezer also emerged at this time and the first range of frozen food became available. The development and widespread ownership of the microwave has introduced a whole new range of food products to the consumer.

The growth of the frozen and cook-chilled food market has been rapid. There is a vast range of frozen and cook-chilled food products which includes ready meals, prepared vegetable dishes, pizzas, soups, sauces, desserts and meat products. In 2005 UK consumers spent £1.6 billion on ready meals. The British are the largest consumers of ready meals in Europe (BBC, 2006). The UK chilled food industry offers the consumer the largest range of products in the world. The trend towards more one person households and busier lifestyles has contributed to this increase in products.

Supermarket own brands

Own brand groceries account for approximately 40 per cent of sales in large supermarkets (IGD, 2004). The success of own brand goods is probably based upon the consumer perception that they are good value for money and that the supermarket has a good reputation for quality products.

Within the retailer's own brand range, many sub-brands have been developed aimed at different consumers. Retailers now offer value ranges, premium ranges, healthy eating ranges and children's ranges of food products.

Premium products and indulgence foods

This is an area of food retailing which is steadily growing. The majority of premium products are expensive when compared to the standard product equivalent. The use of higher quality ingredients and packaging contribute to the cost. Premium products are regarded as special by the consumer. A 'hand-finished Aberdeen Angus' steak pie delivers indulgence and greater choice for some consumers.

Vegetarian and meat alternative food products

Leatherhead Food International (LFI) estimates that the number of vegetarians has remained static at around 5 per cent of the population for a number of years. The largest group of vegetarian consumers are women aged between 17 and 34 years. However, the market for meat-free products is growing as more people are reducing their meat consumption, due to concerns about personal health and animal welfare issues.

The most significant meat-free foods on the market are pastry products, ready meals and products made with meat alternatives – such as Quorn sausages and burgers. Future developments in this market are in the area of meat-free snacks or deli-style ready-to-eat products.

The Vegetarian Society seedling symbol has been an official trademark since 1969. It is the only legally licensed vegetarian symbol in the UK that can be used on meat-free foods. The symbol indicates that a product meets the following criteria:

- free of animal flesh and any ingredients resulting from slaughter
- contains only free-range eggs
- free of genetically modified organisms (GMOs)
- not tested on animals
- not exposed to potential cross-contamination from non-vegetarian ingredients during production.

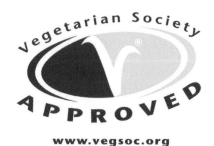

Figure 8.2 *The Vegetarian Society seedling symbol*

Allergy-free products

In the UK 45 per cent of the population has at some point during their life suffered food sensitivities and 2 per cent currently suffer from a food allergy (Allergy UK). The retailing of products for those with food allergies is no longer a niche market. Products which are free from gluten, lactose, egg, soya, nuts and certain food additives are increasingly available.

Functional foods

A **functional food** is a food which claims to have health promoting benefits in addition to the usual nutritional value. Functional foods include a wide range of products. Yoghurt drinks with active bacteria that assist with digestion and sports drinks with added caffeine to boost 'energy' are regarded as functional foods. As consumers become more health aware, there is a greater demand for this type of product and the prediction is that the market will develop further.

Organic food products

Organic food products have been produced without the aid of artificial chemicals or hormones. There are strict guidelines which must be followed in the production of organic foods. They should be produced naturally, using only animal and vegetable fertilizers.

Organic products are often regarded as premium products because they are more expensive than conventional versions. The organic food market is worth £2 billion according to the Soil Association. Spending on organic food and drink grew by 22 per cent between 2005 and 2006, making the UK the third largest organic market in Europe behind Germany and Italy. The sale of organic vegetable boxes and free range eggs has seen the most significant growth. According to the Soil Association in 2006 the sale of free range and organic eggs exceeded the sale of eggs from caged birds.

The Soil Association symbol on packaging (see Figure 4.5) indicates that the product has been produced organically and has met the Soil Association Organic Standards.

Snack products

The choice of snack products has increased tremendously in recent years. The 'healthy' cereal bar has emerged as an important snack product. However, the most common food eaten as a snack in the UK is fresh fruit, followed by hot drinks, crisps and nuts (IGD Consumer Research, 2005). Many consumers are more aware of health issues and the snack market is changing to meet these needs.

Ethical food products

Ethical foods include fairtrade products and food produced with concern for animal welfare.

Fairtrade products ensure disadvantaged producers in the developing world receive a fair price for their products. Fairtrade products may carry the FAIRTRADE Mark (see Figure 4.5) if they meet the trading standards required by the Fairtrade Foundation. Fairtrade products are only a small proportion of food sales but are growing steadily. They tend to be more expensive than conventional products and this may limit purchases by some consumers.

Ethical food can also include food which is produced with a concern for animal welfare. Free range eggs and some meat products belong to this group. They offer the consumer greater choice. The RSPCA set up **Freedom Food** to improve farm animal welfare. The RSPCA's welfare standards cover the rearing, handling, transportation and slaughter of animals based upon the Farm Animal Welfare Council's (FAWC) 'five freedoms'.

The FAWC's five freedoms are:

- freedom from hunger and thirst
- freedom from discomfort
- freedom from pain, injury and disease
- freedom to express normal behaviour
- freedom from fear and distress.

At present they can be applied to the most common animals farmed for food in the UK, if the product meets the standards.

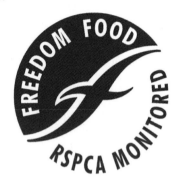

Certification Mark

Figure 8.3 *The Freedom Food logo*

Healthy foods

The range of 'healthy foods' offered for sale has increased. Greater public awareness of the potential risks to health of a high fat diet, a lack of time and possibly knowledge of how to prepare healthy meals have contributed to the rise in 'healthier' convenience food. A wide range of reduced fat, low calorie, sugar-free and salt-free food products exist. The increase in the number of consumers participating in slimming diets and following specialist, low carbohydrate or high protein diets has widened the choice of products further.

Trans fatty acids have been associated with an increased risk of heart disease. Food manufacturers are currently developing a range of own brand products for the major UK food retailers which will be completely free from trans fatty acids.

Ethnic products

Britain is a multicultural society and many foods have been introduced into the UK diet from different cultures. Italian ice creams were sold to wealthy

Victorians in London in the 1850s. Greater opportunities to travel and a wider experience of food from other cultures have created a demand for these products in the UK such as Chinese, Indian, Italian, Thai and Mexican food. According to Active Kids Get Cooking in 2006 nearly a quarter of all ready meals sold were Indian-style dishes.

Locally and regionally sourced food products

Many consumers want locally produced food products. The definition of a 'local' food product varies. It can mean the food is produced within 30 miles of the point of purchase or more broadly that it is a British product. Locally produced meat, poultry, vegetables, fruit, pastries and eggs are appearing on supermarket shelves. The production of locally produced drinks and desserts is a developing market. Consumers are choosing these products as they are perceived to be fresh, better for the environment and higher quality.

The Red Tractor logo is used on several meats, vegetables and dairy products. It indicates conscientiously produced food of UK origin. Red Tractor is managed by an independent, not-for-profit organisation that works alongside industry experts to maintain and improve food production standards. All Red Tractor farmers, producers, processors and packagers are regularly inspected by one of the 450 independent experts who conduct more than 70,000 inspections each year.

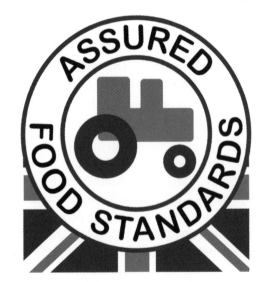

Figure 8.4 *The Red Tractor logo*

Food choices available outside the home

We have already explored the fact that eating out is increasing popular. You will now look at the different places to eat outside the home.

There are many opportunities to eat outside the home and the list below identifies some options:

hotel catering
cafés and tearooms
fast food restaurants
cafeterias at the workplace
vending machine foods
in-store cafes
salad bars and
  delicatessens

restaurant meals
public houses catering
school lunches
friends' homes
roadside catering
aeroplanes
  and cruise ships
takeaway services

Activity 5

Research opportunity
Design a questionnaire to find out about food choice both inside and outside the home.

Research by the IGD identifies the four most popular places to eat out as restaurants, pubs, cafés and fast food restaurants.

Restaurants

Restaurant meals include all meals taken inside hotels, specialist and ethnic restaurants. Research by Mintel on the UK eating out market (2005) found restaurant meals and hotel catering together account for 36 per cent of meals taken outside the home. The research suggested that eating in a restaurant is usually a planned event for a specific purpose such as a special occasion with friends or family.

Public houses

Eating in pubs is very popular. According to Mintel (2005), 23 per cent of meals taken outside the home can be attributed to pub catering. Pubs have changed and are now perceived as inexpensive family-friendly places, with a good choice of food and high quality service.

Cafés

Research has suggested that cafés are emerging as a significant provider of meals away from home. The key development is in the evening café as an alternative to other establishments. The time pressured consumer wants somewhere to eat quickly, with friends or family and that is reasonably inexpensive. This market includes specialist coffee shops selling all day breakfasts, snacks and a range of beverages. The growth of the branded café market has been dramatic. Research by the IGM found that the number of branded café outlets had risen from 778 in 1997 to 2428 in 2005. This represents growth of over 200 per cent in the UK.

Fast food outlets

Fast food outlets remain highly popular in spite of concerns about the consumption of high fat foods. Many fast food restaurants have made changes to their menus in response to consumer demands for healthier foods. However, research suggests it is the preference of children to eat in fast food restaurants and one in four consumers eat in this type of outlet because their children or grandchildren want to (IGM, 2003).

Psychological, social, technological, economic and cultural issues

Initially we learn what to eat from our parents. This learned behaviour will influence meal and snack patterns, acceptable foods, food combinations and portion sizes. It will also affect the manner in which we eat food including the use of cutlery, napkins and fingers. As we grow older the influence of friends and wider factors in society become significant. These may include travel, financial resources, advertising, health and moral concerns guiding our food choice.

Eating habits are the result of both learned behaviours from childhood and wider social influences. These habits develop and may change over a person's lifetime.

There are many factors which can affect the food we eat.

Psychological factors affecting food choice

Psychological factors are concerned with the mental processes and emotional issues which affect our food choice.

Physiological need for food

The need to satisfy hunger drives us to eat. This is a physical requirement and human beings need food to stay alive. The smell, sight and thought of food can stimulate the sensation of hunger and prepare the digestive system for food. The smell of food will really make your mouth water and an empty stomach rumble! After eating the sensation of fullness is felt.

Psychological need for food

For most people, eating food is enjoyable and because food provides enjoyment, it meets an emotional need. People use food to relieve stress and anxiety. Eating food can give us comfort and reassurance. Offering someone who is upset a cup of tea is an example of how food is used as a 'comforting gesture'. The refusal to eat can be used by some individuals to express feelings of unhappiness, anger or jealousy.

Eating preferences

Everyone has unique likes and dislikes concerning foods. These preferences develop over time and are influenced by personal experiences such as encouragement to eat, exposure to a food, family eating habits, advertising and personal values. Parents usually feed their children the food they enjoy which can influence a child's eating preferences for the rest of their life.

Sensory appeal of food

The smell, taste, texture and appearance of food stimulate all the senses. The smell of food is arguably the most powerful sense. Without an aroma food can be tasteless. Smell and taste are closely linked and produce the flavour of food. Taste buds will give the brain some information on the level of sweet, bitter, salt or sour in a product but the smell provides the key information on the flavour. Young children who do not have strong associations between smell and food regard the taste of sweetness as more desirable.

The appearance of food is also important. We expect strawberry-flavoured yoghurt to be pink. We might reject the product if the colour does not meet our expectations. Food processing can remove the colour from food. Food additives can be added to replace this lost colour and make the product more pleasing to the eye. For example, during the canning process peas turn brown and food colouring additives can restore the original colour.

Influence of the media

News reports and documentaries on the television have a major influence on food choice. Reports about the commercial production of GM crops and BSE scares have affected consumer confidence in food production.

Targeted advertising can also affect food choice. Some adverts on television are shown at specific times when the target group will be watching television and such campaigns have been very successful. Restrictions have now been placed on the promotion of 'unhealthy foods' during children's programmes.

Role models in popular culture can influence our food choices if we aspire to their lifestyles. Cooking is a leisure activity for many people. The influence of celebrity chefs on TV has widened the choice of exotic ingredients and specialist equipment available to purchase.

Social factors affecting food choice

Social network

The social network in which a person lives can influence their food choice. It includes family and friends at home and at work. Members of this social network can influence each other's behaviours and values. As we have already discovered, food choices and eating patterns can be instilled from childhood from the family. Friends can affect our food choice, eating patterns and habits. Peer group pressures can influence a person's food choice. The need to belong and fit in with friends can change the individual's attitude towards certain foods.

Activity 6

Group discussion

Discuss occasions when your friends have influenced your eating patterns or food choices.

Geographical location

Where the consumer lives can affect the choice of food. In a large city the choice may be vast but in a rural location it may be limited. Many larger food retailers are situated outside town centres and can be difficult to access without a car. Consumers are increasingly reliant on car ownership when making large food purchases at out-of-town shopping centres.

The changing family and household

More women work full and part time and have less time to spend preparing meals. A possible result of this change is that the choice of convenience foods is increasing. More single person households exist. This has resulted in a wider selection of single-portion foods such as half loaves of bread.

Changes in working patterns

Many people travel greater distances to work. They have less time for breakfast and will eat on the move. Increasingly, food products reflect a more flexible lifestyle – cereal bars, salad tubs and ready-made sandwiches. People who work longer hours may choose to eat more ready meals due to tiredness and a lack of motivation to cook a meal. People working shifts may have different eating patterns from the rest of the household and may take meals to work. The demand for microwaveable ready-made meals and single-portion meals has grown to fit changing working patterns.

Leisure time

Where we live and our lifestyle both affect food choice. Increased leisure time for some families and individuals means that less time may be spent in the home preparing meals. People may eat at different times within a household and opt for convenience such as microwaveable food. More products are available requiring limited preparation – part-cooked meals and stir-in sauces.

Preparation and cooking equipment available

There is a wide variety of food equipment available to make food preparation easier and less time-consuming. Smoothie makers and juicers encourage the consumer to purchase more fruit. Food retailers have introduced products to meet this need – for example, special juicing oranges. Bread makers have led to the development of a range of bread mixes. Stir fry vegetables and ready-made sauces are designed for use in woks. Most significantly, the ownership of microwaves has encouraged the use of ready-prepared frozen and chilled meals.

Income

The amount of money coming into the household will affect the choice of food purchased. The association between poverty and food choice is well researched. The amount of money available affects both the quantity and variety of food which can be purchased. Research suggests more high fat and high sugar foods may be chosen if income is limited. Fruit and vegetables may not be purchased as they can be expensive. Most of the major food retailers offer their own brand of value ranges on key food products. Visiting supermarkets to purchase these products can be difficult for consumers who have to rely on public transport.

Emergence of a social conscience

The introduction of Fairtrade products has extended consumer choice. Ethically produced foods will appeal to some consumers. As demand for these products is increasing, it appears there is greater concern about how food is produced in developing countries.

Increasingly, consumers are demanding more information on what they eat, the production methods, the ingredients and the country of origin. Some food products travel great distances before arriving on supermarket shelves. This can be described as **food miles**. A Farmers Weekly campaign in 2006 stated that 95 per cent of fruit and 50 per cent of vegetables eaten in the UK are imported. The amount of food air-freighted around the world has risen by 140 per cent since 1992 which will contribute to global pollution. In the future there may be a greater demand for food with low food miles and a small carbon footprint.

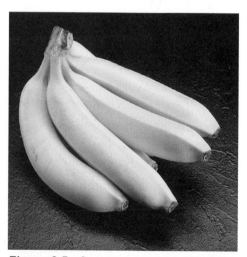

Figure 8.5 *Bananas are consumed in Britain but grown elsewhere*

Health issues

Interest has grown in healthy convenience foods as consumers become more concerned about health and diet. Retailers and manufacturers make food products to meet the demand such as 'low fat' ready meals.

Functional foods such as cholesterol-lowering spreads and probiotic drinks have been introduced, offering greater food choice.

Retailers are more responsive to special diets and label some products accordingly, such as gluten-free. The range and choice of products for those with special dietary needs have increased significantly.

The use of food additives in products aimed at children has decreased as public concern about the possible cocktail effect of additives has increased. The **cocktail effect** is when a combination of food additives is consumed together. Products which contain no artificial additives have emerged.

Technological factors affecting food choice

The ownership of fridges, freezers and microwaves

The increased ownership of fridges in the 1960s and 1970s meant it became possible to keep food fresher for longer. It was not until the 1980s that a significant number of people owned a freezer. Household ownership of microwaves has increased from 55 per cent of households in 1991 to 87 per cent in 2002 (IGM, 2004).

The ownership of these appliances has undoubtedly affected our food choice. The range of chilled, frozen and microwave products is vast. According to the research group Mintel in a report 'Eating habits: improving the appeal of convenience options', published in 2007, ready meals have recorded the fastest growth rate since 2002.

Development in food packaging

Food packaging has provided more food choice. Packaging extending the shelf-life of a product means less frequent shopping trips are necessary. An example is the modified atmospheric packaging for raw meats. **Modified atmospheric packaging** (MAP) has the air changed inside the food package. Oxygen is reduced and carbon dioxide and nitrogen are increased. This allows perishable food to remain fresher for longer, giving the consumer greater choice.

Packaging provides solutions to busier lifestyles such as self-heating cans of coffee. Special plastics and cardboards have been introduced so food products can be cooked in either the microwave or conventional oven.

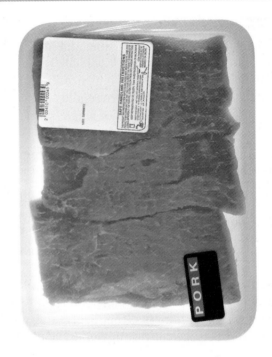

Figure 8.6 *Meat in modified atmospheric packaging*

Development in food products

Mycoprotein is an industrial food material developed to replace meat. It is a fungus which contains high quality protein. It can be sliced, dried and cut into chunks or minced. Mycoprotein can be found in ready-made meals, such as curries, casseroles, sweet and sour dishes and pies, and can also be bought as a raw ingredient for cooking. It offers the vegetarian consumer a greater choice of food products.

Development in food production

The development of commercial fish farms has contributed to the increased supply of salmon, shellfish and trout.

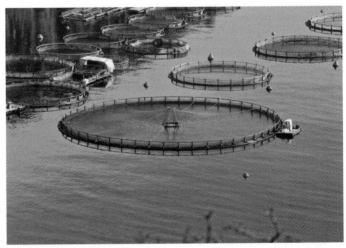

Figure 8.7 *A fish farm*

Technology has allowed food to be fortified. **Fortified food** is when nutrients are added during processing to products such as breakfast cereals and sports drinks. This provides choice for the consumer who may wish to take greater control of their health through food choice, knowing that these foods will provide specific health benefits.

The need for greater convenience has led to the development of spreadable butters and filtered milk. Filtered milk goes through an additional, fine filtration system which prevents souring bacteria entering the milk. This can extend the shelf-life of the milk by up to 45 days in a refrigerator and an average of seven days once opened.

Extrusion cooking involves raw materials such as flour, starches and liquids being mixed into a semi-solid dough. This mixture is heated and then forced (extruded) through specially designed die holes. This product is then dried to produce a range of breakfast cereals, pasta shapes, sweets and savoury snacks.

Accelerated freeze-drying (AFD) is a fast and effective way of drying frozen food. It involves drying food in a vacuum at a reduced pressure. The method offers the consumer more choice and convenience. It is used for soups, fruits, instant coffee granules and dried milk.

Developments in ICT

ICT networks link food retailers to suppliers and can react quickly to increased demand for a food product. The consumer has more food choice as the availability of food products is managed more effectively.

The internet has also affected food choice. Many food retailers offer an online method of purchase. Food products can be purchased from small, specialist producers offering further choice such as wild Scottish salmon.

In Chapter 9 you will explore in greater detail the impact of ICT on food retailing.

Improvements in transport

Rapid transportation of perishable food products in a controlled environment improves consumer choice. Fruit and vegetables can be imported from around the world. Effective transport methods have increased the year-round availability of many foods. Food is no longer seasonal and can be obtained at any time of year.

Activity 7

Group discussion and review

Discuss where the food we eat comes from, who produces it and how it is produced. Draw up a list of some commonly eaten foods and the countries that produce them.

Then on your own keep track of the foods you eat in one day. Find out where the foods are produced or grown.

Using a world map, food labels and images, identify the sources of some key foods.

Economic factors affecting food choice

Advertising and marketing strategies

Advertising in store and on television influences consumer purchases. The use of role models in advertising campaigns has a significant influence on the popularity of the supermarket image/brand.

Activity 8

Group discussion

Think of the celebrities you can associate with a food retailer or a food product.

In-store marketing methods used by food retailers can tempt people to buy certain foods. The careful placement of more expensive branded products at eye level, attractive displays with associated products positioned next to each other and free samples are just some of the strategies used.

Government policies

Government policies and international trade agreements may affect the choice available to the consumer and the cost of products. Britain is a member of the European Union and therefore must support the Common Agricultural Policy.

The **Common Agricultural Policy (CAP)** was set up to avoid food shortages and ensure European farmers received an adequate income for their produce. European farmers were paid (subsidised) to produce food. This led to the overproduction of food during the 1980s. It disadvantaged farmers in developing countries as subsidised food was sold on the world market at a low price. The CAP has kept some food prices high for European consumers. Low income households spend a greater proportion of their income on food so they have been affected most by high food prices. The CAP is being reformed and the link between subsidies and production may be removed.

Fishing quotas have placed restrictions on the type and quality of fish caught. This may affect the choice available to the consumer and manufacturer when developing products containing fish.

Biofuels are fuels produced from oilseeds. These fuels can be used as an alternative to diesel. There is great demand for them. The cultivation of oilseeds to make biofuels on farmland may affect the price of cereals. It could contribute to food shortages and a rise in the price of some cereals such as wheat.

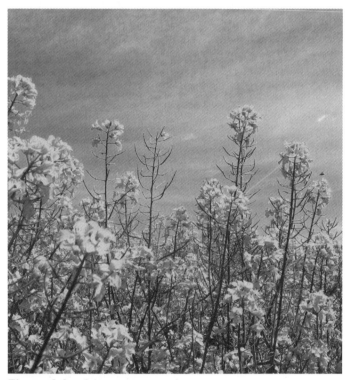

Figure 8.8 *Cultivating rapeseed*

Cultural factors affecting food choice

Hospitality and festivals

In many different cultures, food and drink are associated with hospitality. Food can be used to celebrate events in an individual's life, such as a birth or a marriage.

The Christian festivals of Christmas and Easter have food associations. Christmas is traditionally associated with mince pies and turkey while Easter is associated with Easter eggs and hot cross buns. Retailers seize on cultural occasions by producing food products for the consumer such as a range of Christmas puddings in December.

Other cultural groups celebrate festivals with specific meals and foods. In Islam the end of Ramadan is celebrated by exchanging sweets. In Judaism, Matzo, special unleavened bread, is broken to celebrate Passover.

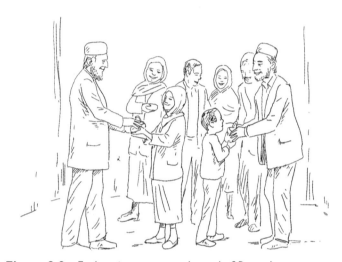

Figure 8.9 *Exchanging sweets at the end of Ramadan*

Cultural and religious groups

Some cultural groups have guidelines regarding acceptable foods, food combinations, eating patterns and eating behaviours. In the UK there are many cultural and religious groups, some of which have special dietary guidelines. Following these guidelines creates a sense of identity and belonging for the individual to the group.

Activity 9

Research opportunity

Select a religious group such as Hinduism, Judaism or Islam. Investigate how religious belief can influence food choice and the celebration of festivals.

Migration

Migration has ensured people bring their food tastes and style of cooking into the community. The arrival of

Polish workers in the UK has swelled the market for Polish food. Specialist Polish delicatessens and supermarket chains are now offering Polish products.

Purchasing food resources appropriate to needs

Food consumption is repetitive behaviour influenced by many of the issues we have explored in the factors affecting food choice. However, the situation or context in which food is consumed can affect purchases. The purchase of food resources usually meets the needs of individuals and households.

You will start this section by exploring the different needs within households. You have already investigated the fulfilment of needs to motivate human behaviour. However, food retailers are capable by shrewd marketing and advertising to create needs and desires in consumers.

Needs that may influence food purchase

Figure 8.10 shows some of the needs that may be considered by individuals and households when purchasing food.

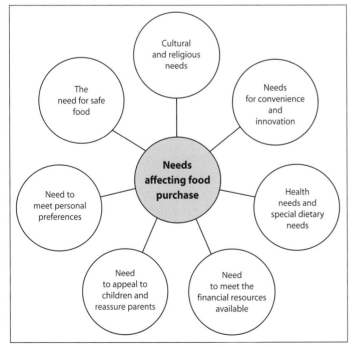

Figure 8.10 *The needs that affect food purchasing*

Need to meet the financial resources available

The average weekly expenditure on food and non-alcoholic drinks was £45.30 for each household in 2005–6 in the UK. The £45.30 spent each week was divided into £12.10 on meat, £3.40 on fresh vegetables, £2.80 on fresh fruit and £3.80 on non-alcoholic drinks (ONS, Family Spending, 2006). Some households will spend more than £45 a week on food and some will spend less. Food purchases are linked to the financial resources available and the needs of the household.

Supermarkets offer a range of food products to suit different levels of income. The popularity of value brands has grown considerably. Discount food retailers, such as Netto and Lidl, can offer very competitive pricing on selected products. This is usually a strategy to entice the consumer into the shop to spend more.

Supermarkets encourage consumers to buy their products in many different ways including special offers, 'Buy one, get one free', 20 per cent extra free or introductory pricing. However, caution is required to assess whether these deals are genuine bargains.

Need to appeal to children and reassure parents

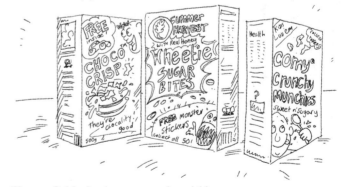

Figure 8.11 *Products targeted at children*

There is a wide range of food products aimed at children and their parents. Food manufacturers produce mini portions of popular ready meals, smaller yoghurts, small drinks cartons and a variety of savoury 'cheese' snacks. These products are ideal for lunch boxes. The national drive to encourage the consumption of fruit and vegetables has contributed to the development of fruit bars, small packets and boxes of dried fruit, smaller apples and easy-peel fruit for children.

Many products are promoted with labels such as 'Free from artificial additives' or 'Organic'. This aims to inspire confidence to the parent that the product is safe. Tamper-proof packaging on jars of baby food also offers reassurance to consumers concerned about the security of the food product.

Need to meet personal preferences

We have already explored the development of food products which meet our moral, environmental and social concerns. The growth of Fairtrade products, vegetarian, organic and freedom foods are an attempt by food manufacturers to meet our concerns.

Some consumers are motivated by the need for indulgence and pleasure. The range of premium products continues to develop, including fashionable salads, delicatessen products, sushi, fresh juices and luxury ice creams.

In the UK there has been significant growth in the proportion of single and two-person households. This has driven a need for smaller packet sizes and single serving portions of many food products. The market for bread is changing with sales of 400 g loaves now growing significantly faster than 800 g loaves.

Health needs and special dietary needs

Health issues have a high media profile and have an immense impact on food consumption decisions. Health issues associated with nutrition, digestion, allergies, obesity and health will influence some consumers. We have investigated the rise of organic foods and allergy-free products early in this chapter.

There is a much greater choice of healthy food. The consumer may choose diabetic products, cholesterol-lowering spreads, bread fortified with omega 3, low salt and low fat versions of many products.

The consumption of fruit and vegetables is at its highest level for 20 years according to the Expenditure and Food Survey by DEFRA in 2007. The choice of fruit and vegetables available is vast and there is much more encouragement to consume them.

Cultural and religious needs

Food retailers now sell a wide range of ethnic products as demand increases. A wider choice of convenience products made with 'Halal' meat is emerging. More adventurous consumers require curry pastes, coconut milk, spices, exotic fruit and vegetables. Travel and cultural diversity are driving the growth of continental and ethnic bakery products such as naan breads, French breads and ciabatta.

Need for convenience and innovation

Consumers are demanding greater convenience from food products. We have already explored the importance of ready meals and ready-made components to address this need, but there are other products which appeal to busy consumers. Grated cheese, chopped salad and washed vegetables save time with meal preparation. Toasting is the most popular snack preparation method. A wide range of bakery products have been developed to meet the demand for snacks.

The packaging of food product is developing. Ring pulls on tins, resealable drink cartons, peelable films on cooked meat packets and stand-up pouches for sauces and soups offer convenience. Increasingly, the consumer requires food packaging that is refillable, easy-to-recycle or biodegradable.

Need for safe food

Consumers want to be reassured that the food they are choosing is safe to eat. Food scares triggered by Bovine Spongiform Encephalopathy (BSE) in meat, salmonella in eggs, and E-coli poisoning have made consumers more concerned about health and hygiene in the food industry. The implementation of new food safety and hygiene regulations has restored some public confidence. Developments are being made in providing clearer food labelling and greater transparency in the traceability of food products. The cattle passport system introduced in July 1996 traces the movements of all cattle born in or imported to the UK. This system aims to secure public confidence in the safety of meat.

The Lion Quality mark seen on egg shells and egg boxes indicates that the eggs are from farms which are concerned about food safety. The Lion Quality mark signifies that the chicken is vaccinated against salmonella, there is careful temperature control of the eggs and the source of the hens and their feed can be traced.

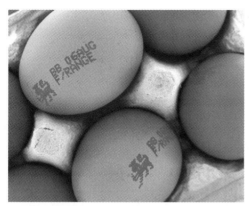

Figure 8.12 *The Lion Quality mark*

The management of resources

In this section you will investigate the management of resources to provide meals. You may wish to refer to Chapter 7 on resources as there is some overlap of knowledge. You will revisit the key principles of resource management and apply them to different contexts, but first we will explore some of the basic principles of meal planning.

Basic meal planning

People have different requirements and needs for food. There are some general factors that should be considered when planning meals:

- age and sex
- lifestyle
- health
- likes and dislikes
- income
- skill and knowledge
- facilities available
- time available
- dietary needs
- type of meal
- climate
- cultural beliefs.

These factors will affect what food is purchased, prepared and eaten. When managing resources these basic requirements must met be first.

Activity 11

Research opportunity
Take each of the factors listed above and produce a web diagram. On the diagram explain briefly how each factor could influence meal planning.

The management of resources can be considered in a variety of contexts, but for this investigation we will focus on a single, elderly person, a student household and a working family with small children. The management of the key resources of money, time and energy will be explored considering their needs. There will be variation in access to resources between these households.

Student households

Students have limited financial resources. Careful meal planning and budgeting can help households with limited financial resources. It will avoid food being wasted and impulse purchasing while shopping. In student households planning meals can save money. Before going shopping it is important to write a list and stick to the list. Planning the meals for each day and beyond can help to avoid impulse purchases which may be unnecessary and expensive. Supermarkets are very effective at marketing food products to increase the likelihood of impulse purchasing.

In a student household it may work out cheaper if everyone eats the same meal. If the meal is cooked and eaten at a set time this can save fuel as there will be no need to heat individual portions later.

Buying food products in bulk can sometimes be cheaper than purchasing individual items separately but it is important to consider whether transporting and storing large quantities is convenient before making these purchases. Tinned goods and dried foods are ideal for purchasing in bulk as they can be stored for many months.

Using vegetables that are in season or on special offer can save money. Washing and preparing vegetables at home is cheaper than buying ready prepared vegetables. Students may have a limited knowledge of food preparation and have limited equipment so meals should be easy to prepare and cook.

A **sedentary lifestyle** has little activity and usually involves a considerable amount of time sat at a desk. Many students lead sedentary lifestyles and this may contribute to weight gain if too many high energy foods are consumed.

All households should choose foods which are healthy but satisfying. Potatoes, pasta and rice are filling and inexpensive. It is crucial that the food purchased is enjoyed by the individuals and households. Any leftovers could be frozen for another meal. Eating in is usually less expensive than eating out. Students can entertain inexpensively by inviting friends round for a meal instead of eating out.

Working households with young children

Some households with young children have insufficient time to prepare nutritious and healthy meals every evening due to work commitments. The use of ready-made components can help these individuals and households. There is an enormous range of meal solutions available in supermarkets which can help the busy parent to provide meals. Families with small children may wish to avoid foods high in food additives, salt, fat and sugar and so should opt for suitable products.

The use of the microwave can help to save time. Food can be defrosted and cooked quickly. This is excellent for working families. A freezer is valuable for food storage. Food purchases can be made weekly or fortnightly and stored safely. Food processors and blenders can save time and some human energy but this should be balanced against the time required to clean the equipment after use. The use of timers on conventional ovens is another way of managing meal preparation to suit the needs of families as meals can be ready when people return from work. A slow cooker can save energy if used on a low setting for a long period and less expensive stewing and braising steak can be tenderised, saving money.

Single, elderly person household

A retired single person may need to save energy when providing meals. Fuel energy can be managed and saved by careful meal planning and use of equipment. Batch baking large quantities of food can save fuel and large quantities can be frozen in small portions and stored until required. Food can be reheated using a microwave quickly and inexpensively. Electrical equipment can also be helpful if the individual lacks the skill or is not capable of completing a task manually due to infirmity. To manage fuel more effectively, use the correct size of saucepan while cooking on the hob with just sufficient water and use a lid. Vegetables should be cut into smaller pieces so they cook faster.

Many elderly people have limited financial resources when shopping for food. Large supermarkets can be more expensive than local markets. The quality of products can vary in a market but the price can be considerably cheaper. It is important to be selective in the food products purchased. High profile brands are more expensive than supermarket own brands. Many supermarkets sell their own value brands which can be considerably cheaper. All consumers should check the date mark before making a purchase and consider whether the food can be stored and eaten before it passes the best before date. Research suggests that many consumers waste food and throw uneaten food away.

Generally, ready meals are more expensive than preparing your own meals. They may also contain high levels of salt and fat. However, a single portion ready meal can be more cost-effective than purchasing separate ingredients and making a meal from scratch for an elderly person living alone.

Buying frozen meat can be cheaper than fresh meat products. Fresh meat from a supermarket can be more expensive than markets and butchers shops. Small quantities are also easier to purchase and can be requested.

A single, elderly person may wish to have a supply of tinned food in case they are unable to food shop frequently. Tinned foods are easy to store, come in small portions and are usually inexpensive.

Activity 12

Practical opportunity

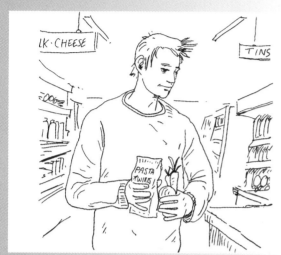

Figure 8.13 *A single student planning a meal*

Plan a day's menu with £6 for a single person.
Prepare the main meal.

Describe how you made savings when purchasing and preparing the ingredients for the meal. Show how you calculated the cost.

Activity 13

Check your understanding

Check your understanding of the meaning of the following key terms:

accelerated freeze-drying	cocktail effect
dashboard dining	deskfast
eating pattern	extrusion cooking
fairtrade products	food miles
fortified food	freedom food
functional food	grazing
meal	meal solutions
mycoprotein	organic food products
ready prepared food	ready to eat food
ready to heat	ready to make
snack	biofuels
common agricultural policy	sedentary lifestyle

Produce a web diagram that includes all these terms.
Give examples of food products where appropriate.

Exam-style questions

1 Describe how the management of resources can provide meals for student households. (10 marks)

2 Discuss how technological, social and cultural factors can affect food choice. (15 marks)

3 Figure 8.14 shows the different methods used to prepare a main weekday meal by respondents.

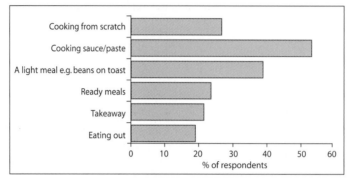

Figure 8.14 *Methods for preparing a main meal: weekday (2004)*

Source: Consumer Unit, IGD

Using the graph, answer these questions:

a. What percentage of respondents used cooking from scratch as the method of preparation for the main meal? (1 mark)

b. Explain the term 'cooking from scratch'. (2 marks)

c. What percentage of respondents used cooking sauces or paste when preparing a meal? (1 mark)

d. Give three reasons for the popularity of cooking sauces. (3 marks)

e. Describe the possible implications of this data on

    i. individual health

    ii. future developments in the food industry. (8 marks)

(Total of 40 marks)

Selection and purchase of household goods

Learning objectives

By the end of this chapter you will be able to:

- explain the rights of the consumer when purchasing goods and services including complaints procedures
- identify the advantages and disadvantages of the range of retail outlets for the purchase of food
- explain ways in which dietary guidelines can influence food purchase and preparation methods
- describe how the management of food resources can meet individual and household needs
- describe the sources of information available to the consumer when deciding which goods and services to purchase
- identify the marketing strategies used in the food retail industry and the methods used to secure loyalty
- describe the food supply chain and changes in food distribution
- understand the technological advances in the distribution and retailing of food.

Introduction

The consumer has rights when purchasing goods and services. A **consumer** is someone who purchases goods or services. There are routes available to the consumer should they need to complain about a faulty good or service. When you buy goods from a **trader**, from a shop or a market stall, you enter into a contract which is controlled by many acts of legislation. This gives both you the consumer and the trader rights.

Legislation exists to protect the consumer from a range of possible dangers. It provides the minimum framework that retailers, manufacturers and producers have to abide by when providing goods and services. Consumers have a right to **redress** if things go wrong when buying goods and services.

Consumer rights

When you buy **goods** or parts you have a right to expect the goods to be of satisfactory quality, fit for their purpose and as described. But you do not have any rights if any of the following apply:

- You were informed of any faults before you bought the goods, or if the fault was so significant you should have noticed it when you purchased it.
- You damage the goods yourself.
- If you made a mistake – you don't like the style or it is the wrong size.
- If you have changed your mind about the goods.
- You want to return the goods because you have seen them cheaper elsewhere.

However, some retailers will issue refunds for unused goods within a time period, whatever the reason may be. This creates additional useful rights for consumers.

When you buy goods privately, you do not have the same rights as when buying from a trader. In this case the law quotes 'caveat emptor' or 'buyer beware'. You have no rights to expect that goods be of a satisfactory quality or fit for their purpose, **but** you do have the right that the goods should be 'as described'.

When you buy goods in a sale you have full rights under the Sale of Goods Act. However, if the goods were reduced in price because of a fault that is brought to your attention or the fault is so large it is obvious, you would not be entitled to your money back later for that particular fault.

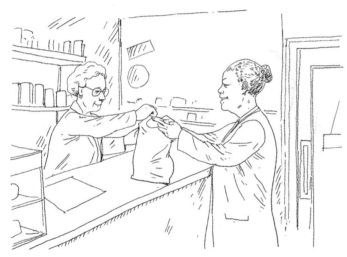

Figure 9.1 *Making a purchase*

You do have rights if the goods are faulty at the time of sale. If the goods are faulty there are remedies which will put it right:

- **A full refund** so you would get your money back in full.
- **Compensation (damages),** which may be based on the cost of repair, or if that is not possible, it may be based on the purchase price with an allowance for usage.
- **Repair or replacement** which must be carried out within a reasonable time and without causing significant inconvenience to the consumer.
- **Reduction in price.**

In most cases, you and the trader can agree to one of these remedies. If you cannot agree, then the courts have the power to choose any of the remedies.

Legislation to protect the consumer

Sale and Supply of Goods Act 1979/1994

There are three main aspects to this Act:

- **Goods must be of satisfactory quality:** This means the goods must meet the standards that a consumer would expect. It should take into account the description, the price and any other relevant information. The goods must also be free from any faults.
- **Goods must be fit for purpose:** The goods must be fit for any specific or particular purpose. If goods do not comply they must be repaired, replaced or the money refunded.
- **Goods must be as described:** Goods should match any description applied to them.

The Sale of Goods Act also applies to second-hand goods.

It protects the consumer by ensuring that the goods sold are for the purpose claimed or shown on the packaging. They are protected from inferior quality items as they have to function correctly for a reasonable amount of time.

Trades Description Act 1968/1972

When a seller describes the goods to the consumer, the consumer must not be misled in any way about the type of goods, the price, quantity, manufacture or the way they have been tested. Consumers are protected because the description of the goods must be accurate and outrageous claims cannot be made about them.

Food and Drugs Act 1955

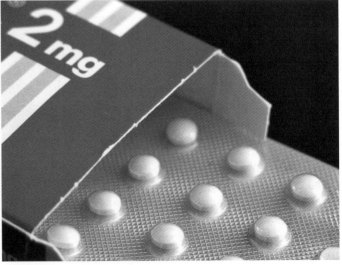

Figure 9.2 *Packaging for drugs*

This Act ensures that food and drugs are named and labelled correctly and that the food and drugs are produced in quality and hygienic conditions. This protects the consumer from being sold food which is unfit, stored or prepared in a dirty environment or is not as described.

Weights and Measures Act 1963

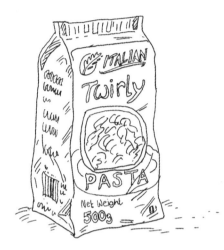

Figure 9.3 *Information about weight on food packaging*

This Act ensures that the weight of a product bought is accurate. It protects consumers from goods being sold in incorrect weights and sizes.

Consumer Safety Act 1978

This Act updated the 1961 Consumer Protection Act and strengthened legislation for goods other than food or drugs. It protects consumers from goods which are dangerous.

The Consumer Protection (Distance Selling) Regulations 2000

These regulations combine with the Consumer Protection (Distance Selling) (Amendment) Regulations 2005. In today's society many of us buy goods and services using the telephone, fax, mail order, catalogue, internet and shopping channels on digital TV. The consumer is protected by this law if the goods do not turn up, or if you do not like them once you have had a chance to look at them. This Act states that you should be given clear information about the order and the trader, a cooling-off period, protection against credit card fraud and the demand for payment of unsolicited goods.

Consumer rights when using services

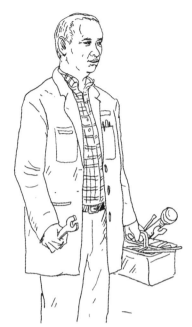

Figure 9.4 *A plumber provides a service*

When you use services you are equally covered by acts of legislation. The word **service** covers a wide variety of work from repairs to a car, building work, having a kitchen fitted, to using a plumber or an electrician.

The most relevant piece of legislation in place to protect the consumer when using services is the Supply of Goods and Services Act 1982.

The Supply of Goods and Services Act 1982

This Act requires a supplier of a service to carry out that service with reasonable care and skill, within a reasonable time and to make no more than a reasonable charge.

If a supplier of a service breaches the conditions of a contract, the consumer has a choice either to claim compensation from the trader for his failure to carry out what was agreed or to cancel the contract. Any goods supplied in the course of the service must be as described, of satisfactory quality and fit for their purpose. If they are not, the consumer is entitled to a repair, replacement or compensation.

Codes of practice

Retailers often belong to trade associations relevant to their business, for example, the Home Builders' Federation (HBF) which is the trade association for house builders.

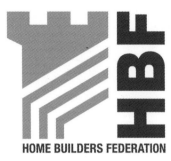

HOME BUILDERS FEDERATION

Figure 9.5 *The logo of the HBF*

Trade associations are groups of companies who offer a guarantee of good practice, and retailers who have joined these associations follow codes of practice to help ensure a good service to consumers. It is worth choosing a company that belongs to a trade association because if you have cause to complain, the trade association can be a useful organisation to ensure your rights are protected.

Requirements of membership of these associations are listed in the codes of practice:
- Servicing and repairs will be speedy and efficient.
- Repairs paid for will be guaranteed.
- There will be details on minimum charges.
- Estimates will be given on request.
- Complaints will be dealt with speedily and fairly.

Activity I

Review

Create a table of all the Acts of legislation which are in place to protect the consumer. Then explain briefly in your table what each Act does and how they each benefit the consumer.

Consumer protection

There are agencies whose role is to protect the rights of the consumer. Some of the agencies that protect consumers include:

The Office of Fair Trading

The Office of Fair Trading has two purposes. First, to protect consumers and explain their rights and second, to ensure businesses compete and operate fairly. It has several main responsibilities. It will recommend to the government where changes in the law or where new laws are needed to protect consumers. It publishes information for the consumer about their rights in leaflets and on its website. It will conduct research into firms where monopoly practices are suspected or when businesses are charging excessively high prices.

The Trading Standards Department

Trading Standards provides information for consumers, businesses and schools. They make sure that consumer goods are safe by aiming to prevent dangerous products reaching the marketplace. They ensure that goods and services are described accurately and that food contains only what it should by checking labels, packaging and advertisements to make sure they are accurate and display all the information required by law. They enforce the Sale and Supply of Goods Act and the Trades Description Act. They check weights and measures are accurate by checking scales, petrol pumps, pub measures and all other weighing and measuring equipment used by traders. They also check farm animals are free from disease and treated humanely at markets and in transit.

The Environmental Health Department

A local authority's Environmental Health Department is responsible for providing a range of services with the purpose of maintaining, improving and protecting the health and quality of life to the community in its area. It deals with environmental health emergencies such as food poisoning, noise nuisance and serious accidents in the workplace.

The Food Standards Agency

The Food Standards Agency aims to protect the public's health and consumer interests in relation to food. It aims to reduce food-borne illness, help people to eat more healthily, promote honest and informative labelling, improve good practice within the food industry and to improve and enforce food laws.

Activity 2

Review

Create a table which lists the agencies whose role is to protect the consumer. Then explain briefly what the agency does and how it protects the consumer.

Figure 9.6 *The logo of the Citizens Advice Bureau*

The Citizens Advice Bureau (CAB) provides free confidential and independent advice from 3300 locations in the UK. It is a registered charity and relies on the help of volunteers. It offers advice on a range of subjects.

Activity 3

Research opportunity

Investigate which are the most common topics that consumers seek advice on from the Citizens Advice Bureau and why.

Activity 4

Review

Answer yes or no to the following questions.

1. I have just purchased a dress and have decided that the colour does not suit me. Can I take it back to the shop and get a refund?

2. The watch I bought is faulty and does not work. I took it back to the shop but the sales assistant pointed to a notice which stated 'No refunds'. Can I get my money back?

3. In the sales I bought some shoes and the heel has come off. When I took them back, the sales assistant would not accept any liability as they were sale items. Is that right?

4. The CD I bought is faulty but I have lost my receipt. The sales assistant says that because I do not have a receipt I do not have any rights. Is that right?

Answer to activity 4

1. No, you are only entitled to a refund if the goods are defective, not as described or not fit for their purpose. However, the trader may be willing to give you a credit note.

2. Yes, traders cannot restrict their liability for faulty goods. Such notices are illegal and the trader could be prosecuted by Trading Standards.

3. No, you have the same rights when buying 'sales' goods as when you buy a brand new item. However, if the item was reduced because of a fault and it was pointed out to you at the time of purchase, or if the

fault was obvious when you bought it, you cannot complain about it.

4. No, you do not have to have a receipt. All the trader will require is proof of the purchase price or the date of purchase. So a cheque stub, bank statement or credit card slip should be sufficient.

Complaints procedures

Consumers have clearly defined rights when purchasing goods and services. But sometimes things go wrong and in these circumstances the consumer should take the following steps to complain effectively:

- Make sure that all the facts are correct.

- Go back to the shop as soon as possible. Take the receipt or some other proof of purchase.

- Explain the problem and say what you expect. Be calm but firm. Show your invoice or receipt but do not part with them as you may need them later. Make a note of what was agreed – what the trader agreed to do and the timescale.

- If necessary, speak to someone in a position of authority and get their name.

- If the shop is part of a larger organisation, write to the head office. Address the letter to customer services or to the managing director or chairman. In the letter describe the item or service, say where it was purchased from and what the costs involved are. Explain the complaint, any action that has already been taken, to whom you have already spoken and what happened. Explain what is expected such as a refund or repair or the job done again. Send the letter by recorded delivery to ensure it is delivered. Keep a copy of any letters sent and do not send original documents such as the receipt. It may also be relevant to take photographs to substantiate your complaint, especially if the complaint is concerning a holiday or sub-standard workmanship.

- If nothing happens within a reasonable time, either send another letter or better still telephone with all the details to hand. Make a note of the date, time and to whom you are speaking.

- If the complaint is still not resolved, it may be necessary to involve other organisations.

- If the trader is a member of a **trade association**, or is covered by a code of practice, write to the trade association detailing the action that has been taken.

- If the outcome is still unsatisfactory, conciliation and arbitration can be considered.

Activity 5

Review

Imagine you have paid for a new patio to be laid. The builders have laid the patio and you notice that the slabs are uneven. Draft a letter of complaint to the building company explaining what action you now require. Quote the relevant legislation to back up your case.

Conciliation

The idea of conciliation is to enable the parties to settle their differences themselves. It does not result in a legally binding decision, and if you are not satisfied with the outcome, you can go to arbitration or to court. Conciliation usually involves trade associations who help resolve disputes and encourage both sides to agree on a compromise. It is free and informal. You should use conciliation if you have a consumer complaint, your opponent is part of a trade association and you are prepared to take the matter to court if the outcome is unsatisfactory.

Arbitration

Arbitration is often a straight alternative to court, in that both sides agree to put their disputes (usually in writing) to an independent arbitrator. The arbitrator then consider the evidence in the same way as a judge and make a decision which is final and binding. The arbitrator will be an expert in the particular field concerned and may be a member of the Chartered Institute of Arbitrators. There are a number of consumer arbitration schemes around for members of specific associations such as ABTA for holiday disputes. This is not free and if you do not like the arbitrator's decision you cannot then go to court. Arbitration can be used if a trade association suggests it, if you are happier presenting your case on paper or you are willing to abide by the outcome.

Court action

This is a last resort if all else has failed. If you are claiming compensation and the amount is for £15,000 or less, you can use the small claims court. The procedure is designed to be used without either side having to go to a solicitor and therefore is inexpensive. However, people are advised not to take action unless you can reasonably prove or back up your claim. Make sure you have receipts and any correspondence. Two of the types of claim most commonly heard in the small claims court are:

- compensation for faulty services provided, for example, by builders, dry cleaners and garages
- compensation for faulty goods, for example, televisions or washing machines which go wrong.

Before you apply to court, it will expect you to make your claim in writing, giving the other person a reasonable time to reply – a month is usual. You should also warn them that you will take court action if they fail to reply. To initiate the court action the claim form needs to be filled in detailing the **claimant's** name and address, the **defendant** and a brief statement of the case. The claim form should be sent or taken to the local county court which will then serve the papers on the defendant. Fees will depend on the amount claimed and these are paid by the opponent if the consumer wins.

If the above measures do not resolve the dispute, the final course of action may be to consult a solicitor.

Activity 6

Review

Fill in the gaps using the words at the end.

Usually when you buy something from a shop you will be satisfied with your purchases. However, sometimes it is necessary to return an item. When this happens the shop —————— should be helpful. If they are not, then it helps considerably if you know your ——————. One of the most common complaints occurs when a consumer returns a faulty good to a shop and an offer is made to —————— or replace it. In many cases this is what the consumer wants. If the goods had actually been faulty though, the consumer has the right to demand a —————— The situation becomes complicated if the receipt for the good has been ——————. This does not mean that you lose your rights. You are still entitled to a refund for —————— goods, but the shop must be satisfied that you actually —————— the goods from them. If you have absolutely no —————— of purchase then it is more difficult to prove you bought the goods from them, so it is better to —————— on to the receipt.

All of this refers to the return of faulty goods. However if you wish to return an item because you have —————— your mind, the shop has the right to refuse a refund or even an ——————. If they agree to either it is an act of —————————— on their part. Most shops do this because they want to build a —————————— for being helpful. Confusion sometimes occurs over goods bought in ——————————. Some people think that they cannot return sale items, yet they can. If a shop decides to —————————— the price of an item in order to sell it more —————————— this does not mean that the consumer does not have rights. They can still demand a refund on anything which is faulty so long as the goods was not —————————— as imperfect in the first place.

advertised	sales	reduce	easily
rights	assistant	reputation	goodwill
exchange	changed	full refund	hold
faulty	bought	proof	repair
lost			

Activity 7

Check your understanding

Check your understanding of the meaning of the following terms:

consumer	conciliation	legislation
consumer	trader	services
redress	goods	trade
association	compensation	claimant
defendant		

Purchasing

Consumers like to make informed choices when purchasing goods in order to gain value for money. If time allows, it can be useful to look in a range of retail outlets or find out information from a variety of sources to be certain that you can obtain the goods that match your needs at the best possible price.

Range of retail outlets available for food

There is a wide variety of retail outlets selling food:
- supermarkets
- the internet
- specialist shops
- local markets
- organic box schemes
- small corner shops.

Provision can vary according to the location you live in.

According to statistics, the number of purchases carried out via the internet is increasing rapidly, and at present it accounts for 3 per cent of total household expenditure.

The most popular retail outlet for purchasing food is a large supermarket. According to Social Trends, household expenditure at large supermarket chains was more than double that at other outlets in 2005–6.

£ per week		
	Large supermarkets	Other outlets
Alcoholic drinks	4.00	2.20
Non-alcoholic drinks	2.70	1.10
Bread, rice, cereals	2.90	1.20
Fresh fruit	2.20	0.70
Fresh vegetables	2.60	0.80
Chocolate and confectionery	1.10	0.80

Source: Adapted from Social Trends 37, Table 6.8

Household expenditure on selected items by place of purchase 2005–6 in the UK

Activity 9

Research opportunity and group discussion

Choose a retail outlet and complete this table by inserting the current price.

	1971	1991	2006	Now
500 g back bacon	37p	£2.35	£3.77	
250 g cheddar cheese	13p	86p	£1.42	
1 dozen large eggs	26p	£1.18	£1.81	
800 g white sliced bread	10p	53p	81p	
1 pint milk	5p	32p	35p	
1 kg granulated sugar	9p	66p	74p	
100 g instant coffee	25p	£1.30	£1.89	
250 g tea bags	n/a	£1.50	£1.49	

Source: Adapted from Social trends 37, Table 6.17

Discuss your findings.

Advantages and disadvantages of retail outlets

Advantages of supermarkets

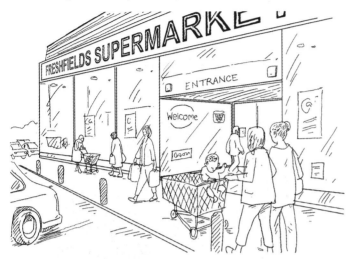

Figure 9.7 *A supermarket*

Busy working people may find supermarkets convenient because they can buy everything they need in one place.

Supermarkets offer a wide variety of food choice at competitive prices, largely because of the scale of their purchasing power.

Loyalty cards are available at many major food retailers which require customers to register in the scheme and then to present their card every time they make a purchase. Each time the card is used, points are awarded which can ultimately be redeemed for discounts off purchases in store, for vouchers which can be exchanged for travel or holiday discounts or admission to tourist attractions and cinemas. Each major food retailer has a slightly different scheme but they all offer discounts that build up when making regular purchases. These cards can also be used to take advantage of further in-store discounts, which is a way of rewarding those consumers who shop regularly enough to participate in the scheme.

Food retailers use the information that they gain from loyalty card schemes to create a huge database of information about their customers' buying habits. This then allows them opportunities to respond more effectively to customer requirements and tailor their goods and services more appropriately to what customers want.

Some supermarkets offer vouchers to enable customers to buy petrol or diesel at discounted prices according to how much they spend in the store.

Families with young children may choose to shop when the children are with a childminder, at school or with a relative. However, if it is necessary to shop with children, parents often choose supermarkets because there are usually some facilities to make the process easier. The facilities include special wide parking places near to the shop entrance with the space to open a car door wide. There are also shopping trolleys with a variety of seating arrangements for babies and young children, including trolleys attached to small cars and ride-in vehicles. Some supermarkets sell children's clothes in addition to all the usual food and household items.

Some supermarkets offer fast-track shopping by allowing customers to scan their own shopping using small hand-held scanners. The information is then downloaded at the checkout and the shopping paid for in the usual way.

Goods are transported to the checkout on a conveyor belt that minimises the handling necessary to progress through the payment system.

A variety of trolleys are available and are designed to be easy to use. These include motorised trolleys for disabled shoppers and new plastic trolleys that are lightweight and designed to steer correctly and run very smoothly.

A ticket system with a corresponding illuminated number ensures that customers are served in order when direct service is necessary, such as when cooked meats are carved.

Some supermarkets offer vouchers for school equipment such as sports equipment and computers.

Facilities are offered in stores to make shopping more comfortable, convenient and enjoyable such as a coffee shop, restaurant, children's play area, toilets and telephone for taxi services.

Supermarkets frequently have promotions where discounted food is offered such as 'buy one, get one free' and 'buy one, get the second half price'.

Disadvantages of supermarkets

Some supermarkets are situated outside main towns so they are easily accessible by road but not as easily accessible by bus. Some supermarkets operate a free bus service but this may not be at suitable times.

Some of the discount schemes such as 'buy one, get one free' may prove too attractive to resist and consumers may buy these products when they do not really need them. If the offer is on a product with a short shelf-life, consumers need to ensure that they will use the product before the use by date expires.

For those consumers concerned about the environment, food miles and carbon footprints, they may find that some products, particularly fruit and vegetables, are flown in from abroad.

It can sometimes be more difficult to buy local produce and support local food producers and farmers in supermarkets.

Supermarkets have been accused of price fixing. Newspapers have reported that the price of dairy products such as cheese and milk have been fixed at a high price.

Some people are concerned about the massive growth of supermarkets and the fact that they have become very powerful organisations and are therefore too well placed to influence our shopping habits.

Advantages of the internet

Using the internet means there is no need to visit a shop, saving both fuel and time. This is useful for busy people. The goods bought are delivered to the door at a set time, usually within either a one or two hour slot.

It is possible to shop for all normal groceries on the internet.

Previous purchases and shopping lists are always saved so each time you shop they are quick to refer back to.

It is very useful for families, particularly with children, when large quantities of food would be bought at one time. It avoids having to push a heavy trolley, loading bags to the car and unloading bags from the car at home.

Some supermarkets offer incentives such as a £10 voucher if they are late delivering your food.

Carrier bags can be returned to the driver for recycling.

Disadvantages of the internet

There are charges made for delivery (on average £5), but with some stores if you choose off-peak times and days, it can cost less.

It is still not a popular method of shopping for most people who prefer to be able to select their goods for themselves.

Sometimes products are unavailable and that is only apparent when the food is delivered, which can be inconvenient.

Access to a computer is obviously essential.

Advantages of specialist shops

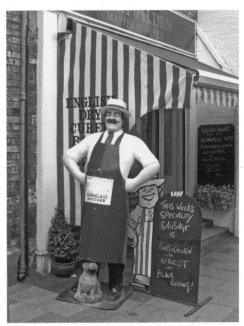

Figure 9.8 *A specialist butcher's shop*

Specialist shops include butchers, bakers, greengrocers, fishmongers, farm shops. They are likely to be situated in small towns or local shopping centres where one trip to the shopping centre can mean that a variety of these shops can be visited.

Many farm shops are diversifying. They are selling a wide variety of local produce and offering facilities such as pick your own produce, coffee shops, toilets and activities for children such as farm walks, treasure hunts, feeding chickens and play parks. This makes a trip to a farm shop a fun activity and provides a pleasurable morning or afternoon.

Specialist shops can offer specialist knowledge and advice. Staff offer expertise, for example, in boning joints and filleting fish.

Specialist shops can offer a more personal service, which many people prefer.

They are more likely to sell local produce therefore supporting local farmers.

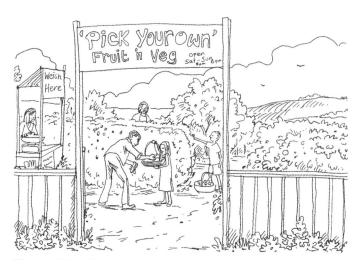

Figure 9.9 *Pick your own produce*

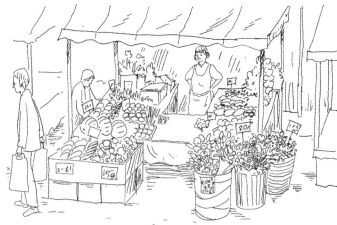

Figure 9.10 *A street market stall*

Disadvantages of specialist shops

Specialist shops can be less accessible because you may have to visit a number of different shops and walk some distance to get to them and then carry heavy bags.

Farm shops are situated in rural areas and generally access can only be gained by car.

There are not as many specialist shops open as there used to be and their trade can suffer if people use the supermarkets for all their purchases.

The problem with small specialist shops is that they tend to be more expensive because they cannot compete with the prices of the major supermarkets.

They are not normally open for long hours and are often closed on Sundays (the exception being farm shops).

Advantages of local markets

Local markets are either farmers markets or street markets. They frequently offer good, fresh produce at reasonable prices. If you live in the country or travel to work on country roads, it might be possible to buy a variety of foods. Eggs, meat and potatoes are most usual and fruit in season direct from a producer operating farm-gate retail sales.

The produce is fresh and detailed information about its production is usually available.

There is less of a carbon footprint and fewer air miles in that the food is not usually flown in from abroad.

This system removes the 'middle man' as the food often comes direct from the producer. This gives the producer or farmer and the consumer a better deal as there are fewer extra costs.

Disadvantages of local markets

Markets are often only available on certain days and for limited hours. This limitation can be a problem for people working long hours. During poor weather, consumers may not wish to visit markets.

Advantages of organic box schemes

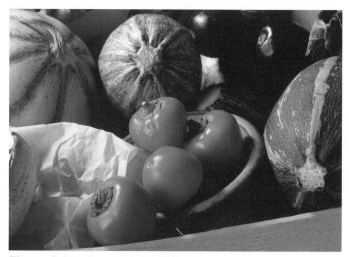

Figure 9.11 *An organic box delivery*

You pay a fixed price for a box of vegetables.

The vegetables are delivered to your door.

The vegetables are organically produced which will mean that chemicals have not been used in the growing process.

Disadvantages of organic box schemes

The vegetables are seasonal and you have to take what is available. This may not suit everyone as there may be vegetables that you do not like, or you may not have the type of vegetables you require for weekly meals.

It can be expensive because you are paying for a product which is organically produced.

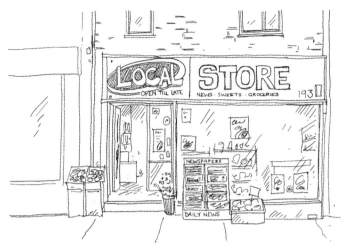

Figure 9.12 *A small 'corner shop'*

Activity 10

Taste testing

Obtain a selection of non-organic and organic foods such as carrots, crisps, chocolate and apples.

Carry out some **difference testing**. Use the table below as a guide and complete one for each food tasted, making comments for each sample about its appearance, flavour, texture and taste.

Food	Sample A	Sample B
Appearance		
Flavour		
Texture		
Taste		

Which sample is the organic sample? Is it A or B? Why do you think so?

Evaluate your findings. What does this tell you about the difference between organic and non-organic foods?

---

hours because of working shifts or at weekends. These shops are usually open seven days a week and some are open until very late at night.

They are very useful for items that might be needed in an emergency.

Local corner stores or petrol station shops are available in most urban areas.

You are less likely to end up buying more than you need because you are less likely to impulse buy or be attracted by offers such as 'buy one, get one free'.

Disadvantages of small corner shops

They usually only stock a limited range of foods.

The foods are generally quite expensive so you pay for the convenience.

They are not usually situated in rural areas.

Activity 11

Research opportunity

Carry out some research on the availability and cost of organic foods at a supermarket of your choice.

Write a report on your findings, considering whether organic foods are economically viable for the average family.

Advantages of small corner shops

Most small corner shops keep very long opening hours, making it possible for people to shop before they go to work, after they finish work, on a day off, at irregular

---

Activity 12

Research opportunity and group discussion

List the range of retail outlets available for shopping in your locality.

Visit one of these outlets and make a note of the following points:

- standards of food safety and hygiene
- friendliness and helpfulness of the shop assistants
- availability of quality produce
- value for money
- convenience in terms of accessibility and opening hours

• any additional services offered to customers (delivery of goods to customers' homes).

Write a report on your findings.

Discuss and compare your findings with the rest of the group.

Activity 13

Review

Summarise in the table below (or draw one up of your own) two advantages and two disadvantages of the following retail outlets

Retail outlet	Advantages	Disadvantages
Supermarkets		
Internet		
Specialist shops		
Local markets		
Organic box schemes		
Small corner shops		

Activity 14

Check your understanding

Check your understanding of the meaning of the following terms:

retail outlet   **organic**   **difference testing**

Dietary guidelines

The aim of dietary guidance is to improve the health of the population. Poor health can be associated with the overconsumption or underconsumption of certain foods. The government issues recommendations on the types of food we should eat and the ideal proportions of those foods.

To help people understand this guidance, foods with similar nutritional values are grouped together. This has been shown as a diagram of a plate of food (the Eatwell plate). The proportions of each food group to be consumed are shown as segments of the plate. The largest segments on the plate show the food groups that should be consumed in the greatest quantity.

The Eatwell plate

The Eatwell plate (shown in Chapter 6) is the new version of the Balance of Good Health plate. The Food Standards Agency produced this updated version with help from health professionals and educators. The Eatwell plate shows how much should be eaten from each food group for meals and snacks.

With two exceptions, the Eatwell plate does not include references to the number of servings or the recommended portion sizes of the food to be eaten. The first exception is fruit and vegetables. The advice is that a wide variety of fruit and vegetables should be consumed and at least five portions a day. The second exception is fish. The advice is to eat two portions of fish a week, one of which should be oily.

People have individual nutritional requirements and it could be misleading to generalise on portion sizes and frequency of consumption.

Many foods we eat are purchased ready to eat such as sandwiches and cook-chilled meals. These products may contain a combination of foods from more than one of the five food groups. They are sometimes referred to as **composite foods**. People need to consider the main ingredients in these products and identify where on the Eatwell plate they should be placed. Products which are high in fat and sugar should not be consumed in large quantities.

The Eatwell plate is divided into five segments. Segment proportions are divided into the five food groups. The percentages are approximate proportions.

Bread, rice, potatoes, pasta and other starchy foods	33%
Fruit and vegetables	33%
Milk and dairy foods	15%
Meat, fish, eggs, beans and other non-dairy sources of protein	12%
Foods and drinks high in fat and/or sugar	7%

Activity 15

Review

Using the percentages above as a guide, draw and label your own version of the Eatwell plate showing examples of foods that you enjoy and eat frequently.

Most people receive all the nutrients they require by eating a variety of foods, in the proportions shown on the Eatwell plate. However, some people require supplements. For example, pregnant women are advised to eat more folic acid to reduce the risk of spina bifida developing in the unborn child. This advice applies to the time before conception and during the early months of pregnancy. **Spina bifida** means 'split spine'. The bones in the spine (vertebrae) do not form properly in early pregnancy. The nerves in the spine may be unprotected, causing damage to the nervous system.

In addition to the Eatwell plate, the government has other guidelines which individuals and households should aim to follow. These are the eight practical tips for healthy eating issued by the Food Standards Agency:

1. Base meals on starchy foods.
2. Eat lots of fruit and vegetables.
3. Eat more fish.
4. Cut down on saturated fat and sugar.
5. Try to eat less salt and no more than 6 g a day.
6. Get active and keep a healthy weight.
7. Drink plenty of water.
8. Do not skip breakfast.

You will now examine how food purchases can meet these dietary guidelines.

Meals based on starchy foods

Starchy foods consist of bread, rice, pasta, potatoes and breakfast cereals. Starchy foods are filling and provide energy. They should be the main part of every meal and chosen as snacks. Starchy foods should make up about a third of the food consumed. As well as providing energy, starchy foods provide fibre, calcium, iron and B vitamins. Wholegrain varieties of starchy foods are an excellent source of fibre and are slowly digested so they help us feel full for longer.

There are several ways to increase the intake of fibre:

- purchase wholegrain cereals such as brown rice
- purchase wholemeal pasta and noodles
- add a portion of wholemeal flour to plain during home baking

- purchase wholemeal or granary type bread
- add pulses such as peas, beans or lentils to stews, soups and casseroles
- purchase high-fibre breakfast cereals such as muesli, bran flakes or porridge.

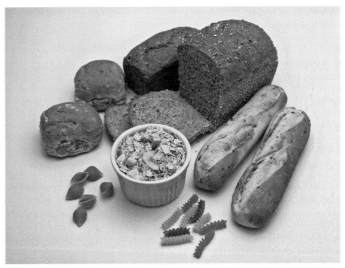

Figure 9.13 *A selection of wholemeal foods*

When choosing wholegrain breakfast cereals, check they are low in sugar. Starch contains less than half the calories of fat. Care should be taken not to add fat when cooking and serving starches because this will increase the energy content.

Eat more fruit and vegetables

It is suggested that five portions or handfuls of fruit and vegetables should be eaten each day. Each portion should be 80 g. Fruit and vegetables provide important vitamins and minerals which have been suggested protect against cancer.

There is a wide variety of fruit and vegetables available and these can be fresh, frozen, tinned, dried or juiced. Potatoes are a starchy food and do not count as a portion of fruit and vegetables.

Activity 16

Research opportunity

Research the range of fruit and vegetables available in your local community in supermarkets and markets.

Then investigate the range of fresh products and the types of processed versions available (tinned, frozen, dried).

Plan and prepare some dishes which demonstrate the versatility of the different types of fruit and vegetables.

There are several ways to increase fruit and vegetable intake:

- purchase a variety including the processed versions and use them in meals and snacks
- eat fresh fruit with the skins left on if possible
- eat fresh vegetables and leave the skins on during cooking
- serve larger portions of vegetables with meals
- prepare dishes with extra vegetables – canned tomatoes, carrots, turnips and mushrooms
- purchase fruit to serve with breakfast cereals – prunes, chopped apple, sultanas.

Fresh fruit and vegetables should not be stored for long periods of time as the vitamin content will fall. There are some preparation methods which can help minimise the loss of vitamins and minerals. Avoid leaving cut vegetables open to the air. Always cover and chill them. Do not soak fruit and vegetables in water because the water-soluble vitamins B and C can dissolve away.

The best cooking method for vegetables is to steam lightly and eat while they are still slightly crunchy. When boiling vegetables always start the process in a pan of boiling water and cover tightly to keep in the steam and speed up the cooking process. Use as little water as possible and save the water once cooking is completed. Use the 'vegetable' water for soup, stock or gravy to benefit from the nutrients dissolved in the water. Do not overcook vegetables. Stir frying and microwaving minimise vitamin loss as they are quick and involve little, if any, water. Serve cooked vegetables immediately. Do not let them stand too long so that they require reheating.

Eat more fish

The consumption of fresh white fish has fallen in recent years. Fish is an excellent source of protein and it contains many vitamins and minerals. Oily fish including sardines, mackerel and salmon are good sources of certain types of omega 3 fatty acids. Omega 3 fatty acids may help to reduce the risk of heart disease.

The guidelines suggest we should aim to eat at least two portions of fish a week, including a portion of oily fish. Guidance for pregnant women is slightly different and they should have a maximum of two portions of oily fish a week (a portion is about 140 g). Marine fish including shark and swordfish should be completely avoided by pregnant women as they may contain mercury. Mercury may harm a baby's developing nervous system.

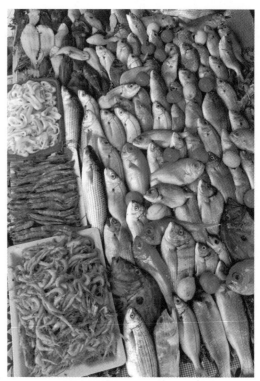

Figure 9.14 *A selection of fish*

Fish can be bought fresh, frozen or canned. Canned and smoked fish can be high in salt so consider this when making purchases. Avoid products in brine.

There are several ways to increase fish intake:

- purchase tuna or salmon for a sandwich filling
- try part-prepared fish products which require grilling or baking – marinated tuna steaks
- add shellfish to a stir fry vegetable dish
- try barbecuing sardines or making fish kebabs
- add cooked salmon or shellfish to a pasta sauce
- try smoked fish in a rice dish – kedgeree
- purchase ready-made fish soups
- use a tinned fish product for lunch – sardines on toast.

When preparing fish you should choose cooking methods which involve poaching, baking or grilling rather than frying. Fried fish has a high fat content.

Cut down on saturated fat

Fats are an important part of a healthy diet. The possible role of fat in the development of coronary heart disease was explored in detail in Chapter 6.

There are two main types of fat:

- **Saturated fat:** Too much saturated fat in the diet can increase the amount of cholesterol in the blood, which increases the chance of developing heart disease. Saturated fat is found in butter, coconut oil, hard cheeses, cream, pastries, cakes and biscuits.

- **Unsaturated fat**: Unsaturated fat can lower blood cholesterol. Fats which are rich in unsaturated fatty acids include sunflower and olive oil, oily fish, avocados, nuts and seeds.

NUTRITIONAL INFORMATION

	Per 100 g	Per 50 g serving
Energy	1669 kJ	835 kJ
Protein	4.6 g	2.3 g
Carbohydrates	81.6 g	40.8 g
Fat	5.5 g	2.7 g
of which saturates	3.4 g	1.7 g
Sodium	0.4 g	0.2 g

Figure 9.15 *A food label showing nutritional information*

The food label can indicate the amount of fat in a product. It is usually expressed in grams (g) of fat present in 100 g of the food product. Some foods state the amount of saturated fat or 'saturates' in the product.

The Food Standards Agency issues the following guidelines to help consumers classify foods according to their fat content.

The total fat content:
- **High** is more than 20 g fat per 100 g.
- **Low** is 3 g fat or less per 100 g.

Saturated fat content:
- **High** is more than 5 g saturates per 100 g.
- **Low** is 1.5 g saturates or less per 100 g.

To meet the dietary guidelines when purchasing food containing fat, try to cut down on products that are high in saturated fat. Choose products that are virtually fat-free or the low fat versions products.

There are several ways to reduce fat intake:
- Eat more white fish and chicken rather than red meat.
- Buy lean cuts of meat and trim off the fat.
- Remove the skin from chicken.
- Use stock cubes or gravy powder to make gravy rather than fatty juices from roast meat.
- In casseroles, soups and stews use less red meat and add more beans, pulses or vegetables.

- Eat less fried or roasted food, but if frying is necessary, use sunflower oil and a minimal amount of oil.
- Invest in a good quality non-stick frying pan as it will reduce the amount of oil required or allow dry frying.
- Use the following cooking methods: bake, microwave, dry roast, dry fry, grill, steam or poach.
- Choose skimmed or semi-skimmed milk instead of full fat.
- Opt for low fat versions of natural yogurt, fromage frais or crème fraiche instead of cream.
- Use tomato or vegetable-based pasta sauces rather than cream or cheese based ones.
- Buy the reduced fat varieties of spread, butter, yoghurt, salad dressings and cheese.
- Cut out or reduce the quantity of takeaway food eaten – burgers, fried chicken.
- Avoid snacks which are high in fat – biscuits, cakes, pastries and chocolate.
- Use spices, herbs, lemon juice and vinegar which are low fat ways of flavouring food, or use soy sauce, Worcestershire sauce, fresh chillies, fresh ginger or garlic to add flavour.

Cut down on sugar

Many people need to reduce sugar consumption. Sugar is found in a range of foods. It is added to cakes, drinks, confectionery and biscuits.

A high sugar intake has been associated with tooth decay. It can cause weight gain if eaten in large amounts and the excess energy is not used by the body. Rather, it will be stored as fat.

To meet dietary guidelines when buying food, always read the label. The labelling of sugar is voluntary unless a product claims to be low in sugar. Sugars which are added to food products during the manufacturing process are known as **non-milk extrinsic sugars**. Non-milk extrinsic sugars are sometimes called added sugars. These are found in cakes, biscuits, fizzy drinks, soups and breakfast cereals, canned food including baked beans, pizzas and pasta sauces. They are more harmful to teeth.

Sugar can also be described as sucrose, glucose, fructose, maltose, hydrolysed starch and invert sugar, corn syrup and honey. If these ingredients appear near the top of the list of ingredients, the food is likely to be high in added sugar.

Research evidence from *Which?*, the independent consumer magazine, found some savoury foods contain more sugar than ice cream. It reported in April 2007 that ready meals such as Asda's sticky chilli chicken and Tesco's crispy beef with sweet chilli sauce contained 19.2 g and 23.1 g of sugar per 100 g respectively. The supermarket own brand vanilla ice cream by comparison contained 17.9 g of sugar per 100 g.

The carbohydrate content on the label can also provide a clue to the sugar content. This is the carbohydrates 'of which sugars' figure on the label. The Food Standards Agency suggests a product should be classed as follows:

- **High** is more than 15 g sugars per 100 g.
- **Low** is 5 g sugars or less per 100 g.

It can be misleading as sometimes the labelling only shows the total 'carbohydrates'. The carbohydrates 'of which sugars' is not shown. This can make it difficult to identify the amount of sugar in the product.

There are several ways to reduce sugar intake:

- Adjust to the taste of hot drinks without sugar or use an artificial sweetener.
- Reduce consumption of cakes, sweets and chocolates.
- Buy fresh fruit instead of ready-made puddings or desserts.
- Cut down on the amount of sugar used to sweeten home-baked dishes.
- Buy foods with less or no added sugar – tinned fruit in natural juices.
- Try sugar-free products in drinks and jellies.

Eat less salt

Salt is added to many processed foods. Most of the salt we eat is already added breakfast cereals, soups, sauces and ready meals. The dietary guidelines suggest we should consume no more than 6 g a day for adults. Eating too much salt can raise blood pressure. This increases the likelihood of developing heart disease or having a stroke.

Food labels often indicate the amount of salt in a food product. This could be expressed as sodium. Once again guidance from the Food Standards Agency indicates how the different levels of salt can be classed:

- **High** is more than 1.5 g salt per 100 g (or 0.6 g sodium).
- **Low** is 0.3 g salt or less per 100 g (or 0.1 g sodium).

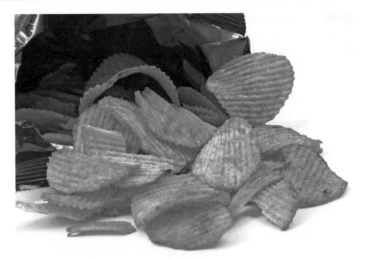

Figure 9.16 *Crisps are high in salt*

There are several ways to reduce salt intake:
- Reduce the amount of salt used in cooking vegetables, stews and soups.
- Use herbs and spices to season.
- Taste before adding to a meal.
- Read labels and purchase the lower salt version if available.
- Try a 'low sodium' table salt.
- Cut down on snacks with a high salt content – crisps or salted nuts.
- Buy low-salt or unsalted butter or spreads.
- Make your own sandwiches, savoury snacks as processed food is high in salt.
- Avoid foods served in brine.

Get active and try to be a healthy weight

We explored the risks associated with obesity in Chapter 6 on health. Being overweight can cause heart disease, high blood pressure and type 2 diabetes. There are many products available to help individuals follow slimming diets and some people find special low fat and sugar products helpful in controlling their energy intake. These products can be more expensive than conventional versions. Eating more wholegrain products which are lower in energy and filling can also be useful. Exercise is important in maintaining a healthy weight as any excess energy from food is used up. The key message is to 'eat less and do more' to help maintain a healthy weight.

Drink plenty of water

We should be drinking about 1.2 litres of water or other fluids every day to prevent dehydration. Water makes up 50 to 70 per cent of an adult's total body weight.

It is important not to consume drinks that are high in sugar. The sale of bottled water has increased dramatically over the past decade. However, the Consumer Council for Water claims that tap water is just as healthy as the bottled variety. It does far less damage to the environment and is at least 500 times cheaper.

Guidelines exist for the consumption of alcohol. The frequent drinking of large quantities of alcohol can cause health problems. In the Chapter 6 you explored these effects in detail. The current guidelines issued by the Department of Health state that women can drink up to two or three units of alcohol a day and men up to three or four units a day, without significant risk to their health.

A unit of alcohol is half a pint of standard strength (3 to 5 per cent alcohol by volume) of beer, lager or cider, or a measure of spirit. A large glass of wine is about two units. Men should drink no more than 21 units of alcohol per week and women no more than 14 units.

When making purchases it is important to consider these guidelines. The consumption of low alcohol or alcohol-free products may be desirable. The latest advice from the government is that pregnant women and women trying to become pregnant should not drink at all.

Do not skip breakfast

Breakfast is regarded as the most important meal of the day by many health professionals. Research has suggested that people who do not eat breakfast are more likely to lead unhealthy lifestyles. People who do not eat breakfast are more likely to snack on foods that are high in fat and sugar, such as biscuits, doughnuts or pastries. Breakfast provides an important boost of energy at the start of the day, as well as important vitamins and minerals.

The selection of food products available to purchase for breakfast is vast. When making these purchases it is important to consider the sugar, dietary fibre, fat and salt content of the products offered.

Breakfast cereals are available to suit virtually all preferences, from high sugar products aimed at children to low fat, cholesterol, sugar and salt products aimed at more health-conscious consumers. Bread and pastry products exist to suit a variety of lifestyles and nutritional demands. These products include a crustless loaf of bread for a busy parent with a fussy child, gluten-free 'pastries' for coeliacs, part-baked baguettes, speciality breads, organic breads and breads with added omega 3.

Activity 16

Research opportunity

Investigate the range of breakfast cereals available in supermarkets. Then consider the potential market and the nutritional claims made.

Draw some conclusions from the products you analyse.

Activity 17

ICT opportunity

Produce an information leaflet or a PowerPoint presentation that outlines the dietary guidelines discussed in this chapter. Offer advice on how to achieve them for a parent with young children.

The management of food resources

We have already identified the current dietary guidelines and described how they can be applied to the purchasing and preparation of food. We will now explain how to put into practice these considerations when managing food for different individual and household needs.

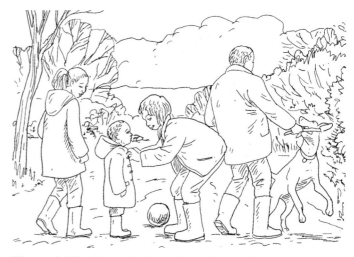

Figure 9.17 *A busy family needs a balanced diet*

In order to achieve the dietary guidelines some people may need to make changes to their patterns of eating. These changes may include eating breakfast every day and reducing the consumption of alcohol.

Achieving a balanced diet in practice for busy families with young children could mean the following meals.

Meal	Food to be eaten	Reason for choice
Breakfast	Puffed rice based breakfast cereal	Starch-based breakfast with no added sugar during processing. Parent adds sugar if required
	Whole milk	Children need energy so whole milk acceptable. Provides fat-soluble vitamin and calcium
	Low fat fruit yogurt	Yoghurt is easy for child to eat and contains calcium and low fat. Different fruit flavours to widen child's palate
Snack	Small apple	Portion of fruit (1)
Lunch	Sliced bread with added fibre	Starch-based lunch. Use bread with added fibre which looks like white bread and may be more appealing to children
	Sunflower spread	Low in saturated fat
	Corned beef	High in iron. High in fat but meets child's energy needs
	Sugar-free jelly in a tub	Easy for child to eat and sugar-free which reduces risk of tooth decay
	Handful of grapes	Portion of fruit (2)
	Water or sugar free squash	Water to drink
Snack	Homemade fruit smoothie	Portion of fruit (3). Use hand-held blender, a homemade version has no added sugar. Children involved in the preparation as they may be more interested in trying new flavours
Dinner	Fish fingers	Portion of white fish grilled. Fish provides protein for growth
	Baked potato wedges	Potatoes provide starch and with skins left on for vitamin retention. Baked without fat
	Peas/sweet corn	Portion of vegetables (4). Microwaved for speed and no salt
	Ice cream and tinned fruit	Portion of fruit (5) in juice not syrup. Ice cream is high in sugar but provides energy if served as part of low energy meal. Ice cream is straight from freezer which saves time. Easy to prepare for busy parent
Snack	Breadstick or rice cake	Low in sugar and fat

Wider issues for the management of food resources

When managing food resources for households and individuals it is important to consider some wider issues.

The time, equipment or storage available may influence food choice and preparation. Those with limited time and equipment may rely heavily on convenience foods.

The financial status of the household or individual is also important. A low income may reduce choice and make meal planning more challenging. Limited transport can restrict access to food and limit choice.

The capabilities of the cook should also be considered. A lack of confidence, skill or knowledge may influence the management of food resources. There could be a greater reliance on ready-made products or takeaway foods.

The health of the individual is very important. Ill health may result in poor management of food resources if consumers are unable to shop and prepare food.

Meeting special dietary needs can add a financial burden to household food expenditure if special gluten-free or soya-based products have to be purchased frequently.

Activity 18

Review and practical opportunity

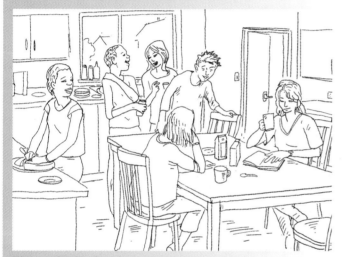

Figure 9.18 *Students in a multi-person household*

Devise a day's meals for each of the following groups:
- a single-person household – the elderly
- a multi-person household – students

Consider the dietary guidelines:
- Base meals on starchy foods.
- Eat lots of fruit and vegetables.
- Eat more fish.
- Cut down on saturated fat and sugar.
- Try to eat less salt and no more than 6 g a day.
- Drink plenty of water.
- Do not skip breakfast.

Consider some wider issues that each household could encounter in their food choices.

Plan and prepare one of the meals or snacks.

Activity 19

Check your understanding

Check your understanding of the meaning of the following terms:

dietary guidelines	non-milk extrinsic sugars
Eatwell plate	starchy foods
spina bifida	composite food

Sources of information

There are many sources of information available to the consumer in order to assist them in making the right choice of product or service.

Media consumer reports

These are becoming more and more widely available to the consumer. They have the advantage that they are more likely to be **impartial** and not **biased** and can be a real help in making a decision. Often a substantial amount of information is documented regarding the **specification** and price or the product. Sometimes comparisons are carried out and products graded against relevant **criteria**. Many specialist magazines will produce the results of recent testing they have carried out, such as *Good Food* magazine, *Practical Parenting* magazine and *Which?* magazine.

Television programmes

Television is available to most families and is a valuable source of information. Sometimes specialist programmes are made regarding certain products and which will inform about 'big' issues that can help you make a decision about your own situation. Information is usually current and accurate. Examples of such programmes are *Panorama*, *Dispatches* and *Watchdog*. *Watchdog* and programmes like *Rogue Traders* flag up and expose disreputable retailers, unsafe items and dishonest tradesmen. The widespread use of cable television also enables consumers to tune into shopping channels. These can be helpful because they regularly demonstrate products so consumers can see what they can actually do.

Internet

More and more people have access to the internet. Consumers can use the internet to research, purchase and view or 'talk' to others in a similar situation and gather relevant information. The consumer can contact manufacturers' sites and receive accurate information concerning specifications and price.

Consumer helplines

Consumer helplines can provide the consumer with a one-to-one discussion and expert advice.

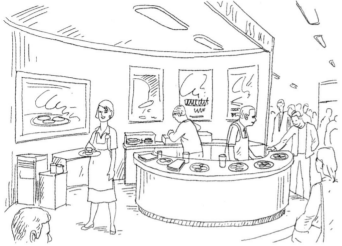

Figure 9.19 *A stand at a consumer exhibition*

Consumer exhibitions

Local and national exhibitions offer specialist advice about a range of items and products that may be of interest to the consumer. These can highlight issues of relevance and offer advice about suppliers within the locality. National exhibitions can be extremely valuable for gathering up-to-date information from a host of suppliers. Special offers are often available and innovative new products are displayed and demonstrated under one roof – for example, the Ideal Home Exhibition or Good Food Show.

Advertising

Advertising is used to encourage people to buy goods and services. It informs consumers about existing and new products and describes and gives details about goods and services. It should be remembered though that advertising, like any form of communication, is aimed at consumers by manufacturers, retailers and providers of services. Their main purpose is to sell goods and services.

Overt advertising is obvious in the form of TV and radio commercials, newspaper and magazine adverts, internet adverts, flyers and programme and film trailers.

Marketing strategies and methods

Food products need to be promoted to generate sales and profits for food retailers. There are two main methods used to promote a food product to a consumer. Within each method there is a range of promotional activities used. First, we will explore the basic methods.

Above the line

This is advertising through independent media. It is expensive and usually involves advertising on television or the radio or in newspapers and magazines. It can be very effective as there may be coverage to a wide audience. Brand loyalty can be built upon and a carefully controlled image of the product can be created.

Below the line

This is promotion by less expensive methods such as direct mail, brochures, flyers, coupons and packaging. It does not involve advertising by the independent media. Various promotional techniques are used by food retailers and manufacturers to build awareness of their products and influence shoppers to purchase.

Both above and below the line promotions can build loyalty to a brand or a retailer. They can also make the consumer more aware of what is on offer and increase the likelihood of shopping around for a promotion seen on TV or in a newspaper.

The type of promotional activity used will be dependent on the product and the target audience. We will now explore some of the popular promotional activities used in the food industry.

TV advertising

The food industry is a key player in television advertising. Food advertising is dominated by the 'big five' products: breakfast cereals, confectionery, crisps/savoury snacks, soft drinks and fast food restaurants. By contrast, the promotion of fresh food including meat, fruit, vegetables, milk and bread is in decline.

The total spending per annum in UK on advertising soft drinks and chain restaurants is £743 million. Of this figure, £522 million is spent on television advertising and £32 million is on children's airtime (OFCOM, 2004). Research has found a significant number of parents tend to buy food products that children want and are susceptible to 'pester power' (TNS Family Food Panel Survey, 2003). There has been considered debate on the impact of television advertising on children's eating patterns and choices.

In April 2007 new rules were introduced that changed the way in which food products can be advertised on TV. These rules are in response to government and public concern about the increase in childhood obesity. TV advertisements for food products that are classed as high in fat, salt and sugar (HFSS) will not be broadcast during programmes that appeal to children up to 16 years of age.

Activity 22

Research opportunity

TV is the dominant media platform, with over £500 m spent on food and soft drinks adverts in 2006, followed by press (£168 m) and outdoor (£62 m). (Outdoor includes billboards, bus stop advertising and sports pitch perimeter advertising boards.)

Investigate these three different types of advertising media. Consider the methods used and how music, role models and image are used to promote a number of different food products.

In-store activity

All food retailers use some in-store methods to promote their products. We will now explore the most popular methods used.

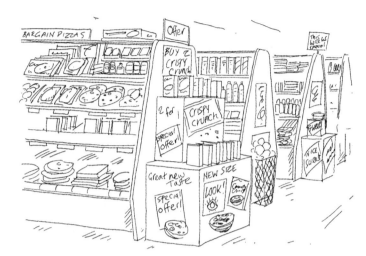

Figure 9.20 *A marketing display in a supermarket*

'Buy one, get one free' offers (BOGOF) are an effective way of encouraging the consumer to try a new product or establish brand loyalty. IGD found 25 per cent of consumers have tried a new product as a result of a BOGOF.

Price reductions will always attract consumers. Discounts off a purchase or a special introductory price can be used to attract the consumer. With coupons printed on the product packaging, consumers can get a discount off a future purchase. Retailers sometimes promote a saving if two different products are purchased together, attracting the consumer. Examples are fresh pasta and a pasta sauce.

Demonstrations and free samples to taste or try in store are another way of introducing a product to the consumer. These methods can sometimes be linked with a money-off coupon if a purchase is made.

Product placement is an important method of in-store promotion. Some retailers place more expensive items at eye level. Retailers also locate commonly purchased items, such as milk and eggs, at the back of the store so consumers have to walk through the entire store to access essential items. During this journey through the store, consumers are more likely to make other purchases. Shelf displays can be used to position associated products together and possibly encourage the consumer to make additional purchases.

In-store displays are particularly important when promoting seasonal items such as Christmas party food and barbeque meats. Dedicated chillers and freezers can be used for more expensive premium products such as luxury ice creams and desserts.

The use of in-store competitions or a contribution to an event or campaign (e.g. computers for schools) could encourage loyalty to a retailer from a consumer.

Announcements during the shopping experience can encourage purchases.

Promotional material including banners, floor adverts and posters can be situated around the store, directing the consumer to a food product.

Packaging

The packaging can be an indicator of the quality of a product. It protects and preserves the food product and can also be used to promote the product to the consumer. The information found on the packaging can attract the consumer's attention. The suggestion that the content contains 50 per cent extra free or the product is free from artificial additives may appeal to a consumer.

The use of persuasive language on the packing can also entice a consumer to make a purchase. The language used can communicate a brand image – high quality products are described as 'finest' and 'premium'.

Methods used to secure loyalty

Loyalty cards

Loyalty cards are available from many food retailers. The market researchers TNS estimate that about 85 per cent of UK households had at least one loyalty card in 2003. The card is presented to the cashier and swiped. Each time the card is used, points are awarded to the consumer. These may be converted into money-off coupons for use in store or used to purchase goods and services from participating organisations.

Loyalty cards can have another role in the retail environment. Basic information, such as name, address, gender and contact details, is provided voluntarily by the consumer when they sign up for a loyalty card. In addition, the application form can extract more personal information about interests and lifestyle which can be used for marketing purposes by the retailer. Consumers can be encouraged to join specialist clubs

such as a food or wine club. The members will receive offers, competitions, advice, extra points and incentives to make more purchases either by email or post.

The retailer is able to monitor consumer purchases. Retailers can identify a consumer's brand loyalties and preferences.

The information can be used to increase sales and expand the range of products with a high profit. Loyalty cards can be an effective way for a food retailer to target consumers with an established buying pattern into purchasing a more expensive alternative. They may post coupons to act as an incentive to try a more expensive but similar product.

In-store facilities

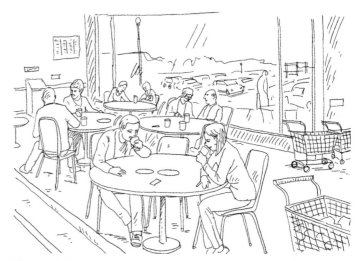

Figure 9.21 *A café in a supermarket*

The facilities and services offered in store can make the shopping experience more enjoyable for the consumer. The facilities and services on hand may include cafés, crèches, toilets, easy parking for families, taxi services, discounted petrol and a variety of trolleys for different consumers. In store there may be a pharmacy, dry cleaning service, photo shop and opticians, all making shopping more convenient for the consumer.

Technological advances in distribution and retailing

You explored how technology has affected food choice in Chapter 8 on food provision. In this chapter the focus is on the distribution of food products.

The food supply chain

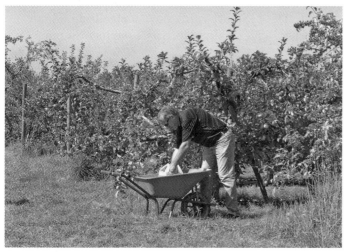

Figure 9.22 *A food producer growing apples*

The food chain involves producers, processors, food manufacturers and retailers. Many food products go through these steps before being purchased by the consumer.

Food producers include farmers, fruit growers and fisheries. Food producers may use a variety of methods to make food ready to eat or ready for the manufacturing process. Common food processing techniques include washing, peeling, pasteurising and spray drying. Food manufacturers make food and drink products using processed products. Wheat is processed by milling into flour and then it is used by food manufacturers to produce baked products. Food retailers sell food and food products to consumers.

The distribution of food is the movement of food through these stages, as shown in Figure 9.23.

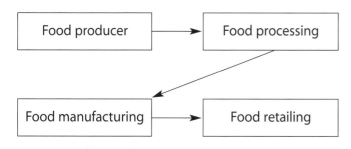

Figure 9.23 *The distribution of food*

Food retailers can deal directly with suppliers, processors and manufacturers.

Food distribution is changing. In the past, large food retailers often preferred to buy the same food products from several different suppliers. This would reduce the risk of disruption if one supplier failed to deliver a food product. It would also promote competition among suppliers, possibly lowering prices for the retailer. However, the trend over the past 20 years has been for food retailers to reduce the number of suppliers and in many cases move to single sourcing.

Single sourcing is when one supplier is the main source of a food or food product for a food retailer. Single sourcing can be very profitable for retailers. A special price can be negotiated for a large, regular order. Many large food retailers now deal with a single supplier for fresh products such as potatoes, root vegetables and soft fruit.

The relative cost of long distance transport has declined in real terms. International trade has become easier, particularly within Europe. This has increased the amount of food imported from Europe. Developments in technology have supported the single source or supplier from a global marketplace.

Benefits to customers

Developments in technology have improved the efficiency of the food distribution and retailing system. This has brought many benefits to consumers. The benefits of constant availability of food products, faster checkouts, efficient pricing, various purchasing and payment options, the traceability of products and more in-store services have made food retail shopping easier and quicker for the consumer.

Greater availability of food products

ICT networks link food retailers to suppliers so they can react quickly to increases in demand for products. Deliveries are scheduled by computer. Rapid replenishment of stock and on-shelf availability is a high priority for food retailers and ICT networks support the need for quick response. This is advantageous to the consumer as there is an increased likelihood that the products they require will always be available to purchase.

Electronic point of sale (EPOS) is a scanning system, used to read a food product code. Virtually all packaged products are marked with a unique 13-digit bar code. When purchasing the product, a laser beam is used to read the barcode at the checkout. The code is then converted by computer to provide the consumer with a product description and price and to provide the store with information to update stock and reorder products if necessary.

Efficient pricing

ICT networks have helped communication between retailers. The development of B2B e-commerce in the food industry has helped retailers widen the geographical search for suitable suppliers and the market price for food products.

B2B e-commerce is business to business exchange of services, information or products. The e-marketplace for food has given food retailers more choice and widened the opportunities to purchase food from different sources. Many food manufacturers and retailers are large enough to have global sources of food products (Tesco, Wal-Mart).

Purchasing options

Many food retailers offer **online grocery shopping** as a method of purchase. Consumers are able to browse a wide range of food products on supermarket websites. The latest research by IGD (Online Grocery set to Deliver, 2007) suggests the £2.4 billion UK online grocery shopping market will more than double over the next five years to reach £5 billion in 2012. Online grocery retailing sales have grown rapidly. This could be due to the significant uptake of broadband technology in the home and increasing confidence in some households in using the technology. Evidence by the IGD has also found that nearly one in ten consumers felt they would not visit a supermarket in five to ten years' time, preferring to do all their grocery shopping online. Online grocery shopping can offer more choice to the consumer as there are retail opportunities for smaller, more specialist food producers.

Payment options

Self-scanning in supermarkets gives the retailer information about purchases and saves time at the checkout. Hand-held scanners allow customers to scan their purchases as they remove them from the shelves. The information from the scanner is downloaded at the checkout and payment made.

Self-scanning checkouts allow customers to scan the items they wish to purchase at the end of their shopping trip. They receive a receipt from the self-checkout unit. They may also pay using a **remote payment terminal**. These terminals will accept electronic payments, credit and debit cards. There is

usually supervision from a member of staff. Electronic payment methods at the checkout have become commonplace. **Smart cards** have embedded chip and pin technology, making electronic payment more secure.

Convenience during shopping

Technology has improved the quality of the shopping environment for the consumer. Automated doors on entry to the store make entrance with a large trolley effortless. The temperature, lighting and air conditioning in the store may be centrally controlled and monitored by computers. Announcements and digital screens showing the latest special offers keep the consumer informed during the shopping experience.

When purchasing fresh fruit and vegetables, **touch screen electronic scales** can be used to weigh and produce a product label. The cashier may also use touch screen technology when processing the goods to be purchased.

Electronic shelf labels allow prices and other information to be displayed electronically and updated easily. **Electronic ticketing systems** exist in many large stores to help manage the queuing system at a delicatessen counter, where one-to-one service is required. **Electronic surveillance tags** are attached to individual products to prevent and detect shoplifting. This tagging is usually associated with bottled alcohol beverages.

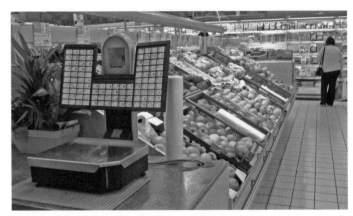

Figure 9.24 *Technology in the supermarket*

Development of the **in-store bakery** has provided the opportunity to purchase freshly baked bread and pastries. Many stores have rotisseries for cooking chickens. Some convenience retailers, such as garage forecourts, offer microwave technology to heat snacks or machines to supply hot beverages.

Improvements in food safety

Developments in ICT have increased the **traceability** of food and food products in long supply chains and made them easier to manage. A supplier can track the movement of a food product more accurately. The new traceability requirements for all EU food and animal feed businesses took effect in January 2005 across Europe (Regulation EC 178/2002). Information on the name, address of supplier, nature of products and date of orders must be systematically stored by each food retailer's or manufacturer's traceability system. This information must be kept for a period of five years.

Technological developments have assisted in the monitoring of temperature during distribution and retailing of food. Some food products require specialist storage – hot, chilled or frozen temperatures. The temperature must be monitored in refrigerators, freezers, cookers, chillers and ovens. Different types of digital probes exist to monitor the temperature in food during cooking, between packs and boxes in storage, and the air temperatures of chillers.

Temperature sensors within the refrigerator, chiller or freezer gather data. This data is then transmitted at regular intervals by radio transmitters to a computer and is logged. If the temperature falls outside the set limits, an alarm is activated.

Faster and efficient methods of transport

Food is transported around the world by plane, ship and lorry. All these methods of transport have become more efficient. The carrying capacity of lorries increased in 2001 to a maximum legal weight of 41 tonnes. The rapid transportation in a controlled environment of perishable food products increases consumer choice. Many food retailers have distribution warehouses where pallet-loads of food products can be collected and distributed nationally.

Developments in stock control

Radio frequency identification tags (RFID) can transmit data to a wireless receiver. These exceptionally small tags can be placed in virtually any product. The tag records more information than the standard barcode, including a unique batch number which can reveal where the food product was manufactured and where it was sold. The 'conversation' between tag and computer reveals an **electronic product code** (EPC) similar to a barcode, except that in this case the information is unique to the item. This helps food

traceability as food products can be identified more effectively. Unlike barcodes, they do not require a direct line of sight to be read.

The use of electronic product codes provides greater opportunities for the retailer to know the consumer. By using tags on food products, it is possible to link the data from the consumer to the purchases made within a supermarket and use the information for more targeted marketing and advertising. This is a much more sophisticated database than loyalty cards can provide.

Smart shelf technology means specially designed shelves which read the radio frequency waves produced by RFID tags. The shelves scan their contents and by the wireless link to the store computer, alert staff when supplies are running low or when a theft is detected. With stock levels being continuously monitored by computers receiving wireless signals from the products themselves, retailers no longer have to rely on staff to monitor the sale of products. Products approaching their use-by date can be identified electronically and located with sufficient time to reduce the items for quick sale. This can reduce losses and wastage.

When a computer senses that stock is running low, it can automatically place an order for more products from the supplier to be delivered. RFID tags can be attached to shipping containers and pallets in an effort to make the location and route of merchandise on its journey from the supplier to the store shelf more efficient.

Developments in food packaging

There have been many developments in the technology associated with food packaging and storage. **Modified atmosphere packaging** (MAP) is a common method used to package fresh meat. Trays are heat-sealed with barrier films and the airspace around the meat is a mixture of carefully composed gases. This process extends the shelf-life of the meat product by preventing discoloration. Vacuum packaging is probably the most widely used form of modified atmosphere packaging for food products.

Controlled atmosphere storage is used in the food industry, usually with refrigeration. It requires the maintenance of certain atmospheric conditions around a product such as reduced oxygen and increased carbon dioxide. This is mainly used for the warehouse storage of vegetables and fruit. Controlled atmospheres are used in the road or sea freight transport of perishable foods.

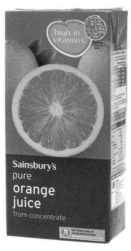

Figure 9.25 *Aseptic packaging*

Aseptic packaging allows a sterile food product to be sealed inside a sterile container made from paper, polyethylene and aluminium in a hygienic environment. The flash heating and cooling used in the aseptic process allows more flavour and nutrients to be retained in the food product. Traditionally, perishable liquid foods can stay unrefrigerated if unopened for up to six months. It is energy-efficient packaging, typically 96 per cent product to 4 per cent packaging by weight. The box-shaped package is a laminate of three materials: high-quality paperboard, polyethylene and aluminium.

Activity 23

Check your understanding

Check your understanding of the meaning of these terms by writing a sentence to describe each term.

aseptic packaging	touch screen electronic scales
B2B e-commerce	below the line
controlled atmosphere packaging	electronic ticketing systems
electronic point of sale	smart shelf technology
electronic product codes	online grocery shopping
electronic shelf labels	traceability
electronic surveillance tags	single sourcing
modified atmosphere packaging	smart cards
radio frequency identification tags	above the line
self-scanning checkouts	remote payment terminal

Exam-style questions

1 Identify four Acts of legislation. (4 marks)

> **ASSESSMENT HINT!**
>
> Identify means to name. So you would select four Acts of legislation and name them.
> Assess is a high order skill. This trigger word will usually appear on an A2 paper and not an AS paper. It means to give your judgement on the merit of something and to put a value on something.

2 Describe one benefit to the consumer of each of the Acts you have named above. (4 marks)

3 What can a consumer expect from a shop when returning faulty goods? (2 marks)

4 Explain why difficulties may occur if you lose a receipt for faulty goods. (2 marks)

5 Explain how shoppers' rights are affected when they buy goods in a sale. (2 marks)

(Total of 14 marks)

Purchasing

6 The table below shows the nutritional value and price of three lasagnes.

Nutritional values per 100 g	Standard supermarket lasagne	Basic supermarket lasagne	Healthy eating option supermarket lasagne
Calories (kcals)	503kJ (120 kcal)	398kJ (95 kcal)	373kJ (89 kcal)
Total fat	5.5 g	2.8 g	2.0 g
(of which is saturates)	2.6 g	1.0 g	0.9 g
Protein	10.1 g	5.4 g	7.8 g
Carbohydrate			
(of which is sugars)	0.7 g	2.5 g	3.0 g
Fibre	1.4 g	2.1 g	1.4 g
Salt	0.8 g	0.4 g	0.6 g
Sodium	0.4 g	0.2 g	0.3 g
Price for each	£1.36 for 400 g	0.79p for 300 g	£1.48 for 400 g

Using the data above, answer the following questions.

a. How much salt does the standard lasagne have?

b. Which lasagne has the lowest KJ or calories and provides the least energy?

c. Which lasagne has the greatest amount of fibre?

d. Which lasagne is the best value for money? (4 marks)

7 Saturated fat intake should be reduced. Give three possible sources of saturated fat in a lasagne. (3 marks)

8 Describe two ways in which the lasagne can be modified to increase the fibre content. (4 marks)

9 The lasagnes are all cook-chill meals. Explain two advantages of cook-chill meals for single-person households. (4 marks)

10 Suggest ways in which families can meet the dietary guidelines to eat less sugar and fat. (10 marks)

11 Evaluate the sources of information available to consumers when purchasing goods and services. (10 marks)

(Total of 35 marks)

Retailing

12 Describe the technological advances in the distribution and retailing of food. (10 marks)

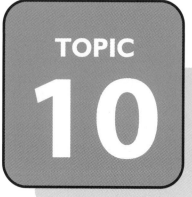

Food preparation and cooking equipment

Learning objectives

By the end of this chapter you will be able to:

- identify the range of labels which appear on equipment
- explain the factors that influence the selection and purchase of household equipment
- list the most common pieces of equipment used in the preparation and cooking of food
- identify the advantages and disadvantages of each piece of equipment
- explain the technological advances in their use and management
- understand how food preparation and cooking equipment are used in the provision of meals for individuals and households in a variety of contexts.

Introduction

This chapter will focus on the selection, purchase and use of food preparation and cooking equipment in the preparation of meals for individuals and households.

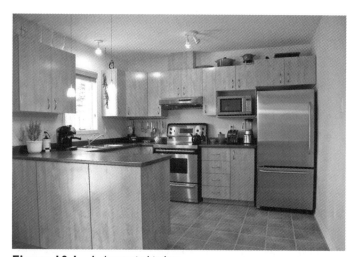

Figure 10.1 *A domestic kitchen*

Equipment labelling

Labels are an extremely informative way in which consumers can find out more about products they wish to purchase. Labelling of equipment is also extremely informative.

There are five distinct labels which can influence our choice of equipment:

- the CE mark
- the British Electrotechnical Approvals Board
- the BSI Kitemark
- the European Union Ecolabel
- the EU energy label.

CE mark

The EU introduced this mark to make trade easier and cheaper between EU countries. It means that a **manufacturer** can claim that its product conforms to the minimum legal requirements for health and safety. It is a self-certification mark applied by the manufacturer to indicate that the product in its view

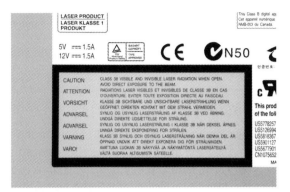

Figure 10.2 *The CE mark*

meets the essential safety requirements. The CE mark indicates that the appliance meets the requirements of European law.

British Electrotechnical Approvals Board

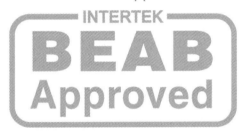

Figure 10.3 *The BEAB mark*

The British Electrotechnical Approvals Board (BEAB) is a guarantee of a product's safety. The mark is given to household electrical equipment that has passed standard electrical tests. These ensure that the consumer will not be exposed to **hazards** such as shocks, burns or mechanical injury. The BEAB is therefore a mark of safety, and confirms to the customer that the appliance has undergone **rigorous** tests covering all aspects of safety.

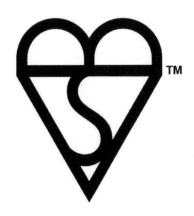

Figure 10.4 *The BSI Kitemark*

BSI Kitemark

The Kitemark is only seen on items which have passed stringent tests. It therefore indicates the standard of performance that might be expected from an appliance, and that it has been made according to the relevant British Standard. It guarantees that the product has been tested for performance and is therefore safe. The British Standards Institution (BSI) is an independent organisation. Once it has confirmed that the product conforms to the relevant standard it issues a BSI licence to the company to use the Kitemark symbol, which is a registered trademark of BSI. The manufacturer pays for this service and the product is tested and assessed at regular intervals. Products are tested for:

- electrical safety
- flammability
- strength.

European Union Ecolabel

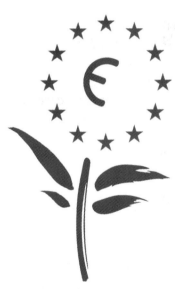

Figure 10.5 *The EU ecolabel*

This label is an official award for products which meet a high environmental standard. Manufacturers can apply to display it on a wide range of household goods including kitchen towels, toilet rolls, washing powder and paint.

The EU energy label

Under this scheme, manufacturers and retailers must tell you about the energy efficiency of many electrical appliances such as washing machines, dishwashers and fridges. It works using a simple scale. Products are rated from A to G, A being the most efficient and G the least. There is also other information on the label, such as noise levels in decibels where the lower the number the quieter the machine.

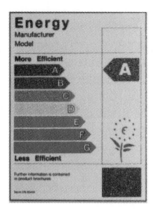

Figure 10.6 *An example of an energy label for an electrical appliance*

Activity 1

Review

Key the above labels into a search engine on the internet.

Make a table which gives you information on the following:

- types of products on which the label appears
- what that label actually tells the consumer about the product.

Using this information create a bulleted list on why the labels are important to the consumer when making a purchase.

Activity 2

Review

Choose a domestic appliance from the following list:
- dishwasher
- washing machine
- tumble dryer.

Describe the features which help to save energy and reduce costs.

Explain how these features can be used to the maximum benefit of the consumer.

Factors influencing selection and purchase

When choosing equipment to buy it is important to choose correctly. Equipping a home will cost money so it is important that the household considers a number of factors prior to purchase. Initial selection is important and the following factors should be considered before each item is purchased.

Price and money available

Finances need to be considered first – how much can the household afford to spend? Once the amount of money to be spent is decided it is a good idea to shop around and compare prices of the same and similar products in a variety of retail outlets or on the internet. Care needs to be taken when discounts and special offers are advertised. If the product is going to be bought on credit check carefully, some retailers also offer interest-free credit.

Design

There are many aspects of design which would need to be considered:
- size
- colour
- shape
- is it **aesthetically** pleasing?
- is it **ergonomically** effective?
- is it a suitable weight for the job?
- is the capacity appropriate?
- is it safe with no sharp edges?
- is it stable and will not tip over?
- is it electrically sound (fuse, cable)?

All of these points are very important to the consumer and should be carefully considered before a purchase is made. Different households may have different requirements and individual taste will also significantly influence choice.

Quality

Generally, price will influence the quality of the product although many economy and budget products represent excellent value for money. Consumers need to shop around and decide on their budget and then select the quality of the item they need. They should look carefully at the materials and finish and test moving parts. The type and nature of the retail outlet may also indicate the quality of the product that is stocked. For example, many department stores have an excellent reputation for selling quality products, whereas some market stalls may sell slightly inferior or seconds quality items.

Fitness for purpose

Consumers need to ensure that the product actually does what it should do. This is especially appropriate with electrical equipment that is becoming more and more sophisticated. It is advisable to research fully the functions of the equipment and decide what is actually required before the sale goes ahead. Even the same products will have different features so it is important to look at the specification to check the product will do exactly what is required.

Advertising and current consumer trends

Most people are influenced by advertising and the perceived popularity of a product. This is clearly visible with the growth of IT equipment, mobile phones and other items of electrical equipment which are used for entertainment or communication.

Energy efficiency

With the current trend towards being environmentally friendly, the amount of electricity or water a product is using is very important to many consumers.

After all this research the consumer should decide upon the best product at a price they are willing to pay.

Activity 3

Review

Using *Which?* magazine, read an article on a product which has been tested.

Then write a report to include the following information:

• the piece of equipment
• which is the best buy and why
• if you were to buy that piece of equipment for yourself tomorrow, which features you would look for and why.

The range of equipment

Many items of food preparation and cooking equipment are designed to save time and/or effort. Therefore if they are used wisely they can make meal preparation and cooking easier.

Activity 4

Research opportunity

Using the two headings of preparation and cooking, list as many pieces of equipment as you can which are used for preparation and cooking.

Alongside each piece of equipment write a sentence on its main use and one advantage and one disadvantage.

You will now look at the most common pieces of equipment for preparation and cooking.

Microwave ovens

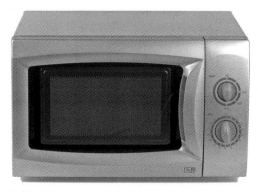

Figure 10.7 *A microwave oven*

Microwave ovens are useful pieces of equipment, used for heating, cooking and defrosting food and cooking frozen ready meals.

The advantages of microwave ovens are as follows:

• Most microwave ovens incorporate a turntable that rotates the food during cooking and reduces the need to stir mixtures or to turn items.

• They use a 13 amp plug socket so that they can easily be plugged in anywhere. They are also portable so they can be moved to rooms other than the kitchen if required.

• They save time and energy because they cook food much more quickly than conventional methods (e.g. baked jacket potatoes). A short standing time is part of the cooking process.

• They can save on washing up if foods are cooked and served in the same dish.

• Microwave ovens are easy to clean and there are no problems of condensation in the kitchen.

• The flavour and colour retention of foods are generally better than conventional methods of cooking due to the quick cooking times.

- Retention of water-soluble vitamins in vegetables is good because liquid used for cooking is minimal.
- Food preparation times can be speeded up if foods are defrosted using a microwave oven.

The following meals and dishes can be prepared successfully:

- vegetables with a small amount of liquid
- fish can be cooked quickly and retains its moisture
- sponge puddings cook well but there will be no colour change
- ready meals
- takeaway meals can be reheated
- foods like chicken portions can be defrosted quickly.

The disadvantages of microwave ovens are as follows:

- Microwave ovens take up kitchen surface space but brackets can be bought to position them on the wall.
- Timing of cooking is critical because food can easily be overcooked and foods like fish can break up.
- A microwave oven does not brown or crisp foods so some foods are unsuitable for microwaving. For example, pastry dishes and biscuits are not good cooked by this method.
- Foods with a high fat or sugar content are best not cooked in a microwave because the temperatures involved can cause combustion.
- Tomatoes and poached eggs if cooked in a microwave must have the skins pierced or they will burst.
- Cold spots may occur if food is not stirred regularly.
- Metal cannot be used in the microwave and nor can some plastics.

Technological advances in microwave ovens

Combination microwave ovens are now available which combine microwaving and browning and crisping – the best of both worlds. These combination microwave ovens can accommodate most containers such as foil, glass and ceramic. Many microwave ovens have an auto cook or auto defrost function which senses weight and moisture content and calculates the cooking or defrost time.

The oven or grill can be set separately to a chosen temperature and so can be used in exactly the same way as a conventional oven or grill.

Activity 5

Practical opportunity

Using a microwave cookbook, find sweet and savoury recipes suitable for a family.

In your next practical lesson, choose one of the dishes and make it.

Alternatively, try this sweet treat recipe.

Easy Chocolate Fudge

100 g good quality chocolate

50 g unsalted butter

1/2 teaspoon vanilla essence

30 ml milk

300 g icing sugar

Method

Line a 18 cm square tin with foil.

Break up the chocolate into squares and cut the butter up into cubes. Place both in a large bowl and melt in a microwave (usually takes between 1 minute and 1 minute 30 seconds depending upon microwave wattage).

Mix in the milk and vanilla essence and beat in the icing sugar a little at a time.

Spoon the mixture into a tin and refrigerate until solid.

Cut into pieces and serve.

Usefulness of microwave ovens

For individuals and households who want food in a hurry, a microwave oven is invaluable. If members of the household come in at different times, or if a member of a household has missed a meal prepared for them, it can easily and quickly be reheated when they arrive home without it losing quality.

Many ready prepared meals and dishes may be bought that simply need heating in a microwave. This is a valuable timesaver for busy people.

Cookers

A cooker usually consists of an oven, a surface heating unit called a hob and a grill. In addition, some cookers have two ovens: a smaller top oven and a large main oven. Cookers can run off a variety of fuels but most are run using electricity or gas. Cookers may be freestanding or ovens may be built in under a work surface.

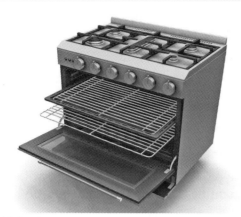

Figure 10.8 *A cooker*

The advantages of cookers are as follows:

- Batch baking, where a number of the same dishes are cooked at once, can be carried out really well in a fan-assisted electric oven as the food is cooked evenly at the same temperature.
- Fan-assisted ovens heat up quickly and maintain an even temperature. They are economical because they cook food more quickly and the temperature required is usually 10 degrees less than a standard oven. Gas ovens have zones of heat so it is possible to cook different dishes requiring different temperatures at the same time.
- Easy-clean ovens with catalytic linings may save time in busy households when the oven is used regularly to cook meals.
- Gas ovens heat up instantly which saves time in a busy household.
- Grills use radiant heat, which cooks food positioned in a grill pan under the heat source. Some grills may incorporate a rotisserie spit. Grilling is a healthy method of cooking because it allows fat from the food to drip away and not to be absorbed by the food.

The vast majority of foods can be cooked successfully in either the oven, grill or hob:

- fruits and vegetables baked in their skins (potatoes and apples)
- casseroles and roasts
- most meat, poultry, fish, eggs and milk dishes
- pasta, rice, vegetables, sauces, stir fry and risotto can be cooked on the hob.
- small fish, chicken joints, lamb or pork chops, sausages, bacon and steaks are suitable for grilling
- some vegetables are also suitable for grilling (tomatoes and mushrooms)
- au gratin dishes and brulées can be grilled.

The disadvantages of cookers are as follows:

- Setting the timer for cooking may be a problem in a warm kitchen and care should be taken if high risk foods are to be cooked in this way.
- In a small house or open plan kitchen, fan-assisted ovens may be noisy.
- Gas ovens which are not fan assisted have zones of heat so the middle of the oven is at the set temperature, whereas the top of the oven will be hotter than the set temperature and the bottom will be cooler.

Technological advances of cookers

Many ovens have electronic auto-timers. These consist of electronic timers which control start time, duration of cooking and end time.

Many electric cookers have ceramic hobs which look attractive and are easy to clean. Some ceramic hobs are Halogen which are designed to give instant heat to speed the cooking time.

Usefulness of cookers

Some cookers have double ovens, a large one and a small one. The small one may be particularly useful for households when not all members eat together or if only one dish needs to be cooked in the oven.

Families may find a large oven very useful when everybody is having a meal together or on festive occasions.

People who enjoy entertaining may find the large oven very useful.

Activity 6

Practical opportunity

Choose a dish which can be made in one pan on the hob such as a Bolognese sauce or a stir fry.

Make your chosen meal in your next practical lesson.

Alternatively, try this recipe.

Risotto

1 tablespoon oil

75 g long grain rice

1 onion

1 red pepper

100 g mushrooms

100 g sweetcorn

450 ml stock

250 g cooked chicken

Method

Make up the stock with one stock cube and 450 ml boiling water.

Chop onion, pepper and mushrooms. Place oil in a frying pan and fry the onion, pepper and mushrooms for about five minutes until soft.

Add the rice and cook for 1 minute.

Slowly add the stock, bring to the boil and simmer until three quarters of the liquid has evaporated.

Stir in the chicken and sweetcorn.

When all the liquid is absorbed, take off the heat.

Optional – garnish with parmesan cheese.

Blenders, liquidisers and smoothie makers

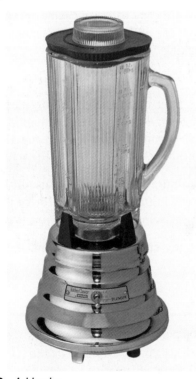

Figure 10.9 *A blender*

A blender or liquidiser is designed to save time when preparing food. The sharp blades that rotate at the bottom of a goblet cut food up and reduce it to a pulp. Smoothie makers operate in a very similar way to liquidisers and **pulverise** fruits and vegetables to produce healthy drinks. Some models are free-standing and some fit on to a food mixer or processor.

The advantages of using this equipment is that many meals and dishes can be prepared far more easily using this equipment:

- puréed baby food, which can be messy and time-consuming if using a sieve instead
- puréed soups or fruit, making breadcrumbs or chopping nuts and crushing ice.

The disadvantages of them are as follows:

- Some models are not designed to cope with very large quantities and the food may have to be pulverised in batches.
- A smoothie maker is specialised and therefore not particularly versatile, so care needs to be taken to ensure it is correctly used.

Technological advances of blenders, liquidisers and smoothie makers

Some attachments can now be washed in a dishwasher. Some models are more powerful and can crush ice.

Usefulness of blenders, liquidisers and smoothie makers

Families with babies or very young children may find this appliance useful to blend nourishing homemade meals and freeze them in batches. It makes families less reliant on commercial baby foods.

Young professionals may use a smoothie maker to make drinks which contain large quantities of fruit or vegetables, making the drink healthy and quick to consume.

Families with children may use a smoothie maker to make fruit smoothies, because they can appeal to children who may find them more palatable than fresh fruit.

Activity 7

Practical opportunity

Find a recipe for soup which needs to be blended or liquidised.

Make your soup in your next practical session.

Practical opportunity

Find a recipe for a fruit-based smoothie.
Make your smoothie in your next practical session.

Food mixers

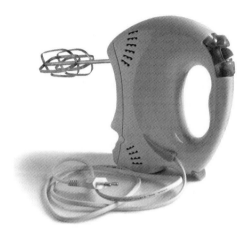

Figure 10.10 *A hand-held food mixer*

There are vast numbers of food mixers available in the shops. They are either hand-held mixers or tabletop machines. Hand-held mixers are designed to mix, whisk, knead or beat small quantities of food. Tabletop mixers are more powerful and are designed to deal with larger quantities of food.

The advantages of food mixers are as follows:
- Mixers are much quicker than mixing by hand and can be used in any bowl or container.
- Hand mixers are particularly useful for whisking egg white to make meringue.
- The tabletop mixers whisk, beat and cream.
- The tabletop version can perform other functions if various blades or attachments are used, such as a dough hook for kneading bread dough and attachments for potato peeling, meat mincing and fruit juice squeezing.

The disadvantages of food mixers are as follows:
- The hand-held machines are sometimes not powerful enough for large quantities of mixtures.
- The tabletop mixers would be useful in a household where a lot of cooking is done but they are expensive and many households would not use one enough to justify the expense of buying one.

- Some tabletop mixers are large and take up a lot of space in a small kitchen.

Technological advances of food mixers

Some models parts can now be washed in a dishwasher. Hand-held mixers are now available with blades which will knead bread dough.

Usefulness of food mixers

These machines are designed to aid preparation by saving time, so a busy person may find one useful. People who enjoy cooking and entertaining may find they speed up preparation time.

Breadmakers

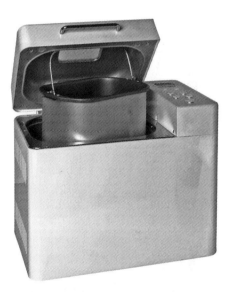

Figure 10.11 *A breadmaker*

These are specialised items of equipment. Their prime use is to make a loaf of bread or prepare dough to make items such as pizzas.

The advantage of a breakmaker is that they can make a loaf of bread from start to finish. All that needs to be done is to weigh the ingredients into the bread pan and set the controls. The breadmaker mixes, kneads and bakes the bread.

As well as making a loaf of bread, some breadmakers can be used to make the following:
- rich yeast mixtures
- sweet breads
- exotic flavoured bread

- dough for bread rolls and pizzas
- jam
- cakes such as gingerbread.

The disadvantage is that breadmaking machines can be quite bulky, but their capacity is small and most of them only produce one loaf which is not usually enough for a large household.

Technological advances of breadmakers

Some models have built-in timers so that they can be set to produce a warm loaf for breakfast. In addition, many machines have other settings so they can be used to make rich yeast mixtures, cakes, gingerbread and jam.

Usefulness of breadmakers

People who enjoy a fresh loaf of bread would find a breadmaker useful, as would those who enjoy cooking. Those living in a rural location may find it too far to travel for a fresh loaf daily so they can make their own.

Steamers

Steaming is a healthy method of cooking because it uses a small amount of water and the food cooks in steam generated from the water used. Electric steamers are thermostatically controlled and the food cannot burn because if the water should evaporate the steamer automatically switches itself off. The steamer lid is tightly fitting to prevent steam escaping and extra levels can be added to cook more food as there are usually two or three tiers.

The advantages of steamers are that it is an easy and economic method of cooking because a number of food items can be cooked at once. It is also a very healthy method of cooking because only a small amount of water is used to cook items, such as vegetables, so the loss of water-soluble vitamins is reduced.

Steaming is suitable for fish, vegetables, desserts such as crème caramel, custard and cake mixture puddings.

The disadvantages is that it can take up a lot of space in a small kitchen because it is quite a tall appliance.

Technological advances of steamers

Most steamers now have timers and are thermostatically controlled so there is no danger when leaving the appliance unattended.

Usefulness of steamers

Steamers would be very useful to someone who likes to eat healthily. For a one- or two-person household a whole meal can be cooked in the steamer – fish, potatoes and vegetables can all be cooked together.

Activity 9

Practical opportunity

Choose a piece of equipment described above.
Prepare one or more dishes to illustrate its value to a single professional person.

Food processors

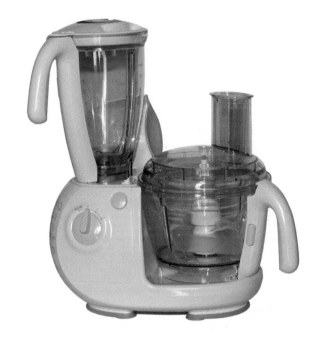

Figure 10.12 *A food processor*

The main functions of a food processor are to chop, liquidise, purée, grate and slice. Exactly how things are cut and sliced depends on the blades that are fitted to the machine.

The main advantage of a food processor is that one machine with various attachments can prepare a variety of foods. They are particularly useful for cutting and shredding large quantities of vegetables. It is very quick and can save time in food preparation.

Food processors can shred cabbage to make coleslaw. They can grate carrots and cheese. They can chop vegetables finely such as onions. They can also rub in fat to flour, make pastry, purée mixtures and make breadcrumbs.

Some machines may also whip and whisk but they are not always recommended for whisking egg white. Because food processors are powerful and the cutting blades revolve rapidly, it is easy to overprocess food unless care is taken and timing is accurate. This can be the case when making shortcrust pastry

Technological advances of food processors

Processors are now very powerful machines. They are also more compact and therefore take up less room in the kitchen.

Usefulness of food processors

These machines are designed to aid preparation by saving time, so a busy person may find one useful. People who enjoy cooking and entertaining may find one useful to speed up preparation time.

Activity 10

Practical opportunity

Use a food processor to make some shortcrust pastry and a quiche.
Alternatively, try this salad using the processor.

Carrot and raisin salad

6 large carrots

75 g raisins

1 tablespoon chopped parsley (chopped in the processor)

2 tablespoons olive oil

1 tablespoon orange juice

25 g sesame seeds

Method

Whisk together the oil and orange juice to make the dressing.

Grate the carrots in the food processor and put in a large serving bowl.

Stir in the raisins, parsley and dressing.

Garnish with sesame seeds.

Contact grills

Contact grills consist of two non-stick plates which can grill foods from the top and bottom.

The advantage of a contact grill is that there is no need to use fat or oil to cook the food because the plates are non-stick. They are time and energy-saving appliances. All models are portable and require no special fitting.

They can be used to successfully prepare the following:
- meats such as steak, bacon, gammon, chops, burgers and chicken breasts
- vegetables such as peppers, courgettes and onions
- toasted sandwiches with cheese, beans and ham fillings.

The disadvantages are that they are quite small pieces of equipment so they are more suited to cooking small amounts of food. Cleaning some models can be difficult. They have quite specific functions so they are less versatile than some other appliances.

Technological advances of contact grills

Some models now have drip trays to collect any fat that comes off the food. This then drains off via a channel. Some have removable plates which can be washed in a dishwasher. Some have a floating hinge which means that any thickness of food can be catered for.

Usefulness of contact grills

For a one- or two-person household they can grill sufficient quantities, but for a larger household it may not cook enough at the same time. They are useful for someone who wishes to cook healthily by grilling and for teenagers or students who want sandwiches as a snack.

Activity 11

Research opportunity

Choose two of the following pieces of equipment:
- microwave oven
- cooker
- blender/liquidiser
- food mixer
- breadmaker
- steamer
- food processor

- contact grill
- smoothie maker.

Investigate the range of meals that could be prepared with two pieces of equipment you have chosen. Which group of people would the equipment most suit and why?

Produce a written report of your findings.

Activity 12

Review

Explain the factors which need to be taken into consideration when choosing equipment for preparation and cooking in the following cases:

- a young couple setting up home
- a family wishing to prepare both economical and healthy meals.

Give examples of specific appliances, dishes and meals.

Activity 13

Check your understanding

Check your understanding of the meaning of the following terms by using them in a sentence:

manufacturer	**hazard**	**rigorous**
durable	**aesthetic**	**ergonomic**
pulverise	**purée**	

Exam-style question

1 Choose three pieces of equipment and discuss with appropriate examples how the equipment has enabled us to produce healthy meals more easily.

(15 marks)

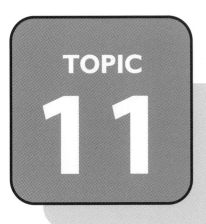

TOPIC 11

Food safety and hygiene

Learning objectives

By the end of this chapter you will be able to:

- explain how food can be contaminated
- identify the different types of micro-organisms responsible for food contamination and food spoilage
- describe the conditions and factors necessary for the growth of bacteria
- identify the sources and methods of transmission of the commonly occurring food poisoning bacteria
- describe the techniques for safe handling of food during storage, preparation and cooking
- describe the incidence and patterns of food poisoning outbreaks in the UK
- name and describe the legislation relating food safety
- explain the current food and hygiene regulations including the Food Hygiene (England) Regulations 2006
- describe the role of an environmental health officer and the Food Standards Agency in monitoring food safety.

Introduction

In this chapter you will explore the ways in which food is contaminated and the sources of food poisoning bacteria. You will investigate food handling and the various ways in which the government monitors and controls the standard of food in the UK.

Food contamination

It is important to protect food from the risk of contamination to prevent it poisoning people. There are three main ways in which food can become contaminated:

Physical contamination

Physical contamination can occur at any stage of food production. Physical contamination includes pieces of metal or plastic entering the food during production. Parts of the food product, which should have been removed during processing including pips, stones, shell, bones or stalks, can contaminate the end-product. Physical contamination includes fragments of food packaging or objects from careless food handling such as plasters, jewellery and hair. Pests can also contaminate food with their droppings, saliva and urine.

Chemical contamination

Chemicals, including metal residues, pesticides, bleaches and cleaning materials, can contaminate food.

The correct storage of cleaning products is important as they can taint food products. The careless use of chemicals in a food preparation environment could contaminate food. Chemicals used in agriculture and farming methods could leave residues in food products such as antibiotics and hormones in meat. The use of food additives in incorrect quantities can pose a risk to health.

Micro-organism contamination

Food changes during storage. This process can affect the colour, flavour, texture and appearance of food. Usually the changes in food are harmless and sometimes they are desirable – softer fruit or tenderising red meat. The changes are caused by micro-organisms and enzymes. **Micro-organisms** are very small living organisms which cannot be seen without a microscope. They include yeasts, viruses, moulds and bacteria.

Food can be contaminated with certain bacteria which will make it unfit to eat and dangerous to health. Bacteria which are harmful to health are known as **pathogenic bacteria**. Food poisoning can be caused by eating food which is contaminated with live bacteria. It can also be caused by eating the waste products, spores or the toxins which bacteria may produce.

Food spoilage by micro-organisms

In this section you will explore the micro-organisms responsible for food spoilage and contamination. There are four types: moulds, yeasts, viruses and bacteria.

Moulds

Moulds are tiny plants or fungi which grow on the surface of food. They produce spores which can travel in the air to generate new growths. They prefer warm, moist conditions to multiply. Mould can be used in the food industry to produce speciality cheeses such as Stilton, Roquefort or Camembert.

Generally, moulds are harmless but some can produce mycotoxins, which can be dangerous. **Mycotoxins** are naturally occurring toxins produced by moulds. Damp cereals may be contaminated with mycotoxins.

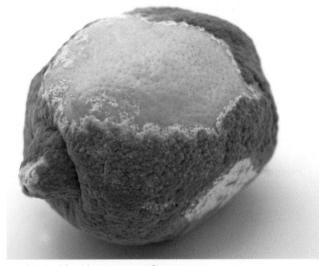

Figure 11.1 *Mould growing on fruit*

Yeasts

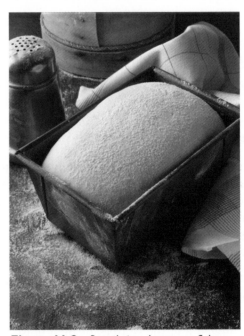

Figure 11.2 *Bread rises because of the action of yeast*

Yeasts do not cause food poisoning, but some types are capable of causing food spoilage. They are found naturally in the environment and require warm, moist conditions to reproduce. Yeasts are essential for the production of bread, wines and beers.

Viruses

Viruses are not usually considered to be living organisms as they consist of genetic material surrounded by a protein coat. They can cause disease as they destroy living cells. Viruses are carried by human beings, animals, birds, water and sewage. Viruses are an increasingly significant cause of food-borne illnesses.

The Hepatitis A virus can be passed on to food products from infected food handlers. The Norwalk virus or Norovirus is an intestinal illness associated with salads, eggs and shellfish. The virus is passed from the faeces of an infected person contaminating food or water. The symptoms are short-lived and so they are not usually reported.

Bacteria

Bacteria are single-celled micro-organisms found in water, air, soil, people and animals. Bacteria have an important role in food production. They are essential in the production of yoghurt and cheese. Probiotic drinks contain 'helpful' bacteria and claim to have health benefits.

Bacteria require specific conditions to multiply, usually food, warmth and moisture.

Spoilage bacteria will over time start the process of decomposition and decay of food products. These bacteria can affect the quality of the food product and sometimes make it unsafe to eat.

Pathogenic bacteria cause food poisoning. Food contaminated with pathogenic bacteria can appear to be perfectly normal. There may be no evidence of decay or spoilage. Pathogenic bacteria include salmonella, staphylococcus aureus and clostridium perfringens. These bacteria will live on food.

A **food-borne disease** is an illness caused by eating food contaminated by harmful substances or by pathogenic bacteria living on the food.

Activity 1

Practical opportunity

You are going to make yoghurt. You will need a special yoghurt maker or a wide-necked vacuum flask. Most commercially produced natural yoghurt can be used as a 'starter'. Whether labelled 'live' or not, most yoghurt contains living bacteria. Only pasteurised yoghurt is free from bacteria.

Yoghurt

½ litre UHT whole milk

Small pot natural yoghurt

Method

Sterilise the equipment you are going to use.

Heat the milk, less 2 tablespoons to 42°C (blood heat) in a saucepan.

Blend the reserved milk with a tablespoon of natural yoghurt until smooth and then stir into the warm milk.

Pour into the pre-warmed, wide-necked flask and leave for six to eight hours or longer.

Turn the yoghurt into a bowl and stand the bowl in cold water. Whisk by hand until the yoghurt is cool.

Cover the bowl, place in a refrigerator and leave for a further four to six hours. It should thicken.

Serve either plain or with a fruit flavour. Adding fresh fruit may produce runnier yoghurt if juice is also added.

Activity 2

Review

What conditions did you create for the bacteria to multiply?

Why might the yoghurt have failed?

Food poisoning

Food poisoning can be caused by pathogenic bacteria, but it can also be caused by viruses, chemicals and metals contaminating the food substance. Food can even be contaminated with poisonous plants and animals. The main focus of this discussion is food poisoning caused by pathogenic bacteria.

There are two ways in which bacteria can make you ill – by eating the live bacteria or eating the toxin they produce.

Eating pathogenic bacteria

When bacteria enter the stomach and intestine, they multiply. This is how the most common pathogenic bacteria – campylobacter and salmonella – cause illness. Some types of food poisoning require the consumption of thousands of bacteria, others including Escherichia coli O157, require the consumption of just a few to cause serious illness.

Eating a toxin

A **toxin** is a poison produced as a waste product by bacteria. Some bacteria, such as staphylococcus aureus and bacillus cereus, produce a toxin when they multiply in foods. In these cases, eating the toxin makes you ill, not eating the bacteria. The toxin causes the unpleasant symptoms.

A **symptom** is a sign or indication of a disease. The body reacts to bacteria or toxins by developing symptoms which include diarrhoea, vomiting, stomach pain, headaches and sweating.

Food poisoning usually begins shortly after eating the contaminated source. The **onset time** is the period of time between eating the contaminated food and the symptoms of food poisoning appearing. Some bacteria will multiply in the intestine and will take at least 12 hours before the symptoms start to appear. Campylobacter takes 24 to 48 hours to multiply, so the meals eaten the day before the illness began are not likely to be responsible. Staphylococcus aureus, Bacillus cereus and Clostridium perfringens all produce toxins. The onset time is much shorter in bacteria which produce toxins and symptoms can appear within a few hours.

Sources of pathogenic bacteria

Food can become contaminated during the production, preparation and retailing. The main sources of bacteria are shown in Figure 11.3.

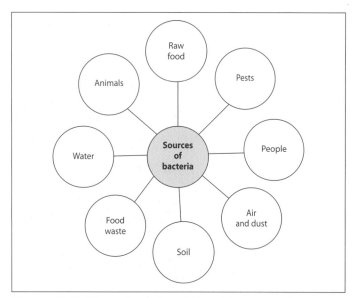

Figure 11.3 *The main sources of bacterial contamination*

Raw food

Raw foods include meat, poultry, shellfish and eggs. These are significant sources of contamination. Food poisoning bacteria can be found on or in many raw foods. Bacteria also live in the gut of healthy animals

and during slaughter these bacteria can contaminate the flesh. The processing methods which follow can spread the bacteria further such as mincing beef for burgers. It is important that all raw food is treated as potentially contaminated and kept separate from cooked and ready-to-eat food.

People

Food poisoning bacteria are found on the skin, in septic wounds, the nose and sometimes the gut of infected people. If food hygiene practices are poor, bacteria can be transferred onto food, where they can multiply and cause food poisoning. Poor food hygiene practices include sneezing, coughing and smoking when handling food. Failing to wash hands after using the toilet and not covering cuts can spread bacteria. Viruses can be carried by infected people and transmitted on food if hygiene practices are poor.

Pests

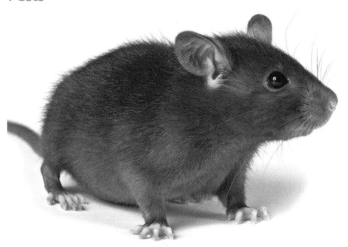

Figure 11.4 *A rat*

Pests include rodents and insects. Rodents are mice and rats. Insects include cockroaches, ants, wasps and flies. These feed and live among faeces, dirt or waste. If a pest enters food premises, it can transfer bacteria onto food intended for human consumption. Some pests have pathogenic bacteria inside their bodies which will spread in their saliva and droppings. During storage, dry food products can become infested with beetles, weevils and mites. Birds and their droppings can also contaminate poorly stored food products.

Animals

Domestic pets and farm animals can be the source of pathogenic bacteria. Cattle, sheep and goats can carry

E.coli in their intestines and care needs to be taken when handling them.

Air and dust

Bacteria can be carried in the air. It is very important to make sure food is covered as bacteria can settle on the surface. Staphylococcus aureus bacteria live in dust, air and sewage.

Water

Poor quality drinking water is often the cause of food poisoning. Some bacteria are carried in untreated water including salmonella and typhoid. By law the water used in the food industry during the processing of food must be potable. **Potable water** is fit for drinking and free from contamination.

Soil

Bacteria and spores can survive in soil. Unwashed root vegetables may carry bacteria. Cereals can be dusty and can carry micro-organisms. Clostridium perfringens is one of several bacteria found in soil and dust.

Food waste

Food waste needs to be disposed of correctly as it can be a source of contamination. Food waste can attract pests which carry food poisoning bacteria.

People at risk

Some people are more vulnerable to food poisoning than others. The vulnerable groups are pregnant women, the very old, young children, the sick or those recovering from a serious illness such as cancer. These groups have a weakened immune system and are less likely to be able to cope with the symptoms of food poisoning. Diarrhoea and vomiting can cause rapid dehydration.

Main types of food poisoning bacteria

The Food Standards Agency had a target to reduce by 20 per cent the number of laboratory confirmed cases of five common bacteria by 2006. The bacteria were Campylobacter, Salmonella, Listeria, E.coli O157 and Clostridium perfringens.

Campylobacter

Campylobacter is the most common form of bacterial food poisoning in Britain. Campylobacter is a bacterium found in the intestines of many types of animals and birds. Birds can contaminate food with their droppings and by pecking. Campylobacter coli and Campylobacter jejuni are the strains usually associated with Campylobacter food poisoning. Less than 500 Campylobacter bacteria are needed to cause infection.

The source of infection is usually contaminated food. Campylobacter is found in most raw poultry and this is believed to be the most significant source of human infection. Inadequately pasteurised milk and contaminated water supplies are responsible for larger outbreaks of the disease.

To reduce the risk of infection we can avoid storing raw and cooked foods together and not using the same work surfaces or utensils when preparing raw and cooked meat. Campylobacter can also come from infected pets and farm animals. Hand washing is very important after any contact with animals. Thorough cooking will destroy the bacteria.

The symptoms of campylobacter include diarrhoea, vomiting, stomach pains and cramps, fever and generally feeling unwell. They begin two to five days after infection and usually only last a week.

Salmonella

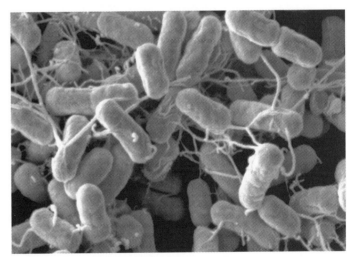

Figure 11.5 *Salmonella bacteria*

Over 2000 strains of salmonella bacteria have been identified. These bacteria are present in the intestines of farm animals and sometimes human beings.

Vegetables, fruit and shellfish can become contaminated through contact with manure in soil or sewage in water. Pets and rodents can carry the bacteria.

The live bacteria are excreted and can be the source of direct food contamination or cross-contamination. The infection usually occurs by eating contaminated food.

Cross-contamination is also possible if raw and cooked foods are stored together. Salmonella can be spread from person to person by poor hygiene. Poor hygiene includes failure to wash hands carefully after using the toilet or after handling contaminated food.

Salmonella causes dehydration and this can be particularly serious in young children, the sick and the elderly. Symptoms include diarrhoea, stomach pain and sometimes vomiting and fever. It takes from 12 to 72 hours for the symptoms to appear. Fatalities or deaths from the disease are rare.

To reduce the risk of infection, proper hand washing is crucial. Cooked food should be kept away from raw food. Raw food should be stored below ready-to-eat food in the refrigerator. You should wash all vegetables before preparation. Salmonella will be destroyed by cooking so ensure food is thoroughly cooked. Avoid drinking water from untreated sources. As salmonella is an infective food poisoning bacteria, you should make sure that toilet areas and personal bedding are kept clean.

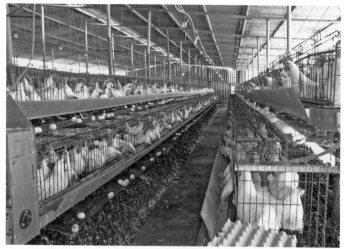

Figure 11.6 *A battery farm producing eggs*

In 1998 a programme was set up to vaccinate all UK laying hens against a common type of salmonella bacteria. This programme has led to a steady decrease in the number of food poisoning cases associated with some forms of salmonella. In one strain known as Salmonella enteritidis, cases are at their lowest level since the late 1980s. In 2004 at least 80 per cent of all laying hens in the UK were vaccinated against Salmonella enteritidis. The 'Lion mark' used by the UK egg industry indicates that microbiological safety and quality standards have been met.

Listeria

Listeria monocytogenes is widespread in the environment. It has been found in soil, sewage, water, animals and people. Two forms exist and healthy adults are likely to experience only mild infection, causing flu-like symptoms or gastroenteritis. However, the more toxic form of listeria can occasionally lead to severe blood poisoning or meningitis. Pregnant women, the elderly and people with weakened immune systems are more susceptible to this form of listeria. Infections during pregnancy can cause miscarriage, premature delivery or severe illness in a newborn child.

Listeria monocytogenes is unusual because it can grow at low temperatures. It will multiply in refrigerators at 5°C. It is destroyed by cooking food thoroughly and by the process of pasteurisation. Foods most likely to be contaminated with listeria are unpasteurised dairy products, cooked meat, pâtés, smoked fish and cook-chill meals. Listeria needs time to reproduce which means that the long storage of susceptible food before consumption increases the risk. Once infected with the bacteria it can take up to 90 days for symptoms to appear. Identifying the source of infection can be a challenge.

To avoid infection, store refrigerated foods for as short a time as possible and follow storage and cooking instructions issued by the manufacturer. Vulnerable groups should avoid eating unpasteurised dairy products. Salads and raw vegetables should be washed before eating.

Escherichia coli 0157

E.coli is found in the intestines of animals and humans. There are many different types, some of which are capable of causing illness. Illness ranges from mild diarrhoea through to very severe inflammation of the gut. The most important toxin-producing strain which can cause human illness is known as VTEC (Verocytotoxin-producing) E.coli 0157. Only a small number of bacteria produce sufficient toxins to cause an illness.

E.coli can be found in raw and undercooked meats, unpasteurised milk, fruit juices, dairy products and raw vegetables.

The bacteria can survive refrigeration and freezer storage, but thorough cooking of food and pasteurisation will destroy them. The symptoms normally take about two days to develop. The main symptom is diarrhoea. In some cases, in young children and the elderly, infection can lead to bloody diarrhoea, kidney failure and sometimes death.

There is a more detailed discussion about the incidence and control of E.coli later in this chapter.

Clostridium perfringens

Clostridium perfringens is found in healthy animals and people. Other sources include raw meat, soil, sewage and manure. When consumed, the bacteria produces a toxin which causes the illnesses. The spores can survive low temperature cooking and they can start to reproduce during slow cooling and unrefrigerated storage.

Food poisoning will occur when food, usually meat, is prepared in advance and kept warm for several hours before serving. The illness will begin within hours of consuming the bacteria. The symptoms are diarrhoea, stomach pain and some vomiting. It is short lived and lasts no more than 24 hours, although elderly people may be more seriously affected.

Other significant food poisoning bacteria

There are some other bacteria which are not the focus of the FSA campaign but are important to explore.

Staphylococcus aureus

Staphylococcus aureus can be found on human skin and mucus linings in the body. It can cause blood and wound infections if there is an opportunity for the bacteria to enter the body. Fortunately most strains of Staphylococcus aureus are destroyed effectively by antibiotics but some are resistant to the antibiotic methicillin. These are called methicillin-resistant (MRSA).

Staphylococcus aureus can cause food poisoning if eaten. Staphylococcus aureus produces a toxin which causes severe vomiting with diarrhoea and stomach pain. These symptoms occur within six hours of infection from the toxin. The sources of infection can be person-to-person contact. Staphylococcus aureus lives on the skin, in the nose or on the fingers of some infected people. Cross-contamination occurs by an infected person handling ready-to-eat foods such as cooked meats. Storage of infected food at room temperature before consumption allows the bacteria to multiply and produce the harmful toxin.

Bacillus cereus

Bacillus cereus is found in soil, cereals and dust. Only a small number of bacteria are required to cause illness. The bacteria will form resilient spores which can survive the cooking process. During cooling time after cooking, the spores will produce bacteria. Bacteria can multiply rapidly at these warm temperatures and produce heat-resistant toxins which will not be destroyed by further reheating.

Bacillus cereus is found in rice and pasta dishes, meat or vegetable dishes, dairy products, soups, sauces and sweet pastry products. Usually these food products have not been cooled or stored correctly. Food which has been inadequately reheated can also be the source.

There are two types of Bacillus cereus: a diarrhoea type with a short onset time of 8 to 16 hours and a vomiting type with an even more rapid onset.

Pathogenic bacteria	Source	Typical symptoms	Average onset time	Special points
Salmonella	Eggs, poultry, cooked meats, unpasteurised milk, insects, sewage	Abdominal pain, diarrhoea, vomiting, headache and high fever	12 to 36 hours	Most common bacteria in the UK. Destroyed by heat above 70°C.
Staphylococcus aureus	Human body, droplet infection, raw milk, meat, meat products	Abdominal pain, severe vomiting	1 to 6 hours	Creates a toxin which causes the illness. High standards of personal hygiene essential.

Pathogenic bacteria	Source	Typical symptoms	Average onset time	Special points
Clostridium perfringens	Raw meat, soil from root vegetables, dust and animal excreta, sewage	Abdominal pain, diarrhoea, nausea	12 to 18 hours	Forms spores which produce a toxin. Spores develop in the danger zone and anaerobic conditions.
Bacillus cereus (i) Vomiting type (ii) Diarrhoea type	(i) Cooked rice (ii) Cereals and cereal products, dust and soil	(i) Nausea, vomiting, diarrhoea later on (ii) Diarrhoea, abdominal pains, rarely vomiting	(i) 1–5 hours (ii) 8–16 hours	Both types produce spores. Toxins from growth of bacteria in food.
Campylobacter jejuni	Raw meat, animal contamination	Diarrhoea, headache, fever, abdominal pain	1 to 5 days	Destroyed by heat. Most common cause of food poisoning in the UK.
Escherichia coli 0157	Raw meats, raw poultry, untreated milk, water, dairy products	Abdominal pain, nausea, diarrhoea, vomiting, kidney failure	12 to 24 hours	Causes gastroenteritis and can be fatal. Sometimes called 'Traveller's Diarrhoea'.
Listeria monocytogenes	Cook-chill foods and ready meals, untreated dairy foods, pâté	Mild flu to serious complications. Can cause miscarriage.	1 to 70 days	Pregnant women, newborn babies, the sick and elderly are at risk. Store food below 5°C and reheat thoroughly. It can survive adverse conditions.
Shigella (bacillary dysentery)	Water, milk, salad, vegetables	Diarrhoea, fever, abdominal pain and vomiting	1 to 7 days	Common among young children although infection occurs in all ages after travel to areas where hygiene is poor.

Summary of main food poisoning bacteria

Activity 3

Use of data

1. With reference to the table above, name two food poisoning bacteria which produce a toxin.
2. Meat is the possible source of which food poisoning bacteria?
3. Which food poisoning bacteria are found in soil? How could you reduce the risk of contamination?
4. Which food-borne disease is dangerous to pregnant women?
5. Name the most common food poisoning bacteria in the UK and identify the symptoms.
6. Which bacteria could come from food handlers?

Conditions and factors for the growth of bacteria

Bacteria can grow very rapidly in the correct conditions. A **bacterium** is one bacteria. A bacterium divides into two by a process called **binary fission.** It needs only 12 hours for a single bacterium to have produced a colony of 16 million.

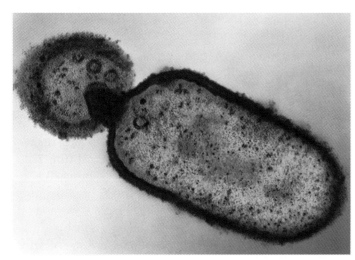

Figure 11.7 *Bacteria growing and budding*

Food poisoning bacteria have four essential requirements: a food source, warmth, moisture and time. Some bacteria also require oxygen.

Food

Bacteria require a food source to reproduce. Food in which bacteria grow rapidly is called **high-risk food.** Bacteria need foods which are good sources of protein. The types of foods on which bacteria can grow easily include:

- cooked meat and poultry
- shellfish and seafood
- uncooked or lightly cooked eggs
- unpasteurised milk and soft cheeses
- gravies, sauces, soups and stocks
- cooked rice and pasta
- prepared salads.

Bacteria will grow in both raw and cooked foods from both animal and vegetable sources. Raw meat and poultry will contain bacteria. Most meat is cooked before consumption and during the cooking process bacteria are destroyed, making the food safe to eat. Contamination after cooking is possible so food should be stored at the correct temperature.

The consumption of foods which are eaten raw, cooked or ready to eat can present a greater risk of food poisoning. These foods may have been handled more during their preparation and production. They are the most important high-risk foods and include ready-to-eat meals, cooked meats, cooked meat products and raw eggs.

Moisture

Without moisture bacteria cannot multiply and cause food poisoning. Dried foods are therefore not usually affected by food poisoning bacteria. Humidity is the amount of water in the air. A kitchen can be a very humid place. Dried foods can be contaminated with moisture in a humid environment. Dried food must be stored in dry, well ventilated and cool areas. Reconstituting a dried food with water or milk will make ideal conditions for bacterial growth.

High quantities of sugar and salt can absorb water from plant and animal cells. Bacteria cannot survive in these conditions so jam making and salting processes preserve food and reduce the likelihood of bacterial contamination.

Warmth

Most bacteria will multiply at ambient temperatures. **Ambient temperature** is normal room temperature and is within the danger zone.

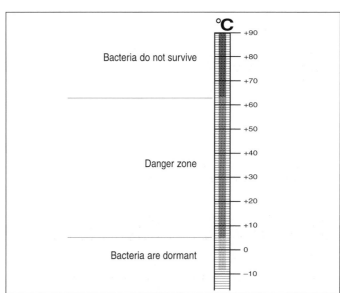

Figure 11.8 *The danger zone for bacteria*

The danger zone is between 5°C and 63°C and will allow bacteria to grow. Between kitchen temperatures

(20°C) and body temperature (37°C) bacteria will grow very fast. At temperatures below 5°C most bacteria are unable to multiply rapidly. They may become dormant. **Dormant** is a period of inactivity when bacteria are unable to multiply. Bacteria can survive the freezing process.

Cooking food at temperatures above 63°C will destroy most bacteria. To ensure the temperature is high enough it is important to check that the core temperature of a food product reaches 70°C for at least two minutes. However, some bacteria are able to form spores and once conditions improve, the spores will become active and start the process of multiplication. Bacteria which can form spores include Clostridium botulinum, Clostridium perfringens and Bacillus cereus.

During the preparation and storage of food it may be in the danger zone. This time should be kept to a minimum.

Sometimes cold food can be combined with warm food (gravies and custards) to warm it up. This topping up of the temperature can bring food back into the danger zone and increase the risk of bacteria multiplying.

Time

When bacteria are left in warm, moist, protein-rich conditions for a length of time, they can reproduce rapidly. Under these conditions the numbers of bacteria can double every 20 minutes. This means that within hours a few bacteria can increase enough to make the food unsafe to eat.

Activity 4

Group discussion

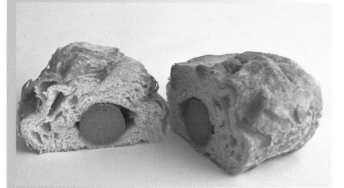

Figure 11.9 *What are the risks when making sausage rolls?*

Consider the process of making sausage rolls in a restaurant. The sausage meat and pastry are delivered

to the kitchen by the supplier in a van. The kitchen is very busy but eventually the preparation of the sausage rolls begins. The sausage rolls are assembled and left. They are baked. Once removed from the oven they are placed in a warming unit (hot holding) in the restaurant. They are held in this unit during lunch.

Can you identify possible contaminants to the ingredients and the finished product?

During the process when are the ingredients and sausage rolls in the danger zone?

How could the risk of food poisoning be minimised?

Acidity or alkalinity

The acidity or alkalinity (pH) of a food will influence the growth of bacteria. The pH of a food is measured using a scale 0 to 14. Acid conditions are pH 0 to 7 and alkaline food are pH 7 to 14. Most bacteria like neutral conditions, a pH value of 7 or slightly alkaline conditions of pH 7.4. Bacteria will not grow in foods with a pH below 4.5, although if bacteria are introduced into an acid food, they may not necessarily die off immediately and could still cause illness. Lemon juice and vinegar can be used as a preservative as they produce conditions which bacteria are less likely to thrive in.

Oxygen

Bacteria vary in their oxygen requirements. Those which need oxygen are called **aerobes** such as Bacillus cereus. Those which do not need oxygen are called **anaerobes** such as Clostridium perfringens. Anaerobes can survive in vacuum-packed food products. Bacteria will grow or survive with or without oxygen including Salmonella and Staphylococcus aureus.

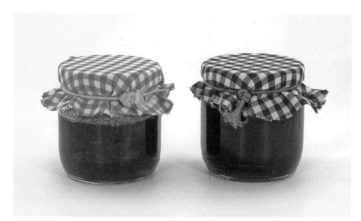

Figure 11.10 *Jams and chutneys are preserved with sugar*

Activity 5

Practical opportunity

Make your own chutney using the recipe below.

Apple, date and ginger chutney

225 g cooking apples, peeled, cored and chopped

500 g chopped dates

15 g piece root ginger, peeled and finely grated

1 clove garlic, finely chopped

300 ml white wine vinegar

½ tsp ground allspice

250 g soft brown sugar

Jam jars with wax-coated paper discs and cellophane covers to seal (or use jam jar lids)

Method

Sterilise jam jars by washing in soapy water and rinsing well. Then place in a cool oven at 130°C/250°F/Gas ½ for 15 to 20 minutes.

Put all the ingredients, except the sugar, in a large saucepan. Simmer uncovered until the dates and apples start to soften.

Stir in the sugar and dissolve.

Simmer gently for 45 minutes until thick and syrupy.

Spoon into sterilised jars, seal and cool. Store in a cool, dark place for at least four weeks, and eat within three months. Once opened, keep in the fridge and use within a fortnight.

Activity 6

Review

Which ingredients will slow down the growth of bacteria?

How can the storage method slow down the growth of bacteria?

Investigate how sugar, alcohol, salt and smoke can preserve food.

Food handling

You will now look at the practical methods for the safe handling of food during preparation, storage and cooking. You will also investigate the incidence of food poisoning in the UK and the possible causes of the outbreaks. You will also focus on E.coli, which has been responsible for several high profile cases of food poisoning in recent years.

Techniques for safe handling during storage

The inappropriate handling and storage of food is one of the most common causes of food poisoning. The correct storage of food should be maintained throughout the production process to the point of sale. The consumer should then continue with good practice at home.

Storage of primary food products

Primary foods have undergone some processing before being used to produce food products. This could include slaughter, harvesting, milling and cleaning. During storage, careless handling and contamination by pests or chemicals can increase the risk of contamination and deterioration. It is very important that people working in these environments recognise the signs of spoilage and monitor the quality of food products regularly.

Storage during transportation

It is important that food requiring temperature-controlled storage is transported in appropriate vehicles. Frozen foods should remain frozen and chilled foods refrigerated. The vehicles used for transportation should be clean. The packaging a food product is stored in should be intact. It should show no signs of rust, leakage or dampness.

Storage in a kitchen fridge

A commercial refrigerator should operate at a temperature between 0°C and 8°C. The ideal temperature is 5°C. Perishable and high-risk foods should be refrigerated. Most bacteria, with the important exception of listeria, find it difficult to multiply in these conditions. Use a fridge thermometer to check the temperature regularly. The refrigerator should be kept clean. Hot food should not be placed in a refrigerator as the condensation it produces can contaminate other food products.

Always keep raw and ready-to-eat food separate. Store wrapped raw meat, poultry or fish near the bottom of the fridge, below any ready-to-eat foods. Protect salad vegetables from any drips from the raw foods by placing them in a lidded box.

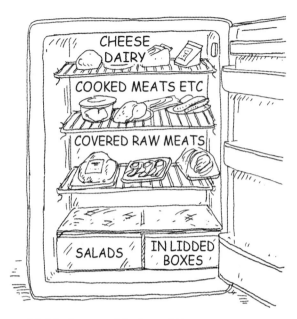

Figure 11.11 *Storage of food in a fridge*

Do not overload the fridge. The cooling air circulating within the fridge needs to flow freely in order to keep the food at a safe temperature.

Freezing

Virtually all bacteria are dormant at temperatures below −18°C. The temperature of freezers should be monitored regularly. Bacterial spores can survive at low temperatures. The defrosting and refreezing of food products may activate spores to produce toxins which could cause illness. It is important that all frozen foods are clearly date marked and wrapped securely.

Dry goods store

Dry goods include many of the food products found in a store cupboard such as flour, milk powder, gravy granules and cereals. Food products should not be stored on the floor but on shelves or pallets. Dry storage areas must be free from spillages and dampness. They should be cool and well ventilated. Packaging should be secure to prevent pests from infesting products. It is important that stock is rotated and date marks checked.

Date marking and food storage

Almost all pre-packed foods must carry a date mark. A date mark is a date on the food packaging which shows the period of time when the food is safe and in the best condition to eat. There are two types:

- **Best before:** This date indicates the period of time during which a food can reasonably be expected to retain its optimum condition. This means it will not be stale or mouldy. The best before date mark consists of the date in terms of day, month and year. The best before date may be accompanied by storage conditions which need to be followed if the food is to retain a reasonable quality until the date shown. This labelling is found on crisp and biscuits packaging.

- **Use by:** Use by date is required for perishable food. This is food with a short shelf-life. Consumption of this food after the use by date could present a risk of food poisoning. The use by date mark must consist of the day and month and the storage conditions which need to be observed (keep refrigerated). It is an offence to sell food past the use by date.

Activity 7

Research opportunity

Make a list of about ten to fifteen food products. Then note whether they use the 'use by' or 'best before' date mark.

Techniques for safe handling during food preparation

Personal hygiene

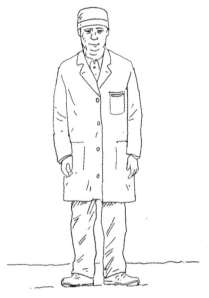

Figure 11.12 *A food worker, appropriately dressed*

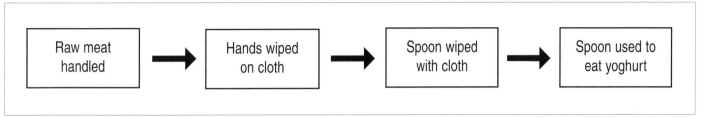

Figure 11.13 *Indirect transfer of contamination*

Food preparation involves a number of stages. During any of these stages food can become contaminated. The personal hygiene of the individual preparing the food may be poor and contamination of the food product could occur. Covering any cuts or grazes on exposed areas with a waterproof dressing is very important. Washing hands with warm water and soap after using the toilet, touching pets or dustbins is essential.

Staphylococcus aureus occurs on the human body – in boils on the skin, the nasal passages and throat. Bacteria can be introduced by an infected person sneezing or coughing over food or failing to cover septic cuts, boils or eye infections (styes) when handling food.

Individuals who are ill or have recently been ill with diarrhoea or vomiting should not prepare or handle food.

It is important to keep handling time to a minimum and wear appropriate clothing when working in a food environment.

Avoiding contamination

There are three types of contamination:

- **Cross-contamination:** Bacteria can move a little but usually they have to be transferred directly or indirectly on to food.
- **Direct contamination:** This is a major cause of food poisoning. The source of the bacteria must be in direct contact with the food. The sources of bacteria are raw food, people, soil, pests, water, air and food waste. It is essential to keep the sources of bacteria separate from ready-to-eat foods at all times.
- **Indirect contamination:** This is the movement of bacteria from a source to a vehicle of contamination. A **vehicle of contamination** can be a person, work surface or object. The transfer vehicle will then contaminate the food. Bacteria in raw food can be transferred to hands, cloths, knives and chopping boards and then on to food. Figure 11.13 shows an example.

To reduce the risk of cross-contamination, the use of colour-coded equipment and chopping boards can be used. There are no legal guidelines suggesting which foods should be prepared on which boards, but the accepted coding system in the UK is as follows:

- Yellow – cooked meats
- Red – uncooked meats
- White – bread and dairy products such as cheese
- Blue – raw fish
- Green – salad and fruit
- Brown – raw vegetables grown within the soil.

If colour-coded boards and knives are not available, avoid using the same knife or chopping board for raw meat and then ready-to-eat foods unless they are cleaned thoroughly between uses.

Activity 8

Review
Explain how each of these sources of bacteria can contaminate the hands:

- soil
- animals
- raw meat
- human waste.

Organising a food preparation area

The cleanliness of the environment should be maintained. Structural damage, including chipped tiles and gaps between units, can attract pests and so should be repaired immediately. Harmful bacteria may multiply in the crevices and cracks on damaged surfaces. Scratched surfaces and chopping boards are harder to clean. Damaged equipment can also be difficult to clean and chipped crockery should be discarded.

Equipment must be in good working order. A poorly functioning refrigerator may not chill food adequately. If it does not work properly, food may not be kept safe. Temperature probes should be checked regularly to make sure their readings are accurate. If the probe is not accurate, it will not give a reliable measure of whether food is stored at a safe temperature.

Wash dishes, equipment, worktops and cutlery with hot water and detergent. Keep dishcloths and tea towels clean and change them frequently.

Organise the preparation of food according to its susceptibility to bacteria. Prepare foods which need refrigeration last and avoid leaving food for longer than necessary at room temperature, as this can allow harmful bacteria to grow.

Activity 9

Review

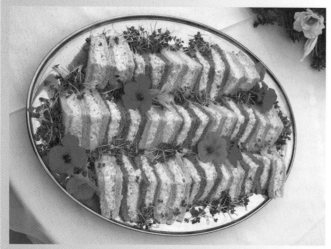

Figure 11.14 *Sandwiches on a buffet*

Imagine you have been asked to organise a sixth form buffet lunch. What advice would you give to the students preparing the sandwiches? Consider the areas of food purchase, personal hygiene, preparation and storage.

Techniques for safe handling during cooking

The best way to avoid food poisoning is to cook your food thoroughly. This destroys the harmful bacteria which may cause food poisoning.

It is important that food is heated thoroughly for all the bacteria to be destroyed. An understanding of the danger zone is important to reduce the risk of food poisoning. The danger zone is between 5°C and 63°C. Food must be cooked and hot food stored at temperatures above this zone. High-risk foods should spend no more than four hours in the danger zone.

Preparation for cooking

Make sure meat and poultry are fully thawed before cooking. Thaw food in a refrigerator or at room temperature. Large items such as a whole frozen turkey can take many hours to defrost and you should never start cooking a turkey before it is completely thawed. The centre of the turkey may still be frozen. The heat from the oven will destroy surface bacteria, but the centre of the turkey will remain in the danger zone – ideal for bacteria to multiply.

Critical temperatures

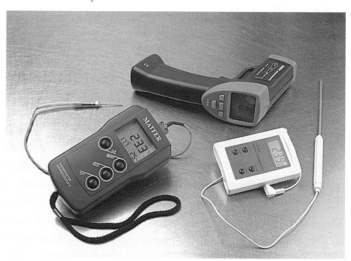

Figure 11.15 *Food temperature probes*

Most bacteria will be destroyed at a temperature above 70°C. To ensure that all the bacteria are destroyed it is important that this temperature is held for at least two minutes.

A temperature probe can be used to ensure food reaches a core temperature above 70°C for two minutes. Special care should be taken with large meat joints or whole poultry, as they are more likely to cook unevenly. To help achieve an even distribution of heat, large joints can be cut into smaller portions, food can be turned in the oven and casseroles and stews should be stirred and boiled.

Measuring temperature

In the food industry the temperature must be monitored and recorded during food production. The use of digital or infrared probes is common. In the home a temperature probe can also be an effective way to ensure core temperatures are above the danger zone and food is safe to eat.

Activity 10

Practical opportunity

Use a temperature probe to do the following:

- Record the temperature of a fridge. Are there any differences between a full and empty fridge? Are there any differences between the top shelf and bottom shelf?
- Check the core temperature of the food you are cooking and cooling. Record your findings. What conclusions about the danger zone can you draw?
- Following the manufacturer's instructions, use a microwave to heat a ready meal. Check the core temperature. Are the instructions correct?

Microwave cooking

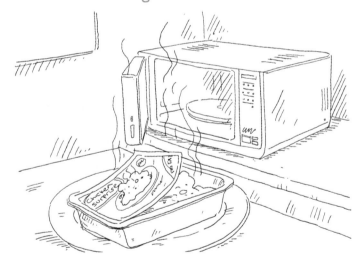

Figure 11.16 *A cook-chill meal reheated in the microwave*

Microwave cooking causes molecules in food to vibrate. The vibration causes friction and creates heat which is not evenly distributed in the food product. Large, dense foods take more time to cook. Most microwaves penetrate only one to two centimetres into the food, so some food may need more than one cooking cycle. The centre of the food is heated by conduction. Conduction is the movement of heat from the outside to the inside of the food. Microwaves do not always cook evenly so food can have hot and cold spots. To prevent this you can re-arrange, cover, stir and rotate the food during cooking.

At the end of the cooking cycle, wait until the standing time is over before serving. The standing time is usually two minutes. The food will continue to cook for a few minutes even when the microwave oven is turned off. Test for completeness of cooking. Juices in chicken, beef, pork and fish should all run clear and the centre of ready meals should be piping hot. Do not reheat cooked food more than once.

Barbecues

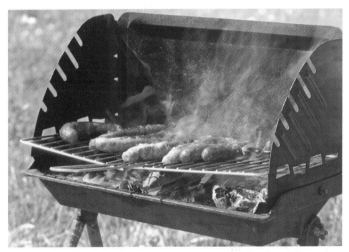

Figure 11.17 *A barbecue*

Poorly cooked meat on barbecues has been linked with food poisoning. Raw meats such as burgers, sausages and chicken can carry pathogenic bacteria. There is a significant risk of illness if raw meats, particularly chicken, are not cooked properly. Raw meat can contaminate surfaces and equipment if it comes into contact with ready-to-eat food. To avoid cross-contamination, do not allow raw meat to touch or drip onto cooked food, wash hands after handling raw meat and use separate utensils for raw and cooked meats. Always check food is evenly cooked and piping hot.

Hot holding

Hot holding is when cooked food is stored at a temperature above 63°C during serving or display for sale. Hot food should be kept at a core temperature above 63°C to stop the multiplication of bacteria. During hot holding it is important to stir or rotate food frequently to maintain a temperature above the danger

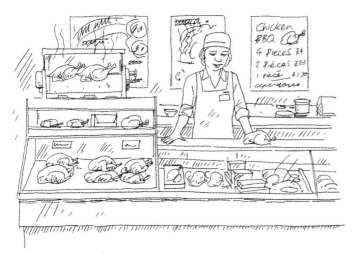

Figure 11.18 *Hot holding of cooked food*

zone. Food may be displayed for up to a maximum of two hours outside the hot holding equipment. It cannot be reheated. Never use hot holding to reheat food. Care should be taken to avoid cross-contamination.

Cooling hot food

Cooked foods which need to be chilled should be cooled as quickly as possible, preferably within an hour. Inadequate cooling is an important cause of food poisoning. During the cooling process, food enters the danger zone, so it is essential to keep the time spent in the danger zone to a minimum. The maximum time cooling food should be in the danger zone is four hours. The aim should be to reduce the temperature to 5°C within two hours, and then it is ready for refrigeration. Stirring and rotating food will contribute to lowering the temperature as it allows air to circulate. Try to protect the food from contamination during cooling. Never put hot food in the refrigerator, as this will raise the temperature of the whole refrigerator and could stimulate the growth of bacteria in other stored products.

Reheating

Leftovers should be used within 24 hours. Store other leftovers in clean, covered containers in the fridge at 5°C. Heat leftovers and pre-cooked food to at least 70°C for two minutes. Food should be very hot and steaming before it is served. Never reheat more than once and if in doubt throw it out!

The incidence and patterns of food poisoning

The food industry takes great care to ensure food is safe to eat. However, the reported incidence of food poisoning has increased significantly since the 1980s. It is possible that the increase is due to a number of factors.

Increased public awareness of food poisoning

There has been increased public knowledge and awareness of the symptoms and signs of food poisoning. This has possibly resulted in large numbers of previously unreported 'stomach upsets' now being reported as cases of food poisoning.

Changing shopping habits

Families and households shop less frequently. Instead of a daily shop, we tend to purchase larger amounts of food less frequently. This means food is stored in the home for longer periods of time. Storage at home may not be adequate and there may be a risk of cross-contamination.

Increased consumption of cook-chill foods

Cook-chill foods require carefully controlled low temperature storage. This may not be provided in the home. They also require cooking thoroughly to destroy any pathogenic bacteria. A lack of understanding of the best way to store and cook these foods has possibly contributed to the increase.

Hot weather and more barbeque food

The number of cases of food poisoning appears to increase during the summer months. It is difficult to attribute this rise to any one cause. It could be due to a greater consumption of barbequed foods which carries an increased risk of food poisoning.

More meals consumed outside the home

As more meals are consumed outside the home the risk of food poisoning is likely to increase. Some establishments may not comply with expected standards of hygiene and food safety.

However, a recent Health Protection Agency survey reported nearly nine out of ten cases of food poisoning in the home occur at dinner parties, barbecues and other events when people cook for larger numbers than usual. Most of these cases were caused by poor hygiene and inadequate storage of larger quantities of cooked food.

More foreign travel

E.coli is the most common cause of travellers' diarrhoea. With increased travel overseas and within the UK, the incidence of this type of food poisoning is increasing. People may return from holiday with food poisoning. Poor hygiene and food handling practices, contaminated food and water supply are the possible sources.

Globalisation of the food market

The speed at which food travels around the globe enables bacteria to survive and spread more easily. More infected food products are brought into the UK by consumers from countries where the standards of food hygiene may not be as high.

Advances in science

New methods of detecting food poisoning bacteria have been developed by microbiologists. The new technology helps to trace outbreaks of disease more swiftly and to intervene earlier. Further advances in microbiology have allowed strains of different bacteria to be identified more effectively. Using sophisticated 'typing' techniques, discrimination between individual strains of bacteria can be achieved.

The emergence of new strains of micro-organisms

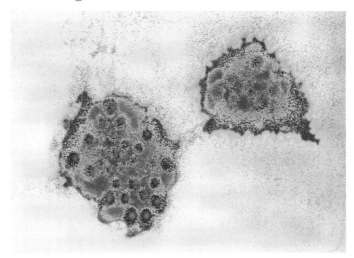

Figure 11.19 *The Norwalk virus*

The first reported cases of E.coli 0157 were in England and Wales in 1982. The Norwalk virus or Norovirus has in recent years emerged as a significant cause of gastroenteritis.

Focus on E.coli

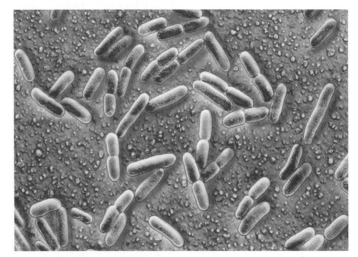

Figure 11.20 *E. coli bacteria*

Escherichia coli (E.coli) are known as enteric bacteria. **Enteric bacteria** can live in the intestines of humans and animals. There are hundreds of different strains of E.coli and many are harmless. However, some strains will cause serious illness. In recent years, microbiologists have identified a particularly dangerous 'VTEC' strain. VTEC stands for Verocytotoxin after the very dangerous toxin (poison) the E.coli strain produces in the intestine. It is also known as E.coli 0157. Several outbreaks of VTEC E.coli 0157 infection have been reported since1985.

How it spreads

It is often spread in faeces, contaminated drinking or bathing water and from touching infected animals and food. E.coli outbreaks have been associated with a wide range of foods: undercooked beef especially beef burgers, contaminated or unpasteurised milk, unpasteurised fruit juices, yoghurts, mushrooms and cross-contamination from infected persons or animals. People working with raw meats, on farms or visiting open farms should pay close attention to good hygiene practices with careful hand washing.

How it causes illness

E.coli produce toxins which enable the bacteria to penetrate the gut lining, causing abdominal pain and severe diarrhoea. Most people fight off the infection within two weeks, but the excretion of bacteria from the bowel continues for longer. Person-to-person infection is an important route of transmission, particularly if poor hygiene practices are followed. Some victims, particularly the old and very young, may go on to develop serious diarrhoea and kidney failure, which can be fatal. Consuming less than ten bacteria can make a person ill.

Control of E.coli

A highly significant outbreak of E.coli poisoning occurred in Lanarkshire, Scotland in 1996. The E.coli food poisoning claimed the lives of 21 people and remains the largest E.coli outbreak in the UK, with 373 cases reported.

The Pennington report published after the outbreak called for the introduction of important measures to reduce the risk of cross-contamination between raw meat and ready-to-eat foods. The recommendations led to the licensing of all butchers handling both raw meat and ready-to-eat food from 2000. A business is not allowed to operate without a licence. Licences are only issued if hygiene standards and staff training are implemented. If standards fall, an environmental health officer from the local authority can withdraw the licence and stop the business from operating.

Some E.coli 0157 outbreaks involving children have been linked with educational and recreational visits to

open farms. This has increased awareness of the risk at open farms from contamination from animals. Young children are at greatest risk of developing complications from an infection. As a result, control measures including hand washing facilities have been introduced. Infection can result from exposure to bacteria from animals or animal faeces and then eating or drinking without first thoroughly washing hands.

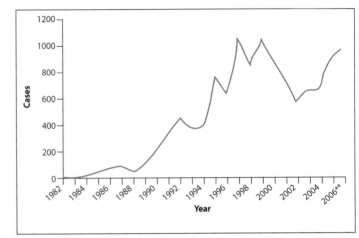

Figure 11.21   *Reported cases of E.coli 0157, 1982–2006*

Source: Health Protection Agency Centre for Infections

Activity 12

The use of data

With reference to the graph above, suggest a reason why the cases of E.coli 0157 began to rise from 1982?

Suggest a reason for the fall in cases in 2000.

Using the internet investigate the high profile cases of E.coli. Find out the source of infection and who was affected.

Activity 13

Review

For each of the following cases of food poisoning do the following:

• Identify the source of the bacteria.

• Suggest how contamination could have occurred.

• Name the type of bacteria which may be responsible.

• How contamination can be avoided.

Case 1

Within a few hours after returning from a holiday overseas, Paula complained of abdominal pain, nausea and diarrhoea. On the last day of the holiday she had been drinking the local tap water and had ice in her drinks.

Case 2

The farm shop sold an excellent range of dairy products, some straight from the field and free from processing. Breakfast the following morning was delicious but within 24 hours of eating it, Robert had a headache, fever, abdominal pain, diarrhoea and was vomiting.

Case 3

The buffet was prepared well in advance and as it was a cold day, the chilled food, although covered, was left ready to eat in the room. There was a good selection of pâté, cooked meats, quiches and meat-based snacks. A week after, people who attended the party and had eaten from the buffet table started to complain of flu-like symptoms. One pregnant woman was very poorly.

Case 4

The supermarket had taken on many students before Christmas to work in the delicatessen. The training covered the very basics of food hygiene. One of the students had been ill with gastric flu but she did not think it was important, so came to work as normal. Later that day customers were developing symptoms of abdominal pain and severe vomiting.

Case 5

The children were very hungry and would not wait. The curry was ready but the rice, which was already cooked and refrigerated, needed warming quickly. The microwave oven was the best option. Within two hours all the children were feeling sick and vomiting. Diarrhoea was to follow.

Activity 14

Check your understanding

Check your understanding of the meaning of the following words:

physical contamination	toxin
binary fission	chemical contamination
symptom	high-risk food
micro-organism contamination	onset time
	dormant
danger zone	yeast
mycotoxins	virus
ambient temperature	mould
campylobacter	aerobes
E.coli	salmonella

food-borne disease	clostridium
anaerobes	perfringens
listeria	date mark
cross-contamination	use by
best before	spoilage bacteria
bacterium	pathogenic bacteria
vehicle of contamination	

Then answer these questions.
1. Name three sources of food contamination.
2. Explain the difference between
   (i) Virus and bacteria
   (ii) Aerobes and anaerobes
   (iii) Use by and best before mark
3. What are vehicles of contamination?
4. Name the method by which bacteria multiply.
5. Explain the danger zone.
6. Which term from the list above is used to describe:
   (i) Inactive bacteria
   (ii) Poison produced by bacteria
   (iii) Bacteria causing decomposition and decay
   (iv) Toxin produced by a mould

Monitoring standards

The Food Safety (General Food Hygiene) Regulations 1995 and Food Safety (Temperature Control) Regulations 1995 have now been replaced with new legislation. The new requirements are set out in new European Community food safety and hygiene laws. This legislation sets the standard required for the safe processing and sale of food across Europe.

Broadly, food legislation can be divided into two areas: general food safety legislation and hygiene legislation.

General food safety legislation
The Food Safety Act 1990

This Act provided the framework for many of the current regulations and is concerned with all aspects of food production and sale. It affects everyone involved in the production, processing, storage, distribution and sale of food. It ensures that all food produced in the food industry is safe to eat. The powers available to local authorities are in the Food Hygiene (England) Regulations 2006.

The Food Safety Act 1990 has been amended but some elements are still applied. In Section 7 it states that it is an offence to render or to make food sold for human consumption injurious to health. A food producer or retailer may not add any substance to food or subject food to any process or treatment which will make it harmful to health. Section 9 concerned with the inspection and seizure of suspected food is also implemented. An environmental health officer (EHO) may at all reasonable times inspect any food intended for human consumption. If the food is regarded as unfit for human consumption, it may be seized.

The legislation provides a defence for food producers, processors and retailers. They must prove that all reasonable precautions were taken to prevent a food safety incident and that they have exercised 'due diligence'.

Failure to take reasonable precautions can result in prosecution. Magistrates' courts may impose a fine, prison sentence or both for offences committed.

General Food Law Regulation (EC) 178/2002

This legislation covers the import and export of food into the European Union. The legislation also covers food safety and presentation. Food is unsafe if it is harmful to health and unfit for human consumption. The labelling, advertising and display of food must not mislead consumers. Food businesses must keep records of suppliers so food can be traced. They must withdraw food which does not meet food safety requirements.

Food hygiene legislation

Food hygiene legislation is based on the following EC Directives and regulations:

- **Regulation (EC) 852/2004** relates to food hygiene.
- **Regulation (EC) 853/2004** provides hygiene rules for foods of animal origin.
- **Regulation (EC) 854/2004** sets out rules for the control of animal products intended for human consumption.
- **Regulation (EC) 2073/2005** sets out the microbiological criteria for foodstuffs.

You will now explore some of the significant legislation.

Regulation (EC) 2073/2005

All food contains some bacteria. This legislation sets out the acceptable microbiological content of food.

Bacteria can be tolerated if the amounts are small as processing will destroy it. The legislation sets out the guidelines for testing and sampling food products to protect the consumer. It provides guidelines on the microbiological criteria for different types of food.

The regulation requires all food business operators to take measures to ensure that microbiological criteria are met throughout the foreseeable life of the product and they must consider the instructions for the use of the product. It is up to the food business to decide any necessary sampling and the testing frequencies. This must be done as part of their procedures based on hazard analysis and critical control points (HACCP) principles, together with implementing good hygiene practices. Microbiological standards are used by food businesses to support food safety procedures. The testing can analyse the acceptability of food during the manufacturing, preparation and distribution.

Food product manufacturers also have an obligation to conduct studies throughout their products' shelf-life to ensure that their foods comply with the microbiological criteria. This is particularly important in ready-to-eat food products that can support the growth of listeria monocytogenes. Food retailers may collaborate in conducting the tests. Specific rules are laid down for sampling and testing and for action to be taken, including withdrawing or recalling products from the market if the tests provide unsatisfactory results. The role of the Food Standards Agency in supporting these tests when product recalls are required will be explored later.

Food Hygiene (England) Regulations 2006

These regulations apply to food businesses and cover all activities involving food. They do not apply to food prepared and stored for private domestic consumption.

The legislation sets out more clearly the responsibility of food businesses to produce food safely and to achieve consistency. For the first time the whole food chain from 'farm to fork' is covered by legislation. Farm to fork means food can be traced through all the stages of production, processing and distribution to the source. The regulations will affect all food businesses – caterers, primary producers such as farmers and manufacturers, distributors and retailers to the sale or placing food on the market.

The regulations do not introduce new hygiene requirements. Food should be stored, handled and processed safely as before. Premises should continue to be kept clean and hygienic. Most of the 'old' requirements relating to cleanliness, the structure of the food preparation environment, provision of equipment and facilities and temperature control requirements remain the same.

The key change is the requirement for a HACCP plan to be put in place. The legislation requires more detailed record keeping. The important documentation includes:

- food safety management procedures
- training records of staff and staff illness reporting procedures
- cleaning schedules
- pest control and waste disposal contracts
- records of checks, problems found and action taken (food temperature logbook)
- list of suppliers.

The Food Hygiene (England) Regulations 2006, specifically Regulation 852 Article 5, introduced the requirement for food businesses to '... put in place, implement and maintain a permanent procedure or procedures based on HACCP principles.'

To meet with the new legislation, all food businesses are required to have written food safety plans in place based on the principles of HACCP.

HACCP stands for hazard analysis critical control point. It is a risk assessment system that has been adopted by the food industry and is widely used in catering and food retailing. It is a system that identifies hazards associated with food and processing and suggests procedures to reduce risks and ensures food is safe to eat. It requires an active approach to reduce risks and hazards.

Implementing food safety management procedures

It is on the HACCP principles that food safety management procedures and plans are based. It is the responsibility of the owner of the business to develop appropriate food safety management systems based on HACCP. These may vary in detail depending upon the type of business, food and processes used and potential risks to food safety and public health.

Food safety plans provide practical steps to identify and control hazards in order to establish and maintain food safety. Many businesses store the food safety plans and monitoring sheets in a folder with other important documentation.

Food safety plans deal with the important stages of food production and food supply. They may also cover staff, equipment and food preparation areas. In a food catering business, they may include many separate plans covering the distinct stages:

purchase and delivery	chilled food
frozen food	stock control
storage and preparation	cooking
hot holding	cooling
reheating	personal hygiene
pest control	equipment and premises
cleaning and maintenance	

The amount of detail included in a plan will depend upon the types of food which are prepared, served or sold by the business. A food safety plan for a business which is cooking or slicing roast meats will need to be more detailed, as the risk of food poisoning is much greater than one for a garage selling crisps and drinks.

Below is an example of a food safety plan for hot holding. **Hot holding** is the process of keeping food hot (above 63°C). The hazard could be that harmful bacteria will multiply if the temperature falls below 63°C.

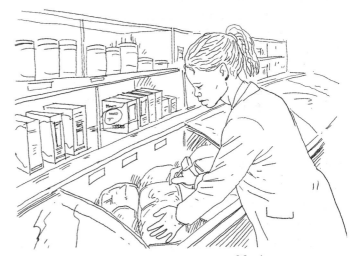

Figure 11.22 *Checking the temperature of food*

In reality, many small businesses produce food safety plans for specific aspects of food production which are relevant to their business. These plans are not very complicated. They identify what will make the food unsafe – the hazards. Then they give ways in which food can be produced safely – the critical control points. Finally, they suggest methods of controlling the hazard – the critical limits.

The plan should give an indication of monitoring the checks and corrective action if necessary.

Safe hot holding

Hazard
- Harmful bacteria can multiply if the temperature falls below 63°C.

Safe hot holding plan
- Cabinet and utensils are clean before use.
- Preheat cabinet before use.
- Keep hot food above 63°C.
- Keep food hot only once.
- Food must be thoroughly and piping hot before hot holding begins (to 75°C).
- Food remains in cabinet and door is closed after use.

Checking hot holding
- Probe the temperature of the food daily. The core should be over 63°C.
- Check the temperature of the appliance is accurate daily.
- Log the temperatures in 'Temperatures Book'.

Corrective action
For example, hot holding cabinet does not maintain safe temperatures for food products.
- Inform the manager if there is a problem.
- Increase the temperature of the cabinet or remove some food.
- If food has been in the danger zone for an unknown time, **destroy food**
- If food has been in the danger zone for less than two hours:
  - cool quickly and refrigerate food below 8°C, ideally between 2°C and 5°C
  - reheat food quickly to 75°C and return to correctly functioning appliance, maintaining temperature above 63°C.
- Ring engineer (number in the folder) and request urgent call.
- Replace equipment if necessary. Supplier contact details in folder.

Who is responsible for these checks?
Name of employee and their training needs.

The plan suggests ways of managing this process and the checks to ensure that the hazards are controlled. As required by the legislation, there is a method of recording the checks.

Food safety plans can demonstrate 'due diligence' if things do go wrong and the business is taken to court.

This may protect the owner of the business from prosecution.

To **prove due diligence** a business must be able to demonstrate that it took every possible reasonable step to achieve safe food. It is likely that the court would demand written records to support the defence. These might include documents from the food safety plans which should be based on the HACCP principles. Other relevant documentation may include staff training records, temperature records, cleaning schedules, supplier specifications, traceability systems, remedial action where food safety problems have arisen and pest control measures.

The role of the environmental health officer

Environmental health officers (EHO) help develop, co-ordinate and enforce public health policies. There are many aspects to their work, but mainly they ensure that people have a better quality of life in a healthier and safer society.

EHOs are employed by local councils and work in specialist areas such as food safety, health and safety at work, housing or environmental protection.

For the purpose of this discussion we will focus on their role in monitoring the quality of food we eat outside the home.

Environmental health officers have the right to enter and inspect food premises at all reasonable hours. EHO do not have to make an appointment to visit premises and can visit without advance notice. They carry out routine inspections of all food premises in their area. The frequency of routine inspections depends on the potential risk posed by the type of business and its previous record. Some 'high risk' premises may be inspected at least every six months, others much less often. EHOs may also visit premises as a result of a complaint.

The inspection

The inspection may start with an initial discussion on the nature of the food business to identify the associated hazards and risks. This should include the identification of all the food-related activities undertaken on the premises, the staff involved and their expertise, the type and quality of food handled and the number and type of consumers involved.

Activity 15

Group discussion

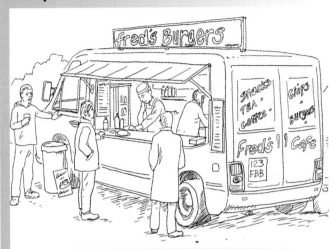

Figure 11.23 *A burger van: high risk?*

Make a list of the different types of food retailers. Talk about the types of premises which are high risk and would require frequent inspections.

During the inspection the officer will wear suitable protective clothing. They will give verbal feedback on the inspection and ask questions to check compliance with the law or good practice.

Inspectors will look at the way the business operates and will identify potential hazards. They will inspect the food safety management system and plans. The EHO will discuss any problems and advise on possible solutions.

At the end of the inspection, the EHO will complete a report of inspection findings which is left at the premises with the manager or owner. This will indicate what enforcement action is to be taken. Enforcement action can range from verbal advice, informal or formal letter and notices through to prosecution.

A formal Inspection letter contains issues that must be addressed to comply with legislation. The EHO will identify which regulations have been contravened and will state the legal requirements as opposed to recommendations. The EHO may revisit to check compliance with the issues in the letter.

An EHO can serve a **hygiene improvement notice** where they have reasonable grounds for believing that a food business is failing to comply with food hygiene regulations. This notice will specify the contraventions, the appropriate remedy and a timescale by which

improvements must be made. Failure to comply with a hygiene improvement notice is an offence which can lead to a fine or imprisonment.

Once one has been served, an EHO will revisit the premises to check that the required work has been completed.

If an EHO believes that there is a significant risk to health or injury due to the condition of equipment, the handling process or the condition of the premises, then a **hygiene emergency prohibition notice** may be served. This immediately stops the use of the equipment or premises or a specified handling process. The EHO will apply to a magistrates' court within three days for a hygiene emergency prohibition order. Photographs of food may be used as evidence. This award if issued must be displayed on the premises in a public place and it can only be removed by an EHO once the issues have been addressed.

To avoid the involvement of a magistrates' court, a food business may elect to closure voluntarily. The EHO will confirm the voluntary closure in writing. During the voluntary closure the improvements will be carried out. However, should the business reopen before improvements are completed, the EHO will serve a hygiene emergency prohibition notice.

The seizure and detention of food

EHOs have the power to inspect and seize food suspected of not meeting food safety regulations. An EHO may take action with a whole batch, lot or consignment of such food. Food is taken if there is suspicion that the food is contaminated and is likely to cause food poisoning or disease. Food which is taken may undergo microbiological examination and testing.

In order to condemn or seize food, the officer must present their findings to a justice of the peace. The justice of the peace will consider the information provided by the EHO and decide whether the food poses a risk to human health and whether or not to condemn the food. If condemned, the cost of destruction falls on the owner of the food.

The owner of food may voluntarily surrender unfit food to the authority as a result of a suggestion by the EHO. This would avoid involvement of the court.

The Food Safety Act 1990 provides officers with powers of enforcement. This will be issued if the law is being broken and will set out certain things that must be completed to comply with the law.

Activity 16

Review by case study

This is an extract from a routine visit by an EHO to a fish and chip shop. Identify the food safety and hygiene issues it raises.

The owner of the premises was working in the shop and greeted the EHO. The owner had a skin complaint and his neck and hands were covered in spots and blisters. He escorted the EHO into the food preparation area. The EHO put on a clean white coat and hat. She washed her hands in a small hand basin; soap, paper towels and cold water were available. It was a hot day and the back door was open. Two long ribbons of fly paper hung from the ceiling. An employee wearing a thin plastic apron was dealing with a delivery of fresh fish and frozen food.

The EHO asked to see the food safety management system. The owner disappeared to retrieve it. Eventually he returned without it, claiming it was at home.

The inspection started with floors, walls and ceilings. There were cracks in the tiles by the sink and paint was flaking from the ceiling above the food preparation area. The light fitting was a fluorescent strip, which was very dusty and a collection of dead flies were encased in the fitment. The touch points including the light switches were greasy.

On one wall there were gaps between the skirting board and plaster, creating deep crevices. Six large sacks of potatoes lay on the floor and were stacked against this wall. A mop bucket was filled with dirty water. Cleaning products were stored by the potatoes.

The premises had two large stainless steel sinks, each filled with used equipment and utensils. Another employee was washing salad and vegetables in a colander under one tap. A saucepan of curry sauce was stored by the sink.

The EHO entered a large walk-in refrigerator. A long strip of cardboard had been placed on the floor. Her temperature probe revealed this was operating at the correct temperature of 5°C. Fresh fish was stored on a top shelf uncovered and next to a tray of cooked pies. All the manufacturers' packaging had been removed from the pies except the coloured tin foil bases. Heavy items including cartons of milk and a plastic bucket of batter were on the floor. The shelves in the fridge were clean but there was evidence of splashing and spillage against the walls.

Next the EHO inspected the hot holding area. The

temperature dial on the hot holding cabinet indicated that it was at 75°C, the EHO's own probe revealed a temperature of 65°C. The cabinet contained a selection of pies, cooked fish and sausages. On a desk near the cabinet was a needle probe which was being used to check the internal temperature of food products.

The EHO went outside the premises. An uncovered vat of used cooking oil was by the back door, awaiting removal by a waste disposal company.

Write a letter to the manager of the fish bar informing him of your concerns. Give him instructions to improve food safety and hygiene.

The Food Standards Agency

The Food Standards Agency (FSA) is an independent organisation. Its main aim is to protect public health in relation to food in the UK. It was set up by the government in April 2000 by the Food Standards Act 1999. A number of high profile cases of food poisoning in the 1990s created the need for unbiased departments to report on issues where farming and food safety were linked.

The FSA is based in London but it has offices in Scotland, Wales and Northern Ireland. The Meat Hygiene Service is a branch of the Food Standards Agency. The FSA debates important issues concerning food safety in the UK. Since 2003 some meetings have been web-cast live. This enables consumers to see the decision-making process in action. Meetings conclude with a questions and answers session in which web viewers can question the FSA directly.

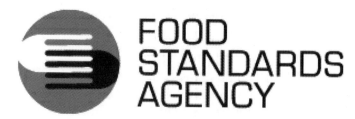

Figure 11.24 *The Food Standards Agency logo*

There are four key strands to the FSA:

- **Policy advice and legislation:** The FSA is accountable to parliament but does not need government approval to act or offer advice. It provides advice to the government on food safety and standards. This information is used by government to make legislation. It represents the UK government on food safety and standards issues in the European Union.

- **Research and surveillance:** The FSA bases its advice, policies and decisions on the best available science. It will commission research and surveillance from its budget. Through research, the FSA identifies areas of weakness in food safety, including concerns over controls on farms, in slaughterhouses and food retailing.

- **General food law enforcement:** Local authorities, including environmental health departments, are responsible for routine food law enforcement (except for meat hygiene). The FSA will monitor and support their role.

- **Public information and education:** The FSA provides public information and develops health promotion and education activities. The FSA provides educational material to help school children learn about healthy eating and safer food preparation. Some resources are aimed at both primary and secondary school children. They provide videos, CD-ROMs, interactive games, the food bus and cookery clubs.

The FSA and farming

The FSA has a key role in preventing contaminated food entering the food chain. It may introduce controls over the movement of animals and will carry out surveillance where disease is suspected. It also monitors the quality of animal feed.

Food hygiene and food-borne illness

The FSA advises the government on all aspects of food hygiene policy and the microbiological safety of food. It issues licences to fresh meat plants to prevent the transmission of BSE.

Outbreaks of food poisoning are still the responsibility of the local authority but the FSA will support their investigation into food-borne illness. It may become directly involved if a significant food poisoning incident extends beyond the local level. The FSA manages large-scale food scares and issues public warnings.

The FSA launched an advertising campaign on television, highlighting the danger of food poisoning caused by barbecues. The adverts showed the dangers of eating undercooked sausage. There have also been advertising campaigns at Christmas showing the food poisoning risk associated with undercooked poultry.

Novel foods and food additives

Novel foods are defined by the FSA as a food or food ingredient which does not have a significant history of consumption within the EU before May 1997. Novel foods include genetically modified foods and cholesterol-lowering foods. The FSA assesses novel food applications in accordance with EU legislation.

The FSA is responsible for all matters concerning food additives and takes action to protect the public if new information about the safety or use of food additives comes to light. Following advice from the Advisory Committee on the Microbiological Safety of Food (ACMSF) in February 2005, the agency announced a recall of products containing Worcester sauce. The products contained the potentially harmful dye Sudan I.

Chemical contamination and radiological safety

The FSA is responsible for checking the chemical contamination of food. It will carry out investigations to find out the intake of contaminated food and the sources of contaminants. It monitors radioactive waste and other sources of radioactivity in the food supply. It will run a surveillance programme for radioactivity in the food chain.

Food intolerance

The FSA provides information to the food industry, caterers and the public on food intolerance. It commissions research into food intolerance. The FSA develops changes to EC labelling rules to ensure that there is greater public awareness of food intolerance.

Food emergencies

The FSA would manage and coordinate a national food emergency from contaminated food.

Food standards and quality

The FSA ensures that the consumer is not misled about the quality and composition of food. It conducts surveillance programmes on food authenticity and monitors food labelling.

Nutrition

The FSA provides balanced information to help the public make decisions on what they wish to eat. The FSA defines a balanced diet and uses it as a basis for health education resources. The Eatwell plate is a resource used to explain the principles of eating a balanced diet. The FSA works with health departments in defining the health education message on nutritional issues and in developing government policy.

The FSA has been involved in the campaign to tighten the rules on TV advertising aimed at children. It devised a nutritional profiling system to assess the amount of salt, sugar and fat in food products, and using this scheme made judgments about food products. In 2007 the TV Regulator OFCOM introduced restrictions on advertising of products which scored poorly under the FSA scheme.

The FSA will propose legislation relating to nutrition such as labelling, health claims and dietary supplements.

Targets

The FSA has had targets to improve many aspects of food safety, hygiene and food labelling. These include reducing food-borne illness by 20 per cent between the years 2001 and 2006. The FSA aims to encourage healthy eating; in particular it encourages consumers to reduce salt consumption and suppliers to provide informative labelling on food products.

Activity 17

Check your understanding

Check your understanding of the meaning of the following terms:

Food Hygiene (England) Regulations 2006	**food safety plans**
due diligence	**Food Standards Agency**
hygiene improvement notices	**farm to fork**
hygiene emergency prohibition notice	**HACCP**
environmental health officer	**hot holding**
	novel foods

Exam-style questions

Figure 11.25 shows the number of recorded (notified) cases of food poisoning in the UK between the period 1985 and 2005.

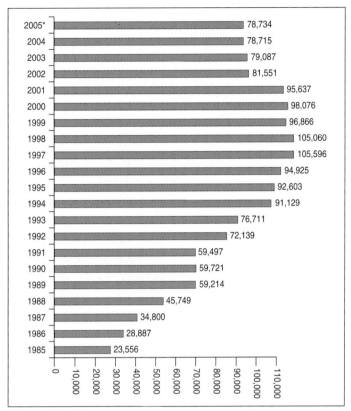

Figure 11.25

Provisional figures for 2005

Source: Health Protection Agency Centre

1 a. How many reported cases were there in 2005?

b. Which year had the greatest number of cases?

c. Describe the trend in the graph.

d. Give three reasons why the number of cases has increased since 1985. (4 marks)

2 Define the following terms:

a. danger zone

b. cross-contamination

c. high-risk food (6 marks)

3 Explain why it is necessary for food handlers to be trained in food hygiene. (15 marks)

4 Discuss the role of the FSA in ensuring food is safe to eat. (10 marks)

(Total of 35 marks)

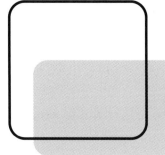

Assessment advice

Learning objectives

By the end of this section you will:

- Understand how the AS units are examined
- Know the definitions of trigger words used in examination questions
- Investigate a variety of ways in which to revise and improve exam performance
- Examine some candidate responses and read a commentary on their strengths and weaknesses.

How the AS is examined

In this section we will examine the purpose of the exam and the structure of the AS papers.

Assessment objectives

The exam must meet the assessment objectives. These objectives are very important and you need to be aware of them before you go into the exam.

The assessment objectives cover both knowledge and skills. Exams are written to find out how much you know about the subject, but also to test your skills when applying the knowledge. Your mark will be based on how effectively you meet both these objectives. The assessment objectives are described below.

AO1 Knowledge and understanding

Demonstrate knowledge and understanding of the specified content.

This is the **knowledge of the subject** you have covered, but you are also expected to demonstrate an **understanding of the subject**. This means that you should not just take everything you have learnt at face value, but be able to see the knowledge in different contexts.

Questions which assess this objective may involve extracting information from data, defining a key term or stating a fact.

AO2 Apply knowledge and understanding and analyse problems

Demonstrate the ability to **apply knowledge and understanding**.

Application is the skill of being able to take knowledge and apply it to different contexts and situations to understand why problems and issues arise. The skill of analysing problems in a variety of situations is important. It is one thing to understand a term or concept; it is another to be able to apply it to a real life situation. Most of the marks are awarded for this objective. These questions may involve describing, explaining or discussing issues.

Structure of the papers

There are two exam papers:
- AS Unit G001: Society and Health
- AS Unit G002: Resource Management

Each paper has **two** sections, A and B.

Section A consists of structured questions, sometimes linked by a common theme provided at the start of the question. Some questions require a very short response and others require a longer response in continuous prose. Section A is compulsory.

Section B consists of questions that are structured in two parts, (a) and (b). These questions are awarded 25 marks, 10 for part (a) and 15 for part (b). These are essay questions which all require answers in continuous writing. You must answer **two** out of **three** questions.

Key words used in examinations

Answering examination questions is a skill. It is something which you can learn and learn to do well. In fact, for final external examinations your technique in answering questions is just as important as the information you have revised and retained.

Throughout the course you will have answered examination-style questions as part of your preparation for the final exam. A crucial skill is to understand what the question is asking. A question will begin with a trigger or key word, which will give an indication of the expected response.

Key/trigger words and their meanings

Analyse – examine minutely, separate into small parts to find out their nature. Find the essence of. For example: Analyse the reasons why fruit and vegetables are so important in the diet.

Assess – give your judgment of something. Put a value on it. Judge the worth of something. For example: Assess the advantages and disadvantages of buying on credit.

Critically assess – assess something, as defined above, but also make a judgement of it, backed by a discussion of the evidence. For example: Critically assess the forms of control over advertising.

Comment on – write concise explanatory notes on. Make remarks on or about a topic. Give an opinion about something. For example: Comment on the government white paper *Choosing Health*.

Compare – point out the differences and similarities between the given items.

Consider – think about in order to understand or

decide. Weigh the merit of something. For example: Consider the main trends in the pattern of family expenditure.

Contrast – point out the differences between two or more given items.

Describe – write out the main feature. Write a picture in words.

Discuss – investigate or examine by argument, from more than one viewpoint, setting out factors tending to support, and those tending to cast doubt on the proposition. It is not always necessary to come to a conclusion.

Evaluate – see also 'assess'. Judge the worth of something by means of stated criteria. For example: Evaluate the usefulness of a microwave oven.

Examine – look at or study closely. Find out the facts. For example: Examine the ways in which a consumer can collect information before making a purchase.

Explain – set out the facts and the reasons for them, make them known in detail, and make them plain or clear. For example: Explain clearly why there is a housing shortage in Britain.

Identify – name and select, pick out. For example: Identify the problems encountered by a homeless person.

Illustrate – make clear by the use of examples. Explain or clarify by the use of concrete examples.

Justify – show adequate grounds for decisions or conclusions. Prove to be right. Give a good reason.

List – set out in the form of a list. One word answers or single sentences are sufficient.

Outline – write out the main points or a general plan, but omit minor details.

State – give only the bare facts, expressed clearly and fully.

Suggest – make a recommendation or selection. For example: Suggest ways of saving money.

Getting ready for your exams

The purpose of this section is to help you achieve a better performance in the exam and to develop your confidence in revising for exams. It covers important study skills and how to prepare for revision. To achieve the grade you deserve, you need to start organising your revision well before the exams. This section also covers improving your examination technique and reviewing candidate responses to exam questions.

Organising revision

Make a timetable

Find out where, when and how many exams you have. Check there are no clashes with two exams scheduled at the same time.

Devise a revision timetable: there are many online templates you can download, or you can just make your own using a calendar. Allocate time for each subject, time to review your revision notes and relaxation time. An effective revision timetable should make provision for reviewing each topic at least twice: first to reinforce earlier learning, and then again just before the exam to consolidate your understanding. Start serious revision at least eight weeks before the exams.

Get the equipment ready

Organise these resources before you start. It is also worth considering if you have missed any lessons and subsequent notes you will need to collect.
- Class notes
- Mark schemes from the OCR website
- Past papers from the OCR website
- Textbooks
- Coloured pens
- Highlighters
- A3 paper
- Revision cards
- Plastic wallets

Environment

The place where you work is very important. You should choose somewhere calm and quiet at home or at school.

You need good lighting and plenty of fresh air. The place where you work should be free from distractions with a desk and comfortable chair.

How to revise

To understand revision and learn how to revise it is important first to grasp the processes of memory and understanding. Just attending lessons and making notes cannot provide understanding of any subject. The information you receive must be worked and used. You must rearrange, rewrite and discuss the subject. It will not be until you have **used the knowledge** that you will feel that you understand it. Connecting the knowledge to what you already know will help. One way of using information and demonstrating that you understand a topic is to produce a web diagram or a mind map.

Constructing a web diagram

1. Take a blank piece of A3 paper, and turn it to landscape.

2. Choose a clear title, e.g. 'Poverty'. Write this in a space about 4 cm–10 cm in the centre of the paper. Use three different colours. Allow the word to create its own shape (do not use a frame).

3. Choose the main ideas associated with your title – no more than eight. These are like the chapter headings in a book. Write them in CAPITALS on evenly sized lines or branches from the centre. The lines are thick and curved, like the branches of a tree connecting to the trunk.

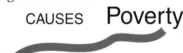

CAUSES   Poverty

4. Start to add a second level of thought. These words are linked to the branch that triggered them. Remember these lines are thinner and the words may be lower case (not capitals).

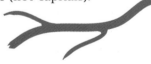

5. Add a third or fourth level of data as thoughts come to you. Use images as much as you can, instead of or in addition to the words. Allow your thoughts to come freely, meaning you 'jump about' the web diagram as the links and associations form.

6. Add boxes around key words or image outlines in colour. Use colour pens, make sketches, and group ideas together. Have fun!

Activity 1

Review

Choose a topic you have studied and produce a mind map.

Tips for effective revision

The key to exam success lies in long term preparation, not last-minute revision. After your lessons you should spend a few minutes checking through your notes. Research suggests that if you do not review work, you forget up to 75 per cent in a week and up to 98 per cent in less than a month.

Knowledge is retained best at the beginning and the end of a revision session. The middle of the revision session is the most difficult part. So if something is hard to understand, don't leave it until the middle of the session – start with it. Keep revision sessions to about 40 minutes – 50 minutes maximum.

The essential review

Most of the knowledge will be lost shortly after the lesson. To avoid this happening follow the stages:

1. Take the original information and spend time re-reading carefully.
   Later in the day, rewrite it into a web diagram or bullet list. Make it visual. This could take 30 minutes.

2. The next day, review the information and try to reproduce the web diagram without looking. Check against the original. This could take 20 minutes.

3. During the same week, review again.

4. During the same month, review again.

5. Each topic should be reviewed several times. To help you remember, use some of the revision techniques mentioned in the next section.

Never try to revise information you don't understand. Ask your teacher to explain the information again.

Revision techniques

Everyone is different and different methods work for different people. Find a technique which suits you.

Here are some suggestions:

1. **Index cards** with summarised notes, definitions and key concepts on them. Jot down what you wish to learn on small cards; keep them in your pocket and use any odd minute to go over the facts again and again and again. These can be carried around and read whenever you have a spare time, e.g. travelling.

2. **Coloured sticky notes** with key words or very brief summaries can be stuck where you will see them frequently. Key factual information could be written on them, e.g. factors affecting standard of living.

3. **Use a glitter pen and highlighters** to make key words and information stand out. Be very selective and avoid highlighting everything. Focus on the harder bits and the things you don't already know.

4. **Work with a study buddy:** you and a friend who have studied Home Economics agree to learn the same topic by a specified deadline. Then get together to discuss it and test each other.

5. **Get an assistant to help.** This does not have to be a subject specialist; it can be anyone! Ask someone to listen to your explanations and ask you questions. They can test your knowledge of factual information and definitions. Do a mini presentation to a friend or even by yourself.

6. **Use the media:** it can help your understanding by widening your experiences and knowledge. Listen to thought-provoking radio programmes, read a quality newspaper, watch relevant television programmes and visit appropriate websites.

7. **Read aloud or record on to a tape and play it back.** This method works because you hear the words as well as seeing them, and so engage different parts of the brain. Read the material dramatically: we remember dramatic things, especially if the voices are outrageous or the really important bits are whispered.

8. **Make a rhyme.** Try putting the information into a verse or to music; you will remember it more easily. Try this with factual information.

9. **Invent mnemonics** which are funny, vulgar or relevant to you. Mnemonics are memory aids. They can be constructed from key words in a topic you have studied. Here are some examples:

Effects of unemployment could be 'HEDGEHOG' Housing (poor)/Homelessness, Escapism (smoking/alcohol/gambling), Debt, Guilt (personal failing), Education (apathy/low expectations), Health (poor diet), Opportunities (New skills/training) and Graffiti (example of urban deprivation)

Causes of unemployment could be 'I AM A STAR' Immigration, Automation, Minimum wage (costs more to employ people), Ageism (old people at greater risk), Service industry (different skills required), Trade agreements (imports cheaper), Agriculture and manufacturing decline and Racism/regional variations (some areas of UK high unemployment and some groups at greater risk)

Food poisoning bacteria are Eating Contaminated Stuff Causes Big Smelly Vomit
E.coli, Clostridium botulinum, Salmonella, Clostridium perfringens, Bacillus cereus, Staphylococcus aureus and Viral food poisoning

10. **Look, cover, write, check.** This method works for some people.
Read it ⟶ Hide it ⟶ Write it out ⟶ Check to see if you got it right

11. **Rote learning:** the lowest order of fixing in the memory. The secret of rote learning lies in constant repetition of the material: by writing it down, saying it out loud, singing it in the bath!

12. **Visualise the situation or the knowledge.** Go over the information in your mind's eye and make a mental picture of it. Making up a story is good for remembering lists. You may be able to 'see it' when you need to during the exam.

13. **Draw mind maps or web diagrams** to summarise topics in a visual way.

14. **Talk about the issues** and think about what you are reading: don't just let your eyes follow the words. Ask yourself questions all the time. Close your folder and see if you can talk about what you have just read.

15. **Review it or lose it.** All topics covered should be reviewed. Do not expect to remember something you have read only once. Start each revision session by reviewing what you learned in the previous session: this should take just a few minutes but is critical to success.

How to do well in examinations

In an exam you are being asked not only to demonstrate your knowledge of a subject, but to apply, assess and evaluate information. Your skill at structuring and expressing a response within a time frame is also examined.

The following points will help you to improve your written work.

Plan your answer

Before you start writing, you may wish to gather your thoughts by producing a mini plan, simple web diagram or a list of bullets points. This process may help you recall associated knowledge and examples to support your response.

Questions which begin with 'discuss' expect you to do more than just recite a list of points in no particular sequence. You are expected to arrange information logically. Examiners are impressed by students who express themselves clearly and are organised.

Structure the response

Begin with an introduction that provides the background to the essay. Sometimes writing the question out again in your own words can help this process of setting the scene. Each point should be clearly explained, and contained in a separate paragraph. The use of examples to support the points made is important. One way of remembering this is to use **PEGEX** for each paragraph.

This stands for **point, example and explanation.**

– **Point:** make sure the paragraph is directed at answering the question

– **Example:** now use some facts to prove the point

– **Explanation:** now explain how the point contributes to the question.

Do not be afraid to add your own opinions and experiences if they are relevant.

Keep to the point

Too often, answers consist of both relevant and irrelevant information from notes. These students make no attempt to answer the question that was asked. Such answers will not be awarded high marks. Underline the key words in the question to help you to focus on the question. When writing the response, re-read the question at least once to check that you are keeping to the point.

Use examples

A good answer will select and introduce examples in order to make points which support a discussion, explanation or descriptions.

Demonstrate knowledge in your answers. Use specific detail, not vague generalities. Statements like 'Many unemployed people have problems including debt' will not score many marks without explaining **how** debt can affect the unemployed and giving examples to support your discussion. Whenever you find yourself writing a sentence that begins (for example) 'Many ...', stop and ask yourself 'What are the important issues?' The inclusion of details and explanations will impress the examiner and earn more marks.

Keep to time

You will have 90 minutes to complete the examination papers at AS. You should try to divide your time between Section A and Section B accordingly. It is difficult to be prescriptive about the length of an answer; the quality is more important than the quantity. However, bear in mind you have 75 marks available and 50 are allocated to Section B so most time should be spent on Section B. In Section B you will also need to allocate some time for planning your responses before attempting the questions. It is not unreasonable for an examiner to expect about two sides of writing in the time allocated, for each essay question. A very brief answer is unlikely to contain sufficient detail to be awarded good marks.

Practise writing timed essays. It is not particularly helpful to try and predict the exact questions, though the specification has to be covered over a fixed period of time. Practising timed essays from past papers may improve your exam technique, and may also reveal gaps in your understanding.

Write legibly

If examiners have to struggle to read your handwriting they may not appreciate the quality and style of your answer.

And finally, have a **positive mental attitude**. See yourself as a successful student and be confident in your ability. Do not allow self-doubt to affect your preparation or success.

Candidates' responses

This is a response from a candidate attempting two Resource Management questions. There is an examiner's commentary with these responses and some suggestions on ways of improving the quality of responses.

Question 1

There is a wide variety of food retailers offering greater choices to households.
  (a) Describe the range of retail outlets available for the purchase of food. (10)
  (b) Explain the current marketing strategies used in food retailing. (15)

Candidate's answer (1a)

There are many different places that you can buy food. These include large supermarkets, small town shops, the internet and markets.[1]

The most common is the supermarket. Large out of town supermarkets offer an excellent choice of products.[2] They provide free parking and there are cafe's were you can eat. The supermarket sells special food products which you may not be able to get elsewhere.[3]

The local town can offer a range of small independent shops. There could be a bread shop, butchers and greengrocers.[4] These shops can be a bit pricey but the customer gets advice and can chat.[5] The local shops can sell vegetables from that area. Some people like to buy local produce.[6]

The internet offers another option for the purchase of food. You can buy special food from different parts of the country e.g. Smoked fish from Scotland.[7] The Internet offer the 'conveinance' of arm chair shopping and for those with mobility problems.[8]

The local market maybe another place where you can buy food. The prices here will be cheap and you may be able to get special deals on clothes.[9] The product range may include vegatables that are in season.[10]

Marks awarded 7/10

Examiner's commentary and advice on (1a)

1. A very good start suggesting straightaway that there are four food retailers to be discussed. This is a wide range.

2. Give an example of the range of products, e.g. frozen foods.

3. The identification of free parking, cafés and specialist products is satisfactory but the question requires an explanation. Specialist products could be linked to gluten-free, organic ranges etc. It would demonstrate deeper knowledge and understanding if the candidate could suggest who would benefit from these services.

4. Shows a good knowledge of the type of retailers available.

5. Two merits are mentioned briefly without explanation.

6. An opportunity to show deeper understanding missed here; the candidate could have suggested why consumers may prefer to purchase local produce.

7. Very good use of a relevant example to support point.

8. Develop further, explain why this is a possible merit.

9. Elaboration required; the link should respond to food not clothing.

10. Explain why this is beneficial.

This is a good response to (1a), it would be at the top of the middle band. The candidate has demonstrated some knowledge and suggested a wide range of retailers, but needs to ensure they describe the points fully. Read the question carefully; a description is required. With a little more practice on technique the candidate could increase the mark to the higher band. Give examples to support the points made; these examples could draw upon personal experiences. The candidate could consider the community where they purchased food.

The discussion is clearly expressed and well organised in distinct paragraphs. The response contains occasional errors of grammar, punctuation and spelling. Think about your expression; avoid colloquiums such as 'a bit pricey'.

Candidate's answer (1b)

Plan
Media attention: TV advertising, billboards and bus advertising.
Buy one get one free
Product positioning in shops such as sweets near the tills and eye level positioning.
Product packaging
Loyalty cards
Free coupons when you spend over a certain amount

There are many types of marketing strategies used in the food retail industry most of which are very successful in gaining customer purchases.

The most expensive type of strategy used by the food retail industry is 'above the line' marketing. This includes advertising on the television, billboards and on buses[1] etc.

When advertising on the television food retailers consider the best time to advertise their products to attract their target audience. If they wanted to promote a new children's product they would advertise in the morning in the breaks between children's programmes, this then means that it catches the child's eye and when they got to the supermarkets or shops with their parents they are likely to remember the product they saw on the television and nag their parents for it.[2]

Some food retailers advertise new products on the side of buses and billboards; this gets the attention of all types of people and has the potential of attracting plenty of buyers. The type of product usually advertised on buses and billboards are products that will appeal to all ages, item such as new chocolates or a new flavour of crisps,[3] or a new brand of food.

Another group of marketing strategies that current food retailers use are 'below the line'. This is were they use advertising and sales promotion without the use of the media. Carefully designed product packaging is also used as 'below the line' marketing strategy. Food retailers use bright, colourful and attractive packaging to appeal to the customer.[4]

'Buy One Get One free' offers are probably one of the most common sales promotion techniques used in the food retail industry. This is where if the customer buys a certain product they will get another of the same product free, or if they buy two they get the third free. This is a very sucessful method of marketing as it does persuade people to buy the product because they think they are getting more for their money, due to the fact that they are getting a free product.[5]

Product positioning is also a very important marketing strategy used in the food retail industry. Food retailers put the expensive goods and most popular goods at eye level so that it is the first thing the customer looks at and hopefully the item that they buy.[6] They also use the same technique when trying to appeal to the younger generations, putting products that would appeal to them at their eye level.

Loyalty cards and money off coupons encourage sales.[7]

Marks awarded 10/15

Examiner's commentary and advice on (1b)

1. Demonstration of good knowledge.

2. State a relevant food product to support the point, e.g. breakfast cereals. Reference to restrictions on 'junk' food advertising would have demonstrated greater knowledge.

3. Good description of a strategy and supported by a relevant example.

4. Not on mark scheme but valid point and credit given. Very good demonstration of knowledge linking to food retailing.

5. Good description of a relevant technique.

6. Satisfactory but could have developed further and described in-store positioning/layout in greater detail. Link to a food product.

7. Too brief, candidate needed to elaborate on both points.

The range of marketing strategies and quality of the explanation was just sufficient to be awarded a mark at the top of the middle band. The candidate demonstrates very good knowledge and uses specialist marketing terms appropriately. The range of strategies explained needs to be more varied for greater marks and more explicitly linked to food products. Poor time management resulted in brief explanations at the end. Practise completing questions in exam conditions, e.g. timed. Make sure you have sufficient time to describe all the points listed on the plan.

There were a few errors of grammar, punctuation and spelling.

Question 2

Each year it is estimated that one in ten people in the United Kingdom may suffer from food poisoning.

(a) Describe the sources and methods of transmission of commonly occurring food poisoning bacteria. (10)

(b) Explain the role of an Environmental Health Officer in ensuring that food is fit for consumption. (15)

Candidate's answer (2a)

Plan
Salmonella
Campylobacter
E-coli
Hands during prep
Badly cooked
Undefrosted
Cross-contamination

Food poisoning can be transmitted three ways; chemically, physically or biologically.[1] Food poisoning is most commonly spread in preparation as the food handler may have not washed their hands before touching the food. This physically puts bacteria on the food making it unsafe to eat. Also cross-contamination can happen this way if someone touches raw meat and then touches some cooked ham then the ham might cause food poisoning if eaten.[2]

On the other hand, food may also be made dangerous to eat by not defrosting it properly before you cook it.[3] Also it may cause food poisoning if it is not cooked thoroughly. Furthermore food should be stored at the right temperature[4] to make sure it doesn't cause food poisoning. The danger zone is from 5 to 63°C, and bacteria grows fastest at room temperature.[5] Fridges and all equipment must be clean to avoid food contamination also.[6]

Food poisoning can occur if chemicals get into the food which might contaminate it e.g. Pesticides used in the growing of vegetables, and dangerous liquids like bleach may contaminate the food if the work surface is not clean.[7]

Usually sources of food contaminating bacteria are E-coli on raw meat, salmonella on poultry and camplybacter.[8]

Marks awarded 6/10

Examiner's commentary and advice on (2a)

1. Good start to distinguish between types of contamination. Supporting examples would have improved response.

2. Descriptions of poor personal hygiene and cross-contamination supported with examples.

3. Describe why food is dangerous if not thoroughly defrosted before cooking.

4. Describe the 'right' temperature.

5. Demonstrates accurate knowledge of the danger zone, maybe could have linked the danger zone to room temperature more pointedly.

6. Describe storage in the fridge with examples of shelf positioning and link to methods of transmission in the question.

7. Good examples to support chemical contamination description.

8. More detail on the sources of these microorganisms is required.

The response is the middle of the middle band.

There is a brief plan of key words, this helped the candidate to organise sentences. Planning is satisfactory.

The candidate has demonstrated some knowledge of the sources and methods of transmission but needs to ensure they explain their points fully. The important points were not fully developed i.e. the sources and methods of transmission. By providing relevant examples to support the description the candidate could increase the mark to the higher band. The description is reasonably clearly expressed.

Candidate's answer (2b)

Plan
Seize all food
Food safety laws
Inspect
Give advice
Close down

The Food Safety legislation[1] gave the Environmental health officers (EHO) power to ensure all food sold in retail is fit for consumption. The EHO's have the power to search premises where food is prepared and/or sold and they can close premises down if it fails[2] any of the HACCAP[3] checks. They check the safety of the food being prepared, the cleaness of the preparation room equipment. They check how the food is stored, whether it's at the right temperature[4] and how it's prepared.[5]

They have the ability to take samples of food to be tested, but they can also seize whole stocks of food if they believe it to be unsafe.[6]

The EHO's also offer advice and support for outlets that supply food such as hygiene training, which helps food retail outlets and restaurants to keep their hygiene when preparing food up to the best standard.[7] They can

suggest staff training courses or make the ultimatum that the employees must have more training. They will revisit to check the changes have been made.[8]

Marks awarded 6/15

Examiner's commentary and advice on (2b)

1. Food safety legislation a bit too vague for AS level.

2. Clear basic explanation of the role of the EHO.

3. HACCP greater accuracy required.

4. 'Right' temperature again, an opportunity to demonstrate knowledge missed here.

5. Explain how the EHO does these checks, e.g. use of probes.

6. Accurate knowledge of the seizure of unfit food.

7. Good knowledge of the role of the EHO in supporting retailers.

8. Could have developed this further with references to Improvement notices, fines.

The response is just at the bottom of the middle band. There is a brief plan of key words but could have supported the response with more detail. Planning is brief and this section carries more marks. The candidate has demonstrated limited knowledge of the role of the EHO. There were only a few examples used to support the explanation and some inaccuracies in the recall of key information. The lack of detail and inaccuracies are the main weaknesses in the response. Revision of key facts is an important priority for this candidate.

Summary of assessment advice

Memory and revision

- Understanding depends upon **working with** and **using information. Connect** the information to what you already know, e.g. use other examples to illustrate it.

- Understanding and memory change over time. You retain information best at the beginning of a learning session.

- A revision period of 2 hours needs breaking into at least two shorter sessions with 10 minute breaks

- Recall is easier if information is in small packages.

- Review is crucial. Review means simply reading the information again; it should take just 10 minutes. You must build in a time to review previous sessions one day, one week and one month after the original session.
- Regular review stimulates understanding of a subject area and helps you to link knowledge from different areas.
- Link information by relationship, repetition or rhyme. Vulgar, vile and very funny items are easier to recall.

Exam techniques

- Never waffle on about everything you know on the topic regardless of its relevance.
- Never ignore the question and answer your own.
- Follow the instructions in the question. There will be one or more trigger words which give exact instructions and these must be followed.
- Read the question carefully and note exactly what you are asked to do – the context and question will set the scene.

- Plan the essay questions. List the content, or make a mind map – do not rewrite this but use it effectively.
- Decide how to order the content after you have planned – use numbers if this helps.
- Maintain an awareness of time. Be strict on yourself: allow half an hour for section A, and half an hour for each of the two essays in section B. You can always return to a question if you have time at the end.
- Try to read through your answers when you have completed the paper.
- As a very general guide, for a 10 mark question you need 5 to 7 well-explained points, and for a 15 mark question, 7 to 9 well-explained points.
- Each point you make in an essay must be well explained. Remember PEGEX: make the point, explain it and give an example.
- Stick to the point – for example, if the question asks you to describe the causes of homelessness, don't write about the effects, or give information about voluntary organisations which help the homeless.

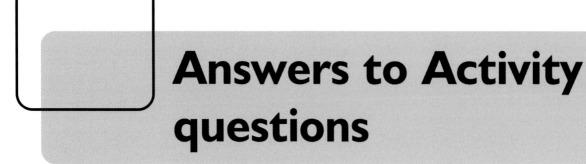

Answers to Activity questions

Chapter 3

Activity 12

It is important to note that decisions are made on the full facts of each case so sometimes the outcomes may vary.

1. Jade is considered at 17 as in priority need and would be housed.
2. Susan is pregnant so is considered as priority need and would be housed as homeless.
3. Derek and Dawn have made themselves intentionally homeless because they used housing benefit to pay off a loan. Therefore they would not be housed as homeless.
4. Sunitta and Harry have means to support themselves and are not considered a priority need so would not be housed as homeless.

Activity 13

These could be other reasons:

- Coming out of an institution such as hospital, prison, residential home.
- Returning from abroad.
- Sleeping rough or in hostels.
- Made homeless by an emergency such as fire or flooding.

Activity 14

Here is an example of a chunky soup recipe which provides both carbohydrate and protein, suitable for a main meal.

Hot sausage soup
½ tablespoon oil
2 onions sliced
1 crushed clove of garlic
Salt and pepper
1 tablespoon tomato purée
75 g tiny soup pasta
1 litre vegetable stock
100 g chorizo sausage

Method
Heat the oil a little and gently fry the sliced onion and garlic for ten minutes.

Add the sausage, pasta, stock, salt, pepper and purée. Bring to the boil and simmer for 10 to 15 minutes, or until the pasta is cooked.

Chapter 5

Activity 2

Here are some starting points for a discussion:
- Meeting the demands of an ageing population.
- The cost of drugs for Alzheimer's disease.
- The cost of new technologies and the price of success – hip replacement, IVF microsurgery, by-pass operations, developments in cancer treatments.
- Postcode lottery – wide variations in costs within and between regions.
- Is spending on preventative medicine too high?
- The future of the family – more reliance on the state and less on the extended family.
- The shortage of qualified NHS staff.
- Out-of-hours provision of GP services.
- Closure of smaller hospitals.
- The distance in rural areas to accident and emergency services and maternity departments.
- The cleanliness in hospitals and the spread of superbugs.

Chapter 7

Activity 9

The graph tells us that the most common method of payment is the use of debit cards. Between 1991 and 2005 there was an eleven-fold increase in the number of payments by credit card. Cash and cheques have seen a steady decline since 1991 to the extent that some shops now no longer accept cheques as a method of payment.

Activity 10

The tables tell us that there are differences in the ways in which debit and credit cards are used in the UK. In 2005 debit cards were used mostly for food and drink outlets, but there has also been an increase in the use of debit cards for a wider range of purchases.

The pattern of usage for credit cards suggests that credit cards are used for more expensive items. In 2005 the average debit card purchase was £41.40, and the average credit card purchase was £60.65.

Activity 14

The graph tells us the following:

- UK households spent an average of £443 a week.
- Transport was the highest category of spending with an average spend of £62 a week. Transport costs include purchase and use of vehicles and transport services such as rail and bus fares.
- The second highest category of spending was recreation and culture at £58 a week. Recreation costs include televisions, computers, newspapers, books, leisure activities and package holidays.
- Food and non-alcoholic drink purchases contributed £45 to the weekly household expenditure of which £10.10 went on meat, £3.40 on fresh vegetables and £2.80 on fresh fruit. Non-alcoholic drinks accounted for £3.80 and £1.80 was spent on chocolate and confectionery per week.

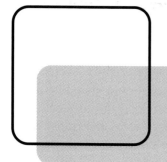

Glossary

Absolute poverty – a state below which it is not possible to live a healthy life, being unable to afford sufficient food, clothing, warmth and shelter.

Accelerated freeze-drying (AFD) – a fast and effective way of drying frozen food. It involves drying the food in a vacuum at reduced pressure (an example is coffee).

Acid rain – rain containing acids that form in the atmosphere when industrial gas emissions (especially sulphur dioxide and nitrogen oxides) combine with water.

Aerobes – an organism that requires oxygen to reproduce.

Ageism – stereotyping against individuals because of their age.

Ambient temperature – room temperature.

Amenities – things that contribute to physical or material comfort.

Anaerobes – an organism that does not require oxygen to reproduce.

Angina – chest pain.

Antioxidant vitamins – vitamin E, C and beta carotene (a form of vitamin A). It has been suggested that vitamin C, beta carotene and vitamin E may offer some protection against coronary heart disease.

Argon gas – can be used to fill the gap in double-glazed units as it transmits heat much less readily than the other gases in air, saving even more money.

Assured short hold tenancy – a type of agreement, usually with a private landlord.

Arterial plaque – consisting of fat globules and cholesterol being deposited on the walls of the arteries.

Atherosclerosis – a disease of the heart caused by the arteries that supply the heart with oxygen becoming narrow.

Auxiliary care – offered in the individual's home for help with gardening, transport and odd jobs.

Baby boom – a sharp increase in births e.g. after the First World War and after the Second World War.

Bacterium – a large group of bacteria.

Best before date – used for long shelf-life products. It is the date up until when the food will remain in optimum condition. After this date the food will slowly deteriorate in quality.

Binary fission – reproduction that involves the splitting of a parent cell into two approximately equal parts.

Biofuels – fuels produced from oilseeds which can be used as an alternative to diesel.

Birth rate – the ratio of total live births expressed as the number of live births per 1000 of the population per year.

Budget – the total sum of money allocated for particular purposes over a period of time.

Burden of dependency – the working population has to pay more tax and national insurance to support those unable to work and provide the services they need.

Campylobacter – the commonest form of bacterial food poisoning in Britain. It is found in most raw poultry and is believed to be the most significant source of human infection.

Care plan – a written document that outlines how the needs of an individual are to be met.

Cavity wall insulation – involves insulating the walls of the home.

Census – a survey every ten years to gather information on the population to help with social planning.

Chemical contamination – the transfer of harmful chemicals to food.

Chilling – involves storing food below the ambient room temperature but not cold enough to freeze the food. It is a legal requirement that high-risk food is stored below 8°C.

Chores – daily or routine domestic tasks.

Civil partnership – a legal relationship, which can be registered by two people of the same sex.

Cholesterol – a waxy substance found in the bloodstream and all body cells. Cholesterol is an essential part of a healthy body because it is used for producing cell membranes and some hormones.

Chronic – lasting for a long period of time or marked by frequent reoccurrence, as certain diseases.

Clostridium perfringens – an anaerobic bacteria (does not require oxygen) that produces toxins which cause food poisoning if eaten.

Cocktail effect – when a combination of food additives are consumed together.

Coeliac – a person suffering from coeliac disease.

Coeliac disease – the main form of wheat intolerance. It is a bowel disease and it is an intolerance of gluten.

Cohabitation – when a couple share an intimate relationship, living together without being married.

Colour coding – a method to identify which equipment should be used in certain areas or for specific tasks, thereby reducing the risk of cross-contamination (e.g. red for raw meat preparation).

Common Agricultural Policy – set up to avoid food shortages and ensure European farmers had adequate income for their produce.

Community nursing care – carried out by community nurses. They provide medical care in people's homes, in GP surgeries and health centres. Community nurses visit people at home to change dressings, give injections and offer advice on home nursing aids and equipment.

Composite foods – may contain a combination of foods from more than one of the five food groups.

Contamination – occurs when pathogenic bacteria are passed from a source of contamination to a high-risk food via a vehicle such as worktops, chopping boards, utensils, hands, equipment and cloths.

Core temperature – the temperature measured at the centre or in the thickest part of a food item or at the bone.

Council Tax Benefit – help towards paying council tax.

Cross-contamination – the transfer of harmful bacteria from a contaminated product to a ready-to-eat food.

Cycle of deprivation – where children are born into poor families with backgrounds of social problems, who then go on to cohabit or marry one another, have children and the cycle begins again.

Dashboard dining – food eaten in a car.

Danger zone – the temperature range within which harmful bacteria can multiply and grow easily (between 5°C to 63°C, the temperature range to be avoided for high-risk foods).

Date mark – a date on food packaging which shows the period of time when the food is safe and in the best condition to eat.

Deforestation – cutting down and clearing away trees or forests.

Demography – the study of the characteristics of human populations, such as its size, growth and vital statistics.

Density – thickness.

Dental plaque – a coating which develops on teeth. If it is not removed by brushing it can cause tooth decay.

Dependency ratio – how many young people (under 16) and older people (over 64) depend on people of working age (16 to 64).

Deskfast – used to describe breakfast that is eaten at a desk, usually at work.

Diabetes – a condition in which the amount of glucose in the blood is too high.

Diet – the usual food and drink of an individual.

Dietary – relating to diet.

Dietary guidelines – the eight practical tips for healthy eating issued by the Food Standards Agency. They are based on starchy foods, lots of fruit and vegetables, more fish, less saturated fat and sugar, less salt, getting active and keeping a healthy weight, plenty of water and not skipping breakfast.

Direct contamination – the route of contamination is direct from the source to the ready-to-eat food (when raw meat touches cooked meat).

Disability Discrimination Act 1995 – makes it unlawful to discriminate against disabled people in connection with employment.

Discrimination – the unfair treatment of a person or group on the basis of prejudice.

Disposable income – what is left over for saving or spending after taxes are subtracted from income.

Domestic care – offered in the individual's home for help with garden maintenance, equipment repairs, laundry, cooking, shopping, cooking and cleaning.

Dormant – inactive bacteria.

Draught-proofing – blocking the gaps to stop the draught entering the home.

Due diligence – must be demonstrated by a businesses to avoid prosecution for contravening food safety legislation. To prove due diligence a business must be able to demonstrate that it took every possible reasonable step to achieve safe food.

Durable – capable of withstanding wear and tear or decay.

Eating pattern – described as where, when and how you eat.

Eatwell plate – shows how much should be eaten from each food group for meals and snacks. It aims to make healthy eating easier by showing the types and proportions of foods we need to have a balanced diet.

E.coli 0157:H7 – one of the many strains causing illness in humans. It is usually associated with eating unwashed vegetables and contaminated meat.

Economically active – people aged 16 years or over who are either employed or are unemployed but want to work.

Economically inactive – those aged 16 years or over who are out of work, and are either not seeking work or unavailable to start work.

Employment – a person's regular trade or profession – in other words the job that they do.

Employment Service Adviser – gives advice to an unemployed person usually at a job centre.

Enteric bacteria – can live in the intestines of humans and animals.

Environment – the combination of external physical conditions that affect and influence the growth, development and survival of organisms, and the circumstances or conditions that surround us.

Environmental health officers – enforce food safety legislation and have the right to enter and inspect food premises at all reasonable hours.

Equitable – even.

Expenditure – the money paid out; an amount spent.

Extended family – usually consists of three generations living together in the same household or living very close to other family members. They have frequent daily contact with other family members and support each other.

Extrusion cooking – involves raw materials such as flour, starches and liquids mixed into a semi-solid dough and heated. It is forced (extruded) through tiny holes to make a range of products (pasta shapes).

Fairtrade products – ensure disadvantaged producers in the developing world receive a fair price for their products.

Family – can be defined as a social unit connected by blood, marriage or adoption.

Farm to fork – food can be traced through all the stages of production, processing and distribution to the source.

Fertility rate – the ratio of live births and is expressed per 1000 population per year.

Flat – a room or set of rooms located in a larger building.

Food-borne disease – an illness caused by eating food contaminated by harmful substances or by pathogenic bacteria living on the food.

Food desert – a poor urban area where residents cannot afford to buy or have a limited choice of healthy food.

Food miles – the distance a food product travels from the producer to the consumer.

Food safety plans – provide practical steps to identify and control hazards in order to establish and maintain food safety.

Food Standards Agency – an independent organisation, whose main aim is to protect public health in relation to food in the UK.

Fortified food – when nutrients have been added during processing.

Freedom Food – a voluntary code for producers to follow established by the RSPCA to improve welfare of farmed animals.

Free radicals – unstable molecules produced as by-products of normal body processes.

Functional food – a food which claims to have health-promoting benefits in addition to the usual nutritional value.

Global warming – an increase in the average temperature of the earth's atmosphere.

Glucose – a monosaccharide (single) sugar, occurring widely in most plant and animal tissue. It is the principal circulating sugar in the blood and the major energy source of the body.

GP – stands for general practitioner, a family doctor.

Grazing – used to describe the practice of eating snacks throughout the day instead of meals.

HACCP – a hazard analysis critical control point is a food safety system which involves identifying all steps in the activity of the food business that are critical to food safety.

Hazard – a possible source of danger.

Health – defined by the World Health Organization in 1948 as 'A state of complete physical, social and mental well-being and not merely the absence of disease or infirmity.'

High density lipoproteins (HDL) – can carry fatty acids and cholesterol to the liver to be broken down. They are sometimes referred to as producing HDL-bound cholesterol or 'good cholesterol' as they remove cholesterol from the bloodstream.

High-risk food – food which without temperature control might support the growth of harmful bacteria or the formation of poisons (toxins) such as cooked meat products and prepared ready-to-eat food.

Home helps – people who help with domestic tasks including cleaning and cooking. There are charges for this service.

Homeless – having no home or haven.

Hormone – a substance produced by one tissue and conveyed by the bloodstream to another to affect physiological activity, such as growth or metabolism.

Hot holding – the process of keeping food hot (above 63°C).

Household – can be defined as one person living alone or a group of people who share the same address and living arrangements.

Househusbands – men who have taken over the traditional female domestic role.

Human needs – food, warmth and shelter are essential for life and these needs must be satisfied first. But we have other needs, the need to feel safe, be successful and be satisfied with life: these must also be addressed.

Hygiene emergency prohibition notice – may be served if an EHO believes that there is a significant risk to health or injury due to the condition of the equipment, the handling process or the condition of the premises of a food business. The notice immediately stops the use of the equipment or premises or a specified handling process.

Hygiene improvement notice – may be served where an EHO has reasonable grounds for believing that a food business is failing to comply with food hygiene regulations.

Hysterectomy – the surgical removal of part or the entire uterus (womb).

Immigration – the migration into a place or a country of which you are not a native in order to settle there.

Incinerated – waste which is burnt. This is also called energy from waste.

Income – the total amount of money earned from work or obtained from other sources over a given period of time.

Income Support – available to people aged 16 to 59 years who cannot work and do not have enough money to maintain a reasonable standard of living.

Infant mortality rate – the death rate during the first year of life.

Informal care – care provided by a relative or friend.

Insulin – a hormone made by the **pancreas** which controls the level of glucose in the body.

Intervention – to involve oneself in a situation to alter an action.

Job Grants – designed to help with the costs of moving from unemployment into work. The grant is a one-off payment which is free of tax and available to claimants of JSA and Income Support.

Job Seekers' Allowance (JSA) – available for those under retirement age who are out of work or working less than 16 hours a week on average. To qualify, claimants must be available for work, able to work and actively seeking work.

Key worker – someone who works in the public sector in an area where there is a high demand for housing.

Land-filled – means waste which is buried in the ground.

Leisure – the time used at a person's own discretion in a variety of ways once they have completed various duties such as study, domestic chores and work. It is the time left over.

Life expectancy – the number of years that an individual is expected to live as determined by statistics.

Lifetime Homes – have sixteen design features that ensure the home will be flexible enough to meet the existing and changing needs of households, e.g. the need for wheelchair or pushchair access.

Lipoproteins – cholesterol that combines with protein in the blood stream.

Listeria monocytogenes – food-poisoning bacterium, unusual because it can grow at low temperatures. It is destroyed by cooking food thoroughly and by pasteurisation. Foods most likely to be contaminated are unpasteurised dairy products, cooked meat, pâtés and smoked fish or cook-chill meals.

Lone parent family – formed from a single male or female parent and dependent children living together. The most common reason for a lone parent family is divorce, separation or an unwillingness to marry or cohabit from one partner.

Low density lipoprotein (LDL) – combines with cholesterol in the bloodstream. It tends to stay in circulation and may over a period of time start the formation of plaques associated with heart disease. This is sometimes referred to as LDL-bound cholesterol or 'bad' cholesterol.

Low e or low emissivity glass – has a special heat-reflective coating between the two panes of glass that will reduce heat loss through the glass by nearly half.

Maisonette – an apartment or flat on two levels with internal stairs, or which has its own entrance at street level.

Malabsorption – the defective or inadequate absorption of nutrients from the intestinal tract.

Manufacturer – a person or enterprise that makes or processes something.

Maslow's Hierarchy of Needs – a pyramid structure of needs with the most basic needs at the bottom and the highest needs, which are most difficult to fulfil, at the top.

Meal – an eating occasion which usually takes place at a specific time and place.

Meal solutions – consist of a range of food products that can be combined to make a meal, including some products which are ready to make, ready prepared or ready to eat.

Menopause – the period marked by the natural and permanent end of menstruation, occurring usually between the ages of 45 and 55.

Methane gas – created when organic waste breaks down. It has the potential to be explosive and is also a significant greenhouse gas which can contribute towards global warming.

Micro-organism – an organism that is only visible through a microscope. Micro-organisms include bacteria, moulds and yeast and viruses.

Micro-organism contamination – the transfer of harmful bacteria to food.

Migration – the movement of persons from one country or locality to another.

Mortality rate – the ratio of deaths expressed per 1000 population per year.

Mortgage – a loan from a bank, building society or finance company, used to buy a home.

Moulds – tiny plants or fungi which grow on the surface of food. They produce spores which can travel in the air to generate new growths.

Multidisciplinary care – where care is provided by a range of different agencies and professional carers.

Multifactorial disease – a disease which has many factors increasing the risk of it.

Mycoprotein – an industrial food material developed to replace meat. It is a fungus which contains high quality protein.

Mycotoxins – naturally occurring toxins produced by moulds. Damp cereals may be contaminated with mycotoxins.

Myocardial infarction – a heart attack.

New Build HomeBuy – allows families or individuals to buy a share of a property, typically 50 per cent, from a housing association and pay rent on the rest.

New Deals – a wide number of schemes for different groups of people who are unemployed and claiming benefit. They offer intensive support to find work, give subsided employment opportunities and specialist training.

NHS – a government-run service which provides doctors (GPs), hospitals and community health services which meet health care needs of individuals.

Non-milk extrinsic sugars – sometimes called hidden sugars found in cakes, biscuits, fizzy drinks, soups, and breakfast cereals, canned food including baked beans, pizzas and pasta sauces.

Novel foods – defined by the FSA as a food or food ingredient which does not have a significant history of consumption within the EU before May 1997. Novel foods include genetically modified foods and cholesterol lowering foods.

Nuclear family – a family which lives a considerable distance from other family members. They do not have regular frequent daily contact with other family members; contact becomes a matter of choice. The nuclear family usually consists of two generations living together: parents and children.

Obesity – a BMI (body mass index) of 30 or above.

Occupation – a person's job or profession.

Omega 3 – essential fatty acid (EFA).

Onset time – the period of time between eating contaminated food and the symptoms of food poisoning appearing.

Open Market HomeBuy – a government supported scheme. It aims to help certain groups of people who cannot afford to buy a home on the open market to purchase a home. It provides access to additional money called an equity loan, which runs alongside a conventional mortgage.

Organic food products – foods produced without the aid of artificial chemicals or hormones.

Osteoporosis – a diet-related condition which involves the thinning of the bone, involving loss of organic matter and bone mineral.

Owner occupier – a person who owns their own home or is in the process of buying it.

Ozone layer – a layer in the stratosphere (at approximately 20 miles) that contains a concentration of ozone sufficient to form a protective shield against most ultraviolet radiation from the sun.

Pancreas – a gland lying just behind the stomach which produces insulin.

Passive smoking – breathing in someone's cigarette smoke.

Pathogenic bacteria – a bacteria or other micro-organism that can cause illness or disease.

Personal care – offered in the individual's home for help with bathing, toileting, dressing, companionship, hairdressing, manicure and feeding.

Pharmacists (chemists) – experts in medicines.

Physical contamination – the presence of any unwanted matter in food such as hair, nails and bolts.

Population – the people inhabiting a specified area.

Poverty – the state of being poor and lack of the means of providing material needs or comforts. It is a situation where resources are insufficient to meet needs.

Poverty trap - once in poverty, it is difficult to get out of it.

Premature – unexpectedly early.

Preventative – a remedy that slows or prevents the cause of an illness or disease.

Primary care – provided by health professionals at the first or primary stage of health care. Much of the health care provided remains in the primary care stage.

Pulverise (purée) – to rub food through a strainer or process it in a blender.

Ready prepared – parts of a meal that have been prepared by the manufacturer.

Ready to eat food to go/hand snacks – includes hot or cold food ready for immediate consumption, and suitable for eating on the move.

Ready to heat – a complete meal at least part-cooked by the manufacturer (frozen or chilled meals).

Ready to make – raw ingredients that are made or prepared in the home bought by the consumer.

Reconstituted (step) family – a family unit in which one or both parents have previously been married and have children from that relationship. There will be a step-parent for the children.

Recycling – the processing of waste-manufactured products to provide the raw material to make new ones.

Registered Social Landlords – independent and non-profit-making landlords. They receive some government funding to build homes and provide specialist housing for vulnerable groups.

Relative poverty – having resources below the average individual or family, so that one is in effect excluded from what we would consider ordinary living patterns and activities.

Replacement level – the number of births per woman required to replace the existing population.

Repossession – when the lender reclaims the property due to failure by the borrower to pay mortgage instalments.

Residential care homes – registered with the Department of Health's Commission for Social Care Inspection. The staff in a residential home can help with personal care such as washing, going to the toilet, taking a bath, getting up or dressing. All meals are provided and there are activities and outings.

Rigorous – rigidly accurate; precise.

Salmonella – a rod-shaped bacteria that causes typhoid fever and food-borne illness.

Sanitizer – cleaning products which combine the functions of a detergent and a disinfectant in a single product.

Saturated fat – usually from animal sources that is solid at room temperature and whose fatty acid chains cannot incorporate additional hydrogen atoms.

Scapegoat – a person or group of people who are blamed for something that is not their fault.

Sedentary lifestyle – a lifestyle with little exercise.

Sheltered accommodation – flats or bungalows designed for elderly or disabled people. There is usually some type of warden system allowing people to live as independently as possible.

Secondary care – provided if a health condition requires further treatment, which is not possible to offer in primary care.

Snack – consists of a small amount of food or beverage taken between meals to relieve hunger.

Social HomeBuy – allows social housing tenants to buy a share in their current home at a considerable discount or to buy outright.

Social housing – the term used to describe affordable homes provided by councils and Registered Social Landlords.

Socialisation – the process by which a child learns to fit into their social environment. This process can take many years but starts at home with parents.

Social services – a wide range of support and care services which look after our health and welfare. They are also referred to as social care services.

Social support and surveillance – offered in some communities. It may include visiting, companionship, social events, trips out and pet care. These services can be supplied by voluntary organisations.

Social stigma – severe social disapproval of personal characteristics or beliefs that are against cultural norms.

Societal factors – factors in society which can influence health, such as housing.

Spina bifida – means 'split spine'. The bones in the spine (vertebrae) do not form properly in early pregnancy. The nerves in the spine may be unprotected, causing damage to the nervous system.

Spoilage bacteria – the process of food gradually becoming inferior caused by bacteria.

Standard of living – defined as a measure of the goods, services and luxuries available to an individual or household once the basic necessities are met.

Starchy foods – consist of bread, rice, pasta, potatoes and breakfast cereals. Starchy foods are filling and provide energy.

Statutory – imposed by law.

Stock rotation – the practice of using a product with the shortest shelf-life before using a similar one with a longer shelf-life.

Sustain – to keep in existence or maintain.

Sustainable community – used to describe a place where needs are met and opportunities provided. In these communities there will be a sense of belonging, trust and inclusion.

Symptom – a sign of a disease or condition.

Tartar – hardened tooth plaque. Both tartar and plaque are acidic and will dissolve away the protective enamel coating of the tooth, creating cavities if left unchecked.

Temperature control – the use of temperature as a control measure to stop a hazard from arising. The use of heat (cooking, hot holding) and refrigeration are the main ways of temperature control.

Tenant – a person renting a property.

Tenure – used to describe the type of property held or lived in; this could be owner occupied or rented.

Tooth decay – caused by sticky deposits called plaque collecting around the gum line and in crevices between teeth. The plaque consists of food remains and bacteria in the saliva. It is acidic and will start to dissolve the tooth enamel.

Toxin – a poisonous substance produced by some bacteria and fungi.

Trans fatty acids – usually produced by processing fats and oils to produce food products. This may make them harmful and consumption should be reduced.

Type 1 diabetes – also known as insulin-dependent diabetes (IDDM). It usually develops in childhood when the body becomes unable to produce insulin.

Type 2 diabetes – also known as non-insulin-dependent

diabetes (NIDDM). It develops when the body produces some but not enough of the insulin it needs, or when the body is not able to use the insulin properly.

Unemployment – the lack of employment; the inability to find work.

Use by date – used for perishable high-risk food. The date up to which the food may be safely used if stored properly. Foods must not be used after the expiry of the use by date.

Vehicle of contamination – the route of food contamination by harmful bacteria.

Very sheltered housing – housing for people with disabilities or the very frail who feel unable to live completely independently

Villi – tiny finger-like projections which normally provide the very large absorptive surface of the small intestine.

Virus – DNA surrounded by a protein coat. Unable to replicate without a host cell, viruses are typically not considered living organisms.

Voluntary organisations – non-statutory bodies, set up and run by their members rather than by government. They complement state provision of health and social care services.

Waste – what people throw away because they no longer need it or want it.

Waste hierarchy – specifies the following order of preference for dealing with our wastes, with those towards the top of the list more desirable than those towards the bottom. In order, the hierarchy is reduce, reuse, recover, recycle, compost, recover energy, disposal.

Welfare benefits – financial support from the government if you are unemployed and looking for work. Benefits are also used to provide additional income when earnings are low, or if someone is retired, bringing up children, caring for someone, ill or has a disability.

Welfare state – a system supported by the government or state that attempts to provide economic security for people when they are unemployed, ill or elderly, such as the NHS and state benefits.

Welfare to work – a range of strategies to help the unemployed into work and off benefits.

Workless households – contain at least one person of working age but no one is in employment.

Yeast – a fungi reproducing by budding.

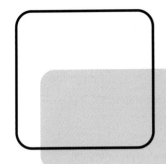

Index